Orthodontic Functional Appliances

Orthodontic Functional Appliances

Theory and Practice

Dr Padhraig Fleming BDent Sc. (Hons.), MSc, PhD, MOrth RCS, FDS (Orth.) RCS, FHEA

Senior Clinical Lecturer/Hon. Consultant
Barts and The London School of Medicine and Dentistry
Queen Mary University of London
Institute of Dentistry
Whitechapel
London
UK

Professor Robert Lee BDS, MDS, FDS, MOrth RCS (Eng.)

Hon. Professor/Consultant
Barts Health NHS Trust
Barts and The London School of Medicine and Dentistry
Institute of Dentistry
Whitechapel
London
UK

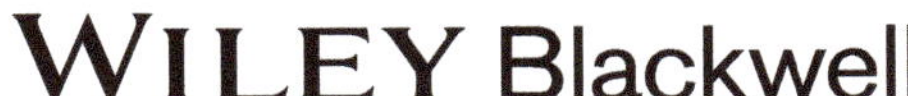

This edition first published 2016

Registered Office
John Wiley & Sons, Ltd, The Atrium, Southern Gate, Chichester, West Sussex, PO19 8SQ, UK

Editorial Offices
9600 Garsington Road, Oxford, OX4 2DQ, UK
The Atrium, Southern Gate, Chichester, West Sussex, PO19 8SQ, UK
1606 Golden Aspen Drive, Suites 103 and 104, Ames, Iowa 50010, USA

For details of our global editorial offices, for customer services and for information about how to apply for permission to reuse the copyright material in this book please see our website at www.wiley.com/wiley-blackwell

Library of Congress Cataloging-in-Publication Data

Names: Fleming, Padhraig S., author. | Lee, Robert, 1947 July 26– , author.
Title: Orthodontic functional appliances: theory and practice / Dr. Padhraig Fleming, Professor Robert Lee.
Description: Chichester, West Sussex; Ames, Iowa : John Wiley & Sons, Inc., 2016. | Includes bibliographical references and index.
Identifiers: LCCN 2016007082 | ISBN 9781118670576 (hb) | ISBN 9781118670545 (Adobe PDF) | ISBN 9781118670569 (epub)
Subjects: MESH: Orthodontic Appliances, Functional | Malocclusion–therapy | Orthodontics, Corrective
Classification: LCC RK521 | NLM WU 426 | DDC 617.6/43–dc23
LC record available at http://lccn.loc.gov/2016007082

A catalogue record for this book is available from the British Library.

Wiley also publishes its books in a variety of electronic formats. Some content that appears in print may not be available in electronic books.

Set in 9.5/12pt Minion by SPi Global, Pondicherry, India

1 2016

Contents

List of contributors

Dr Andrew DiBiase
BDS, MSc, MOrth RCS, FDS (Orth.) RCS
Consultant Orthodontist
East Kent Hospitals NHS University Foundation Trust
Department of Orthodontics
William Harvey Hospital
Kent
UK

Dr Colin Larmour
BDS, MSc, FDS RCPS, MOrth RCS, FDS (Orth.)
Consultant Orthodontist
University of Aberdeen Dental School and Hospital
Aberdeen Royal Hospitals
Aberdeen
UK

Mr Kieran McLaughlin
MSc, Adv Dip Dent Tech
Orthodontic Technician
Barts Health NHS Trust
Barts and The London School of Medicine and Dentistry
Institute of Dentistry
London
UK

Dr Peter Miles
BDSc, MDS, FCID
Senior Lecturer
University of Queensland School of Dentistry
Queensland
Australia

Visiting Lecturer
Seton Hill University Center for Orthodontics
Pennsylvania
USA

Professor Peter A. Mossey
BDS, PhD, MOrth RCSEng, FDS RCSEd, FFD RCSI
Professor of Orthodontics
Division of Oral Health Sciences
Dundee Dental Hospital and School
Dundee
UK

Preface

Orthodontists are united in a quest to achieve functional, aesthetic and stable outcomes compatible with optimal health and stability of the dentition. While the focus on aesthetics has intensified in recent years, the scope to alter facial growth, and in particular aesthetics, with orthodontic appliances has been disputed. Functional appliance therapy offers the possibility of modifying growth, producing potentially more meaningful facial as well as inter-arch change. The skeletal and soft tissue variations in individuals are the main limiting factors in our ability to achieve the perfection we desire. The use of functional appliances has been one of the more contentious areas within orthodontics for decades. Paradoxically, these appliances have been relied on to produce skeletal change, dental change or a combination of both in pre-adolescent, adolescent and indeed mature individuals for a century. While users of these appliances have often harboured inconsistent objectives, the popularity of the appliances, while subject to regional variation, has been sustained and relatively consistent.

This book would not have been possible without the inspiration of early developers of functional appliance therapy and more recent innovators including the likes of William Clark, who have been integral in the refinement, simplification and popularity of functional appliances. The authors have used functional appliances successfully both throughout our training and within our orthodontic practices in growing Class II patients. Our aim within this textbook has been to highlight the rationale, indications and implications of this approach. While a number of chapters are intended to have a clinical and practical focus, we hope to have maintained an evidence-based underpinning throughout. In particular, while we are aware of the limitations of much of the evidence pertaining to appliance therapy, irrespective of design, we emphasize best available evidence in the form of randomized studies.

Allied to the research focus, however, we attempt to supplement theoretical concepts with practical elements. We are unapologetic in relation to our emphasis on the Twin Block, as this has proven a reliable, effective and user-friendly appliance within our respective practices. However, we endeavour to embody contemporary and universal approaches to functional treatment in an unbiased fashion, particularly by devoting chapters to both flexible and rigid fixed functional designs. We therefore hope that a clinician without experience of either removable or fixed functional appliances will be capable of identifying appropriate patients, designing a suitable appliance and managing the care of a functional case effectively on the basis of this textbook. To this end, we have documented a significant number of personally treated cases to augment the theory behind the biological basis and indications for functional treatment.

We would like to express our gratitude to a number of people who have influenced our lives and our professional careers. In particular, we would like to pay tribute to our families, Caroline, Oliver, Sophie, Anne and Johnny Fleming, whose endless love and support are always appreciated. We would also like to recognize Norma Lee and her children for their unlimited patience and understanding, and Dr Margaret Collins for encouraging and recommending this publication. We are indebted to Dr Peter Miles, Dr Andrew DiBiase and Professor Peter Mossey for agreeing to write chapters within this book and for adding an extra dimension to our efforts. Finally, we would like to acknowledge Mr Kieran McLaughln for his technical expertise and passion in fabricating and describing the technical aspects of a range of removable appliances.

Above all, we hope that you enjoy the book and that our efforts and approach have a bearing either on your treatment or on your expectations of treatment with functional appliances.

Dr Padhraig Fleming
Professor Robert Lee

CHAPTER 1

Biological basis for functional appliance therapy

A functional appliance is one that uses the facial muscles and masticatory muscles to produce changes in the position of the individual teeth or arches. Any oral appliance causing a change in the forces of occlusion and alteration in muscular activity is likely to produce displacement of individual teeth or arches. Therefore such appliances can be either removable, inducing a displacement of the mandible by a process of interference or by stimulating an avoidance reflex, or fixed, involving the use of a mechanism causing the mandible to be held in a different position for function.

Facial growth

Maxillary growth occurs primarily by intra-membranous ossification with surface remodelling, resulting in a downward–forward displacement of the maxilla at an angle of approximately 40 degrees to the cranial base.[1] Growth of the maxilla is complex and may be affected by alterations in the sutures of the maxillae. Resorption on the superior surface and the apposition of bone on other surfaces affect the position of the maxillary dento-alveolar complex, with resorption of the anterior surface being typical during the downward–forward growth of the basal bone. However, while apposition of bone occurs on the inferior surface of the palate, resorption occurs on the superior surface, resulting in a net downward displacement (Figure 1.1).

Björk and Skieller's tantalum implant studies have shown that mandibular growth in children and adolescents occurs mainly as a consequence of an increase in condylar length in a posterior and superior direction due to endochondral ossification.[2] Elsewhere mandibular growth is a product of surface apposition and remodelling. Appositional growth does not occur anteriorly at the chin, with chin growth being expressed chiefly at the lateral aspects. Mandibular growth otherwise manifests as remodelling of the alveolus and of the bony areas with muscular attachments. Growth of the ascending ramus primarily occurs posteriorly, with resorption on the anterior aspect (Figure 1.2).

The mandible is not directly attached to the skull, but rather held in position by the muscles, ligaments and tendons, with the condylar head of the mandible being placed in the glenoid fossa within the temporal bone. The synovial articulation between the condyle and the temporal bone is classified as a ginglymoarthroidal joint, as both a ginglymus (hinging) and arthroidal (sliding) element exist, permitting the required mandibular opening and excursive movements during function. Changes in the position of the glenoid fossae will have consequent effects on the position of the mandible.

Orthodontic therapy involving functional appliances therefore might be expected to produce changes in the position of both the maxilla and the mandible, and combinations of growth restraint and growth induction would result in clinical changes in three dimensions. Detailed information on facial growth has been presented by Enlow[1] and Björk and Skieller.[2]

While increases in the absolute mandibular dimensions outstrip those of the maxilla during adolescence, this does not normally result in occlusal improvement in Class II malocclusion without active orthodontic intervention.[3] Based on longitudinal data from growth studies, some straightening of the profile and reduction in facial convexity may occur during the pubertal growth phase,[4] although this has not been a universal finding[5] and little change in the skeletal profile occurs in late adolescence.[6] Foley and Mamandras[7] noted that twice as much mandibular as maxillary growth arose in Class II males and females from 14 to 20 years old based on a North American Caucasian sample. However, a greater increase in absolute mandibular length is to be expected, as its overall dimension is greater than that of the maxilla, with the percentage difference in the increase between mandibular and maxillary less significant; mandibular length also incorporates a profound vertical element, while maxillary growth is usually measured from ANS (anterior nasal spine) to PNS (posterior nasal spine) and is therefore essentially horizontal. Positive occlusal interdigitation may also limit changes in inter-arch relationships. Moreover, in an analysis of patients with skeletal 2 patterns aged 8 to 18 years and increased overjet who had no orthodontic treatment, 4 mm more forward growth of the mandible than the maxilla was observed, but the occlusion and overjet remained unchanged into adulthood; this lack of change was attributed to the cuspal interdigitation.[8]

The rate of craniofacial growth, particularly of the maxilla and the mandible, is believed to undergo a pre-pubertal peak. The rate of growth is generally limited prior to this period, although a transient juvenile peak in growth rate has been

Orthodontic Functional Appliances: Theory and Practice, First Edition. Padhraig Fleming and Robert Lee.

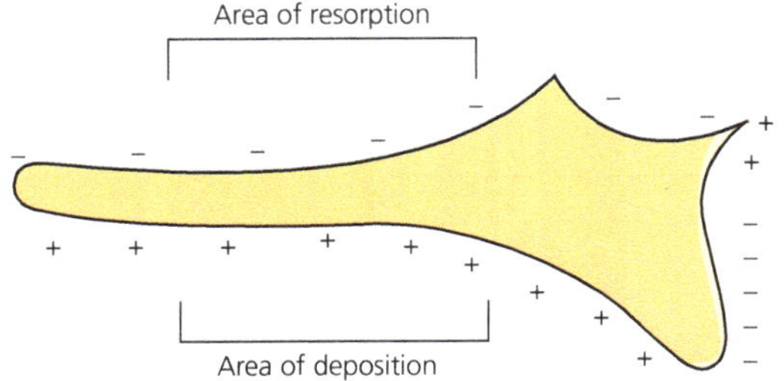

Figure 1.1 Resorption on the superior surface of the maxilla accompanied by deposition on the palate surface leads to an inferior displacement.

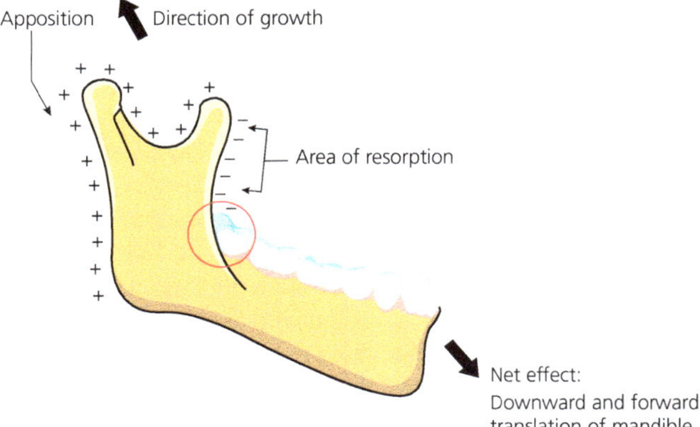

Figure 1.2 Mandibular growth occurs via condylar growth in a posterior and superior direction resulting in downward and forward displacement. Resorption on the anterior surface of the ascending ramus combined with resorption on the posterior surface leads to forward movement of the ramus.

described in females. Riolo et al.[9] described an annual rate of increase in the length of the mandibular body (Gonion–Pogonion) of 1.7 mm and 2.5 mm, respectively, in 8-year-old males and females. The corresponding figures at 13 years were 2 mm and 1.8 mm. Intuitively, therefore, treatment involving growth modification is ideally timed during a period of maximal growth. However, while this sounds relatively simple, a range of techniques directed at timing treatment have been developed and trialled, with limited success (Chapter 4). For example, while the rate of mandibular growth is thought to mirror increases in statural height, there is significant variation.[10]

Arbitrary use of chronological age, typically 10 to 13 years in females and 11 to 14 years in males, continues to be an accepted method of estimating the timing of most efficient and effective growth modification in Class II subjects. However, little difference has been demonstrated in the relative skeletal effectiveness of functional appliances in subjects of mean age 10 years relative to a group treated just after the onset of puberty (mean age 12 years 11 months).[11] Moreover, Pancherz et al., who in earlier research highlighted an increase in condylar growth rate in harmony with increases in statural height,[12] have since reported on the use of the Herbst appliance in skeletally mature patients with demonstrable, albeit limited, skeletal changes based on magnetic resonance imaging of the temporomandibular joints.[13]

Function and craniofacial morphology

Craniofacial growth is believed to be capable of a certain degree of morphological adaptation subject to functional requirements, with function known to be required for normal homeostasis and cellular turnover.[14] This theory is based on the work of Van der Klaauw, subsequently popularized by the American anatomist Melvin Moss.[15] According to the functional matrix theory, facial growth, final shape and dimensions are governed by the role of resident organs and tissues, specifically the senses, and essential functions including eating, cognition and breathing. Moss believed that the properties of important organs were related to underlying skeletal components. In particular, two major functional elements (cerebral and facial) were described with unique tissues and spaces. Moss hypothesized that expansion of each capsular matrix was accompanied and facilitated by bone growth via endochondral and intra-membranous ossification to preserve functional spaces. These hypotheses were supported by experimental evidence demonstrating altered skeletal growth following separation from soft tissue elements, while the presence of enveloping soft tissues led to the observation of normal growth patterns. Applying Moss's concepts to the potential for modification of growth with functional appliance therapy, it could be argued that postural changes with associated soft tissue alteration may be accompanied by a redirection or indeed acceleration of skeletal growth. Moreover, correction of abnormal soft tissue patterns and behaviour was a tenet for the pioneers of functional appliance therapy, many of whom advocated its use to restore normal function and development. Moreover, in animal models altered masticatory function and associated changes in muscular loading have been shown to affect condylar cartilage thickness and chondroblast differentiation.[16, 17]

The malleability of cranial shape following the application of continuous forces during the process of cerebral growth and skull development has been demonstrated in tribal groups. This is apparent in the skulls of indigenous people in South America, where the bandaging of the skull from shortly after birth resulted in significant alteration in the shape of the cranium (Figure 1.3). It would appear that the overall size of the brain has been maintained while the shape of the supporting cranium is significantly altered. Similarly, dramatic changes have been observed in long bones and as a result of other local practices including foot binding, which reduces foot size to an extent by repositioning the bony elements.

Orthodontists involved in changing the facial shape of those with malocclusion would wish to alter similarly the directional growth of the mandible in relation to the maxilla. Positional change in these relationships could be sufficient to correct sagittal, vertical and transverse occlusal discrepancies. It has been recognized that skeletal II discrepancies are primarily related to the position of the mandible relative to the maxilla rather than the overall size of the underlying bones (Figure 1.4).[18–20] McNamara, in an analysis of a North American Caucasian group, has, for example, shown that 49% of skeletal II patterns presented with SNA (Sella–Nasion–A point) values below 81

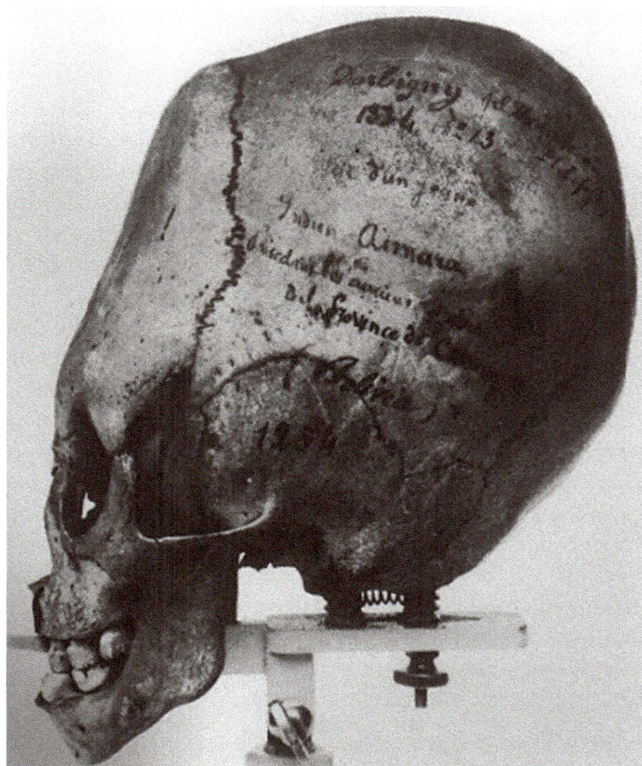

Figure 1.3 An example of the effects of cranial binding in a South American female from the Atacama desert. Typically, binding is undertaken for a relatively short period (approximately 6 months) in infancy; the effects are marked and persist into adulthood.

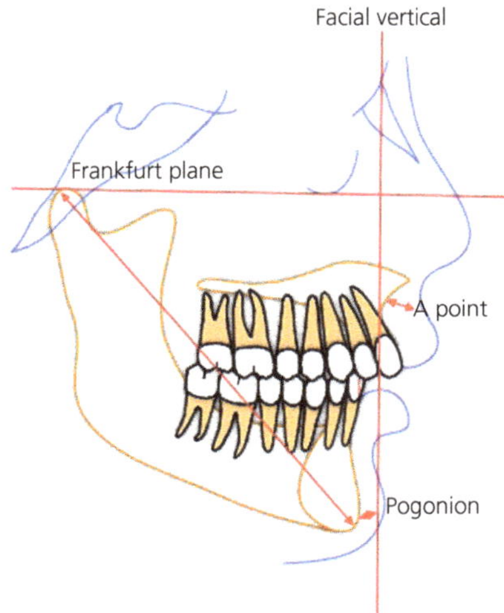

Figure 1.4 Skeletal II discrepancy is typically related to mandibular retrognathia rather than maxillary protrusion. However, analysis of the Burlington, Bolton and Ann Arbor samples demonstrated that 49% of skeletal II patterns were associated with SNA values below 81 degrees. Moreover, SNB was below 78 degrees in 82% of the sample.[19] Therefore, much of the focus of growth modification has been on the propensity to effect lasting change on mandibular position and dimensions. McNamara subsequently developed a cephalometric analysis involving a facial vertical line drawn perpendicular to the Frankfurt plane.[20]

degrees. Moreover, the SNB (Sella–Nasion–B point) was below 78 degrees in 82% of the sample.[19] Consequently, the majority of experimentation and clinical efforts have been centred on the ability to produce permanent change in mandibular position and dimensions.

Forward mandibular posture appears to concentrate stresses within the mandibular condyle. Finite element analysis has indicated that stress levels within the condyle are doubled with flexible fixed functional appliances, for example.[21] Moreover, Gupta et al.,[22] in an experimental model, have reported accumulation of tensile stresses in the postero-superior aspect of the condyle with sustained mandibular forward posture. Similarly, tensile forces arise in the glenoid fossa within the posterior connective tissues. It is postulated that these mechanical changes might correlate with enhanced cellular differentiation. While clinical research, most recently in the form of randomized trials, has become the mainstay of this experimentation, laboratory-based experimentation on primates and rodents provides much of our theoretical knowledge on the biological basis for growth modification and functional appliance therapy.

Experiments on primates

The condylar cartilage is a secondary cartilage capable of regional adaptive growth, contrasting with primary long-bone epiphyseal articular cartilages. Secondary cartilage appears later in embryonic development, with chondrification of the condyle thought to begin around week 9 *in utero*, and has a distinctive pattern of organization and proliferation with appositional growth, while primary cartilage grows interstitially (see Chapter 3). Primary cartilage is thought to respond to systemic growth stimuli such as hormones, while secondary cartilages only secondarily react to these stimuli. Moreover, while hypertrophic chondrocytes tend to be arranged in columns in long bones, they are organized haphazardly in condylar cartilage; this may favour a multi-directional growth pattern in response to mechanical stimuli. Furthermore, condylar cartilage is not loaded by body weight but by sporadic and intermittent forces applied during mastication, swallowing and parafunctional activity. Mechanical loading and stimuli are prerequisites for normal condylar growth, inducing specific biochemical responses in chondrocytes and pre-osteoblasts. Decreasing the load on the mandibular condyle by reducing occlusal contact has been implicated in a thinner, less dense condylar cartilage layer.[23]

Postural changes have long been considered capable of producing occlusal change, with for example Andreasen highlighting marked occlusal changes with his eponymous appliance, the Andreasen Activator. However, the ability to produce significant skeletal change has been contested primarily since the advent of cephalometry, when evidence began to emerge that orthodontics may be restricted to inducing dento-alveolar change and the concept of the immutability of the skeletal pattern became accepted.[24]

Extrapolation of animal experimentation to the human form is complicated by a range of factors. A specific problem in studying mandibular growth in animals is the nature of the mandible in each species, with unique patterns of attachment of the muscles into the condyle, individual shaped discs and glenoid fossae and specific types of mastication. In an effort to explore growth changes in mammals most comparable to human primates, a number of studies have been undertaken on various species of Macaque monkeys. Nevertheless, there are accepted and influential differences in the pattern and rate of growth between these species and humans, with Macaque, for example, being skeletally mature by the age of 3 years. Moreover, their metabolism is believed to outstrip the rate of human metabolism by a factor of approximately 4 and associated cellular turnover is markedly more rapid than in humans.

In an analysis of Rhesus monkeys, Moyers et al.[25] studied the effects of anterior mandibular displacement produced by occlusal overlay splints at the equivalent of 6 years of age in humans. After 3 months of treatment, a skeletal III pattern was produced with associated overcorrection of the molar relationships to Class III. Treatment-related changes included an increased growth rate at the maxillary tuberosity allied to restraint of vertical maxillary growth in the molar region. In addition, accelerated posterior and superior condylar growth occurred during the treatment period. Dental changes were more limited, with some mesial movement of the lower molars observed. The mandibular growth acceleration was confirmed, as posterior manipulation of the condyles was not possible under general anaesthesia.

An early study by Stöckli and Willert[26] examined the condyle and glenoid fossae of the Macaque *irus* monkeys. Two of the animals had no intervention and six of the experimental animals had 5 mm forward displacement of the mandible with a cemented splint; the animals were sacrificed at different periods to compare the nature of the growth at pre-specified intervals. The conclusion was that the condyle had a characteristic pattern of growth. The condyle was shown to have an outer surface, the articular surface, formed primarily of fibrocartilage. The layer immediately underneath is referred to as the intermediate cellular proliferative layer. This area is cartilaginous in nature, with thickening induced in the layer of cartilage and an increase in the number of cells in response to prolonged mandibular displacement. The third layer of hyaline cartilage is essentially a cartilage being replaced gradually by bone with consolidation. The overall effect of this forward displacement of the mandible was increased length in the bone, which was greater than expected in the non-intervention group. The proliferative area was shown to be increased up to five times more in experimental animals and it was also noted that an increased layer of cellular proliferation occurred in the glenoid fossae.

Further studies by McNamara et al.[27–29] in Macaque monkeys incorporating tantalum implants have identified similar changes and highlighted the relevance of treatment timing of the treatment, based on reported changes in the electromyographic (EMG) activity in the lateral pterygoid muscles. Observation was made of the length of time required to produce additional bone rather than cartilage, with the latter being a less permanent structure. It was concluded that the mandible should be advanced in a step-wise way with gradual advancement rather than single-step activation, with the objective of repeated activation of the lateral pterygoid muscles being postulated to result in additional growth of the condyles. However, Sessle et al.,[30] in a study with a sample of just 4, suggested that the impact of progressive advancement (1.5–2 mm every 10–15 days) on activity within the lateral pterygoid, masseter and anterior digastric was not markedly different to that associated with larger, one-step activation.

A limitation of these studies is that the overall effect of functional therapy in normal primates is to produce a frank reversed overjet with a true skeletal III relationship, as the selection of skeletal II animals is not possible. These changes arise primarily as a consequence of an elongation of the mandible. A study involving implants and electromyographic sensors using Herbst appliances on primates found that occlusal correction was predominantly (70%) attributable to skeletal change from a combination of maxillary restraint, mandibular condylar growth and glenoid fossa remodelling, with 30% of the change due to dental movement. Despite the apparent limitations of animal-based research,[31] these findings have since repeatedly been corroborated within clinical research.[32, 33]

Other animal studies

A number of studies have been undertaken on the condyle of rodents, particularly rats. Apart from the obvious morphological differences (Figure 1.5), significant key growth-related differences exist that complicate extrapolation into humans. For example, using collagen X expression and capillary endothelium as surrogate measures of maximal mandibular growth, growth rate may peak as early as days 38–56 in the rat.[34] Furthermore, rat alveolar bone tends to be denser than in humans and bone plates are without marrow spaces; there are also marked differences in the arrangement of periodontal fibres.[35] Although rat condyles also have a specific arrangement, with a different discal attachment and very much larger lateral pterygoid muscles, it has been possible to evaluate the treatment-induced changes histologically with various types of functional appliances. Petrovic et al.[36, 37] highlighted the presence of prechondroblasts in the proliferative layer beneath the surface fibrous capsule. These prechondroblasts tend to proliferate and are increased in number when a functional appliance is placed and the animal has the mandible actively postured forwards. Surgical incision of the lateral pterygoid muscle was shown to prevent this change from occurring; the lateral pterygoid muscle was, therefore, identified as a critical active component inducing additional condylar growth. This finding lent further support to the concept that the muscle should be activated incrementally to ensure that additional growth was maintained throughout the functional phase. It has been noted, however, that the lateral pterygoid muscle in rats has a greater bulk and more extensive attachment than that of primates.[38] Nevertheless, further work on

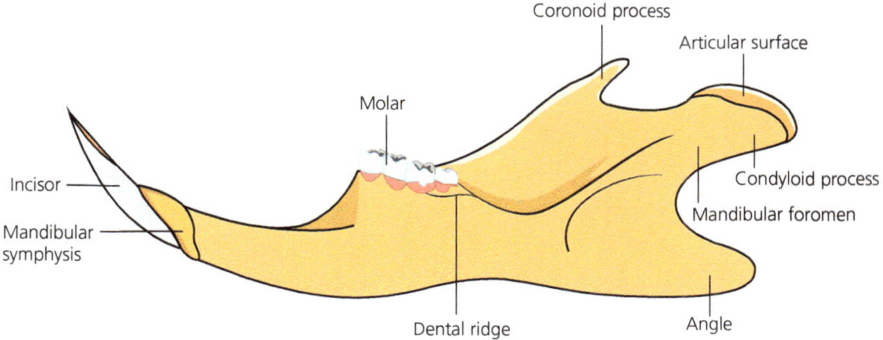

Figure 1.5 Schematic representation of the mature rat mandible. The rabbit and mouse mandibles have a similar morphology with a short ramus and relatively pronounced angle.

the rat model by Petrovic et al. has highlighted that mandibular advancement induced a significant time-related thickening of the prechondroblast–cohondroblast layer, with bone deposition along the posterior border of the ramus inferior to the condylar cartilage over a period of 6 weeks.[39]

Further *in vitro* research by Rabie[40] and co-workers produced detailed information on the cellular changes occurring in the condyles, highlighting the biochemical cascades induced by stimulation of the lateral pterygoid muscle resulting in vascular infiltration into the retrodiscal tissues, and also provided details on the regulation of collagen synthesis. They also observed the requirement for Type II collagen in the cartilage to be regulated by the agent Sox9 resulting in Type X collagen, which is required prior to the ossification of the cartilage. It was observed that this ossification took approximately 5 months to occur from placement of the experimental appliances. This 5-month phase in the rat is likely to be indicative of a much more prolonged period in humans or primates. These authors, therefore, advocate incremental stimulation of the lateral pterygoid muscle to induce meaningful additional bone growth at the condyles, resulting in supplemental growth beyond that which could be anticipated during normal maturation. A pivotal role for Sox9 and the development of collagen II and X has also been highlighted in a mouse model,[41] with their upregulation and secretion shown during condylar regeneration subsequent to experimental condylectomy.

Rabie et al. further investigated the expression of vascular endothelial growth factor (VEGF) secondary to incremental advancement in an allied study[42] on bony apposition posteriorly in the glenoid fossa. VEGF expression was found to increase and to coincide with new bone formation; increases in both were observed in the experimental group. It appears, therefore, that sustained postural change induces a series of tissue responses producing increased vascularization and bone formation, and that this pattern may be attributable to candidate biochemical markers. Moreover, using similar methodology Tang and Rabie have identified a pivotal role for Runx2, a transcription factor required for chondrocyte maturation and osteoblast differentiation, in the regulation of endochondral ossification following mandibular advancement.[43] A further analysis involving Sprague–Dawley rats has highlighted upregulation of fibroblast growth related factor (FGF8) following mandibular advancement over periods ranging from 3 to 30 days.[44] Cellular enlargement and differentiation were observed in both the condylar cartilage and the glenoid fossa during treatment with bony apposition by endochondral ossification in the condyle and intra-membranous ossification in the glenoid fossa.

Further research on a rabbit model has highlighted the role of matrix-metalloproteases (MMPs), particularly collagenases such as MMP-1 and MMP-13, on removal of extra-cellular matrix, inducing chondrocyte enlargement and differentiation required for bony apposition.[45] MMP expression following forward posture may be amplified by exogenous local administration of transforming growth factor beta and insulin-like growth factor in the inferior joint space. Experimental research of this nature using exogenous hormone delivery in the animal model directed at supplementing mandibular growth has yet to be translated into humans.

The visco-elastic theory

A particular type of activator appliance was developed by Harvold[46] (Figure 1.6) involving activation with an increased vertical dimension very much beyond the rest position, with the objective of stretching the facial musculature and soft tissues. This appliance was underpinned by a different philosophy, with Harvold postulating that changes in mandibular growth could be induced by this passive stretch; the family of appliances that this spawned became known as myotonic appliances.

Woodside et al.[47] evaluated the effects of a fixed functional appliance again in an animal study on Macaque monkeys, finding that increased activation of the appliance by 7–10 mm resulted in forward movement of the mandible without significant growth in its length. These changes arose due to marked cartilage proliferation in the glenoid fossa, which was most apparent in the growing juvenile. Subsequently, the changes achieved with Twin Block and Herbst appliances were

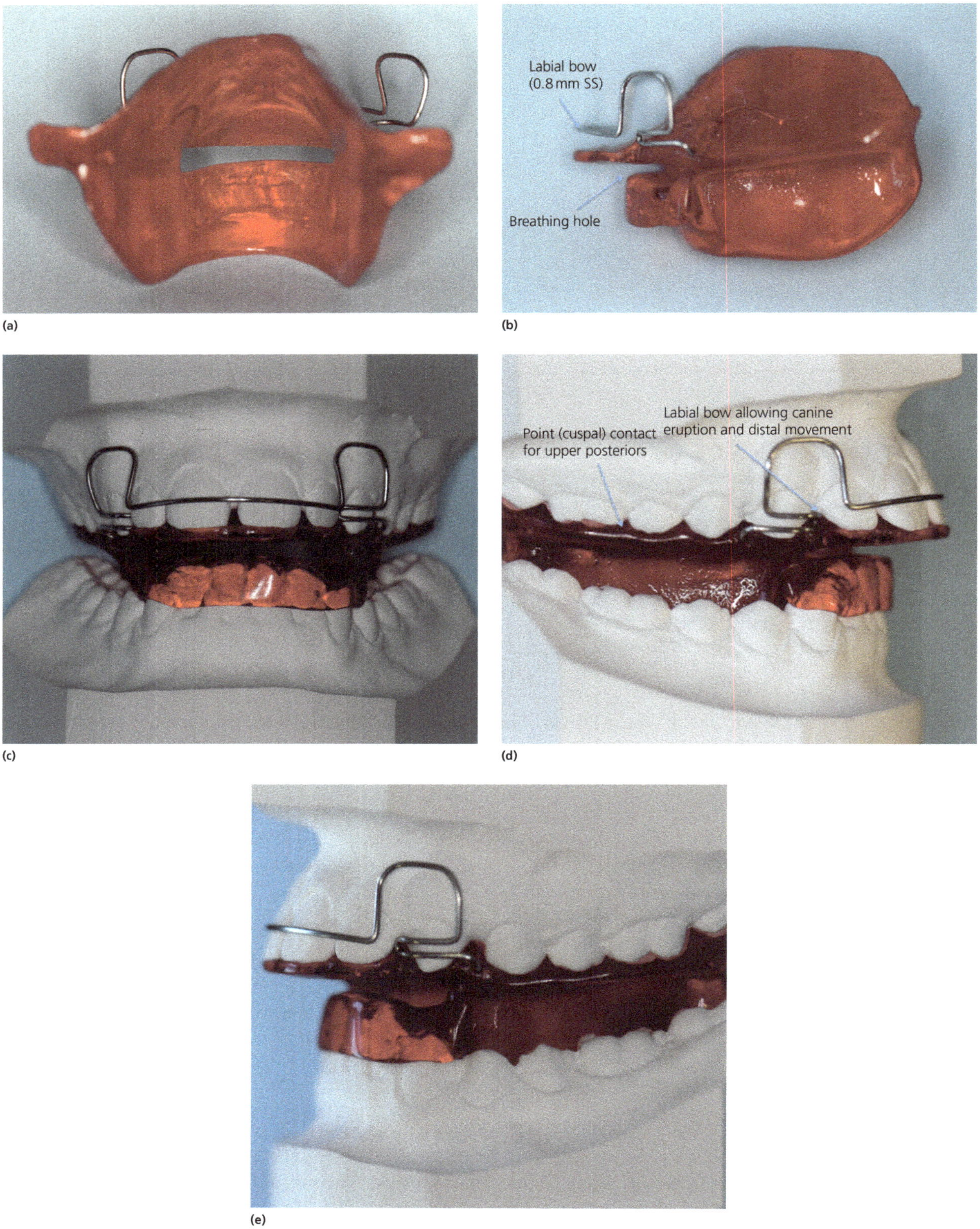

(a)

Labial bow
(0.8 mm SS)

Breathing hole

(b)

(c)

Labial bow allowing canine eruption and distal movement

Point (cuspal) contact for upper posteriors

(d)

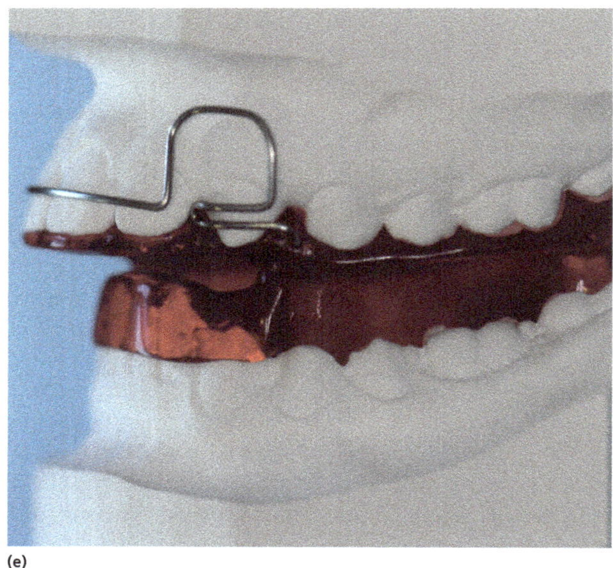

(e)

Figure 1.6 Harvold activator (a–e). The inter-maxillary force should theoretically be concentrated on both the maxillary dentition and palate, while the forces are transmitted to the lingual aspect of the mandible rather than the lower teeth. Consequently, well-extended lower impressions with adequate lingual depth, in particular, are required. The postured bite is taken 8–10 mm beyond the freeway space with near maximal protrusion, this degree of vertical opening allows the inclusion of an anterior breathing hole. During fabrication, extensive plaster relief is important in the lower posterior region to promote full eruption and lower arch levelling, while restricting unwanted lower incisor proclination with extension of the lower anterior acrylic onto the labial aspect of the mandibular incisors (c). The molars are afforded space to erupt, particularly in the lower arch to facilitate arch levelling and overbite reduction. An upper labial bow in 0.8 mm spring hard stainless steel may be added to facilitate retention, although more flexible wire may be used where space closure in the upper anterior region is planned. The labial bow should permit eruption and distal movement of the maxillary canines where required. The relief for the upper posteriors is such that it provides cusp tip contact with the upper acrylic plate with no interference, which might inhibit distal movement of the upper posteriors (d, e). These elements are usually introduced during the fabrication stage, with chairside trimming not usually required. The upper anterior aspect of the acrylic plate should extend to the incisal edges of the maxillary incisors to facilitate three-dimensional control, and a relief chamber is provided palatal to the incisors to facilitate intrusion without retraction.

attributed to visco-elastic stretching forces[48] and these authors described three growth stimuli: displacement, visco-elasticity and referred force from the condyle to the glenoid fossa. They termed this pattern the growth relativity hypothesis. Further investigations by Voudouris et al.[31, 49] involved application of Herbst treatment to Macaque monkeys and identified statistically significant additional growth of the glenoid fossa and condyle in juveniles, with reduced electromyographic postural activity and evidence of comparable levels of growth within the condyle and glenoid fossa. These researchers highlighted the fact that the transition from cartilage to bone was not complete until 18 weeks of therapy. Withdrawal of the postured bite at an earlier stage was subject to antero-posterior relapse. Similar changes in a human subject would require a longer period due to the greater duration of adolescence and slower rate of growth. Voudouris further reported that new bone formation at the condyle and glenoid fossa is related to age and is associated with decreased postural EMG activity of the masticatory muscles, including the lateral pterygoid, masseter and anterior belly of the digastric.[49]

Treatment duration

Fixed functional appliances and removable functional appliances that are worn on a full-time basis will usually correct the overjet and molar relationship within 6 months, but relapse on withdrawal of the appliance is a common finding.[50, 51] A study on rats by Chayanupatkul et al.[52] reported on the histological changes when functional appliances were removed early or following more protracted periods of treatment. The authors found that bone formation is not complete at the condyle following 5 to 7 months of treatment with a Type III collagen remaining. Type III collagen is known to be unstable, leading to emergency-type bone that is less resistant to reversal during function and mastication. The researchers recommended that the treatment time should be doubled to allow replacement bone to be established at the condyle. Extrapolating these laboratory findings to the clinical scenario, it may be reasonable to suggest that at least 1 year of full-time therapy is required to allow establishment of additional bone at both the condyle and glenoid fossa.

Maxillary restraint

All functional appliances used in Class II correction involve either stimulation of the masticatory or facial muscles or stretching of the tissues, which results in transmission of forces to the upper dentition and maxilla. Early animal experiments alluded to restraint of maxillary growth with full-time wear of functional appliances.[29] McNamara et al. also noted occlusal plane changes associated with growth restriction, with the occlusal plane tipping upwards anteriorly secondary to appliance therapy.[29] Consistently in clinical studies with fixed functional appliances, it is noted cephalometrically that reduced forward growth of the maxilla occurs in comparison with untreated subjects. Numerous studies have reported remodelling and an associated change in the position of the glenoid fossa.[48, 50, 53, 54] Some clinicians have designed appliances with the objective of training the mandible to posture forward with an avoidance reflex and the objective of avoiding dento-alveolar movement of the upper and lower dentition,[55–57] but inevitably a degree of dental movement of the upper and lower incisors and reduced maxillary forward movement are evidenced on cephalometric radiographs. Moreover, restraint of vertical maxillary growth has been attempted to encourage a more horizontal vector of forward mandibular growth by restricting downward–backward mandibular rotation. In particular, variants in appliance design in high-angle cases allowing adjunctive use of orthopaedic headgear, such as the Teuscher or van Beek appliance, have been used particularly in Europe. This approach involves high force levels of up to 1 kg directed through the centre of resistance of the maxillary structures, which has been estimated to be apical to the premolars for the maxillary dentition or at the postero-superior region of the zygomaticomaxillary suture for the maxilla.[58, 59] The impact of these appliances in terms of control of vertical growth, however, remains largely unclear, although short-term benefits have been highlighted in non-randomized studies.[60]

Summary

Functional appliances used in the correction of Class II malocclusion have been employed successfully for more than a century. What they have in common is that they all utilize a forward posture of the mandible to transmit forces from the muscles and soft tissues attached to the mandible to produce a more normal occlusion. Developments in appliance design have resulted in a reduced appliance bulk or the ability to fix the appliance to the dentition to allow better patient compliance and more prolonged periods of wear.

Animal experiments point to histological changes that are apparently stable, leading to the development of increased mandibular length. In clinical treatment, however, the same degree of change cannot be expected due to a more gradual rate of biological change and the overall extended duration of human skeletal development. While the emphasis on skeletal effects persists among researchers focusing on both animal models and clinical treatment, it appears increasingly likely that the changes resulting from functional appliance therapy are predominantly dento-alveolar in nature. Nevertheless, important short-term changes in condylar growth manifesting as an increase in mandibular length are likely to result in an improvement in the skeletal II deformity, assuming that the rate of mandibular growth outstrips that of the maxilla. An increase in the lower anterior facial height is also a consistent finding with functional appliance therapy.

References

1. Enlow DH. Facial growth. Philadelphia, PA: WB Saunders; 1990.
2. Björk A, Skieller V. Normal and abnormal growth of the mandible. A synthesis of longitudinal cephalometric implant studies over a period of 25 years. Eur J Orthod. 1983; 5: 1–46.
3. Lux CJ, Burden D, Conradt C, Komposch G. Age-related changes in sagittal relationship between the maxilla and mandible. Eur J Orthod. 2005; 27: 568–78.
4. Lande MJ. Growth behavior of the human bony facial profile as revealed by serial cephalometric roentgenology 1. Angle Orthod. 1952; 22: 78–90.
5. Stahl F, Baccetti T, Franchi L, McNamara JA Jr. Longitudinal growth changes in untreated subjects with Class II Division 1 malocclusion. Am J Orthod Dentofacial Orthop. 2008; 134: 125–37.
6. Baccetti T, Stahl F, McNamara JA Jr. Dentofacial growth changes in subjects with untreated Class II malocclusion from late puberty through young adulthood. Am J Orthod Dentofacial Orthop. 2009; 135: 148–54.
7. Foley TF, Mamandras AH. Facial growth in females 14 to 20 years of age. Am J Orthod Dentofacial Orthop. 1992; 101: 248–54.
8. You ZH, Fishman LS, Rosenblum RE, Subtelny JD. Dentoalveolar changes related to mandibular forward growth in untreated Class II persons. Am J Orthod Dentofacial Orthop. 2001; 120: 598–607.
9. Riolo ML, Moyers RE, McNamara JA, Hunter WS. An atlas of craniofacial growth. Ann Arbor, MI: Center for Human Growth and Development, University of Michigan, 1974: 14–21.
10. Woodside DG. In: Salzmann JA, ed. Orthodontics in daily practice. Philadelphia, PA: JB Lippincott, 1974.
11. Baccetti T, Franchi L, Toth LR, McNamara JA Jr. Treatment timing for Twin-block therapy. Am J Orthod Dentofacial Orthop. 2000; 118: 159–70.
12. Pancherz H, Hägg U. Dentofacial orthopedics in relation to somatic maturation. An analysis of 70 consecutive cases treated with the Herbst appliance. Am J Orthod. 1985; 88: 273–87.
13. Ruf S, Pancherz H. Herbst/multibracket appliance treatment of Class II division 1 malocclusions in early and late adulthood. A prospective cephalometric study of consecutively treated subjects. Eur J Orthod. 2006; 28: 352–60.
14. Bouvier M. Effects of age on the ability of the rat temporomandibular joint to respond to changing functional demands. J Dent Res. 1988; 67: 1206–12.
15. Moss ML, Rankow RM. The role of the functional matrix in mandibular growth. Angle Ortho. 1968; 38: 95–103.
16. Hichijo N, Kawai N, Mori H, Sano R, Ohnuki Y et al. Effects of the masticatory demand on the rat mandibular development. J Oral Rehab. 2014; 41: 581–7.
17. Hichijo N, Tanaka E, Kawai N, van Ruijven LJ, Langenbach GEJ. Effects of decreased occlusal loading during growth on the mandibular bone characteristics. PLoS ONE 2015; 10: e0129290.
18. Moyers RE, Riolo ML, Guire KE, Wainright RL, Bookstein FL. Differential diagnosis of Class II malocclusions: Part 1. Facial types associated with Class II malocclusions. Am J Orthod. 1980; 78: 477–94.
19. McNamara JA Jr. Components of Class II malocclusion in children 8–10 years of age. Angle Orthod. 1981; 51: 177–202.
20. McNamara JA Jr. A method of cephaloemtric evaluation. Am J Orthod. 1984; 86: 449–69.
21. Chaudhry A, Sidhu MS, Chaudhary G, Grover S, Chaudhry N, Kaushik A. Evaluation of stress changes in the mandible with a fixed functional appliance: A finite element study. Am J Orthod Dentofacial Orthop. 2015; 147: 226–34.
22. Gupta A, Kohli VS, Hazarey PV, Kharbanda OP, Gunjal A. Stress distribution in the temporomandibular joint after mandibular protraction: A 3-dimensional finite element method study. Part 1. Am J Orthod Dentofacial Orthop. 2009; 135: 737–48.
23. Basdra EK, Huber LA, Komposch G, Papavassiliou AG. Mechanical loading triggers specific biochemical responses in mandibular condylar chondrocytes. Biochim Biophys Acta. 1994; 1222: 315–22.
24. Brodie AG, Downs WB, Goldstein A, Myer E. Cephalometric appraisal of orthodontic results: A preliminary report. Angle Orthod. 1938; 8: 261–5.
25. Moyers RE, Elgoyhen JC, Riolo ML, McNamara JA Jr, Kuroda T. Experimental production of Class 3 in rhesus monkeys. Rep Congr Eur Orthod Soc. 1970; 46: 61–75.
26. Stöckli, PW, Willert HG. Tissue reactions in the temporomandibular joint resulting from anterior displacement of the mandible in the monkey. Am J Orthod. 1971; 60: 142–55.
27. McNamara JA, Carlson DS. Quantitative analysis of temporomandibular joint adaptations to protrusive function. Am J Orthod. 1979; 76: 593–611.
28. McNamara JA. Functional determinants of craniofacial size and shape. Eur J Orthod. 1980; 2: 131–59.
29. McNamara JA. Neuromuscular and skeletal adaptations to altered function in the orofacial region. Am J Orthod. 1973; 64: 578–606.
30. Sessle BJ, Woodside DG, Bourque P, Gurza S, Powell G. et al. Effect of functional appliances on jaw muscle activity. Am J Orthod Dentofacial Orthop. 1990; 98: 222–30.
31. Voudouris JC, Woodside DG, Altuna G, Angelopoulos G, Bourque PJ, Lacouture CY. Condyle-fossa modifications and muscle interactions during Herbst treatment, Part 2. Results and conclusions. Am J Orthod Dentofacial Orthop. 2003; 124: 13–29.
32. Bishara SE, Ziaja RR. Functional appliances: A review. Am J Orthod Dentofacial Orthop. 1989; 95: 250–58.
33. O'Brien K, Wright J, Conboy F, Sanjie Y, Mandall N et al. Effectiveness of early orthodontic treatment with the Twin-block appliance: A multicenter, randomized, controlled trial. Part 1: Dental and skeletal effects. Am J Orthod Dentofacial Orthop. 2003; 124: 234–43.
34. Shen G, Hägg U, Rabie AB, Kaluarachchi K. Identification of temporal pattern of mandibular condylar growth: A molecular and biochemical experiment. Orthod Craniofac Res. 2005; 8: 114–22.
35. Ren Y, Maltha JC, Kuijpers-Jagtman AM. The rat as a model for orthodontic tooth movement: A critical review and a proposed solution. Eur J Orthod. 2004; 26: 483–90.
36. Petrovic A, Stutzmann J, Lavergne J. Mechanism of craniofacial growth and modus operandi of functional appliances: A cell-level and cybernetic approach to orthodontic decision making. In: Carlson DS, ed. Craniofacial growth theory and orthodontic treatment. Craniofacial Growth Series, vol. 23. Ann Arbor, MI: Center for Human Growth and Development, University of Michigan; 1990: 13–74.
37. Petrovic AG, Stutzmann JJ, Oudet CL. Control processes in the postnatal growth of the condylar cartilage of the mandible. In: McNamara JA Jr, ed. Determinants of mandibular form and growth. Craniofacial Growth Series, vol. 4. Ann Arbor, MI: Center for Human Growth and Development, University of Michigan; 1975: 101–53.

38. Houston WJ. Growth of the muscles of mastication in the rat. Trans Eur Orthod Soc. 1974; 50: 85–90.
39. Charlier JP, Petrovic AG, Stutzmann J. Effect of mandibular hyperpropulsion on the prechondroblast zone of young rat condyles. Am J Orthod. 1969; 55: 71–4.
40. Rabie ABM, Hägg U. Factors regulating mandibular condylar growth. Am J Orthod Dentofacial Orthop. 2002; 122: 401–9.
41. Fujita T, Nakano M, Ohtani J, Kawata T, Kaku M et al. Experssion of Sox 9 and type II and X collagens in regenerated condyle. Eur J Orthod. 2010; 32: 677–80.
42. Shum L, Rabie AB, Hägg U. Vascular endothelial growth factor expression and bone formation in posterior glenoid fossa during stepwise mandibular advancement. Am J Orthod Dentofacial Orthop. 2004; 125: 185–90.
43. Tang GH, Rabie AB. Runx2 regulates endochondral ossification in condyle during mandibular advancement. J Dent Res. 2005; 84: 166–71.
44. Owtad P, Potres Z, Shen G, Petocz P, Darendeliler MA. A histochemical study on condylar cartilage and glenoid fossa during mandibular advancement. Angle Orthod. 2011; 81: 270–6.
45. Patil A, Sable R, Kothari R. Genetic expression of MMP-Matrix-metalloproteinases (MMP-1 and MMP-13) as a function of anterior mandibular repositioning appliance on the growth of the mandibular condylar cartilage with and without administration of insulin like growth factor (IGF-1) and transforming growth factor-B (TGF-B). Angle Orthod. 2012; 82: 1053–9.
46. Harvold EP, Vargervik K. Morphogenetic response to activator treatment. Am J Orthod. 1971; 60: 478–90.
47. Woodside DG, Metaxas A, Altuna G. The influence of functional appliance therapy on glenoid fossa remodelling. Am J Orthod Dentofacial Orthop. 1987; 92: 181–98.
48. Voudouris JC, Kuftinec MM. Improved clinical use of Twin-block and Herbst as a result of radiating viscoelastic tissue forces on the condyle and fossa in treatment and long-term retention: Growth relativity. Am J Orthod Dentofacial Orthop. 2000; 117: 247–66.
49. Voudouris JC, Woodside DG, Altuna G, Kuftinec MM, Angelopoulos G, Bourque PJ. Condyle-fossa modifications and muscle interactions during Herbst treatment, part 1. New technological methods. Am J Orthod Dentofacial Orthop. 2003; 123: 604–13.
50. Wieslander L. Intensive treatment of severe Class II malocclusions with a headgear-Herbst appliance in the early mixed dentition. Am J Orthod. 1984; 86: 1–13.
51. Lee RT, Kyi CS, Mack GJ. A controlled clinical trial of the effects of the Twin Block and Dynamax appliances on the hard and soft tissues. Eur J Orthod. 2007; 29: 272–82.
52. Chayanupatkul A, Rabie ABM, Hägg U. Temporomandibular response to early and late removal of bite-jumping devices. Eur J Orthod. 2003; 25: 465–70.
53. Vargervik K, Harvold EP. Response to activator treatment in Class II malocclusions. Am J Orthod. 1985; 88: 242–51.
54. Pancherz, H. The Herbst appliance: Its biologic effects and clinical use. Am J Orthod. 1985; 87: 1–20.
55. van Beek H. Combination headgear-activator. J Clin Orthod. 1984; 18: 185–9.
56. Teuscher U. A growth-related concept for skeletal class II treatment. Am J Orthod. 1978; 74: 258–75.
57. Bass NM. Dento-facial orthopaedics in the correction of class II malocclusion. Br J Orthod. 1982; 9: 3–31.
58. Teuscher UM. An appraisal of growth and reaction to extraoral anchorage: Simulation of orthodontic-orthopedic results. Am J Orthod. 1986; 89: 113–21.
59. Stöckli PM, Teuscher UM. Combined activator headgear orthopedics. In: Graber M, Vanarsdall RL, eds. Orthodontics: Current principles and techniques. St Louis, MO: Mosby; 1994.
60. Lagerström LO, Nielsen IL, Lee R, Isaacson RJ. Dental and skeletal contributions to occlusal correction in patients treated with the high-pull headgear-activator combination. Am J Orthod Dentofacial Orthop. 1990; 97: 495–504.

CHAPTER 2

Development of functional appliances

The development of orthodontic functional appliances paralleled the ongoing refinement of fixed appliances, with the latter evolving from earlier removable appliances chiefly designed to produce arch expansion.[1] The biological basis for growth modification was proposed by Wilhelm Roux, a German zoologist who concluded that bone adaptation was a 'quantitative self-regulating mechanism'.[2] Roux suggested that bone development was secondary to both nutrition and functional stimuli. Consequently, the possibility that environmental changes including alteration in jaw posture might induce bony changes became more tenable.

Step changes in appliance design were taken in the early twentieth century stemming from Edward Angle's pioneering work, culminating in the Edgewise appliance heralded by the inventor as the 'latest and the best' in 1928.[3] However, fixed appliances were directed at introducing changes within the confines of the periodontal ligament; functional appliances were intended for more significant dento-facial changes. While some of the earliest pioneers of the concept of facial orthopaedics were American, most of the developments related to functional appliances in the twentieth century emanated from Europe, as US orthodontists continued to be influenced by Angle's school, which concentrated on fixed appliances. Moreover, prior to the introduction of cephalometry, there was a popular misconception that orthodontic treatment with fixed appliances combined with elastic traction was capable of inducing significant skeletal change.

During the first half of the twentieth century precious metals were in short supply in Western Europe and indeed the use of precious metal alloys in dentistry was banned in Nazi Germany; consequently, fixed appliance use, which relied heavily on precious metals at that time, was curtailed throughout much of Europe. Furthermore, a significant amount of orthodontics was provided by non-specialists at that stage in European countries with developed social welfare systems; hence, there was an emphasis on improvement of malocclusion for large population groups without a quest for perfection. Against this political backdrop, functional appliances provided an attractive and ultimately cost-effective and efficient solution.

An early form of functional appliance was the bite jumping plane appliance, developed by Norman Kingsley in New York in 1880.[4] This appliance was held in place by a succession of ligatures passing between the teeth and a vulcanite bite plane, causing the mandible to be displaced forward in occlusion. This is similar to an anterior inclined plane, which was to become established in Europe as a popular removable appliance design. Kingsley had earlier been responsible for the development of occipital headgear.[5] Even Edward Angle, who focused exclusively on the use of fixed appliances later in his career, developed a modification to molar bands by introducing interlocking rings, which served to posture the mandible forward in an effort to address Class II occlusion.

Pierre Robin, based in Paris, is credited as the first clinician to undertake functional orthopaedics therapeutically. Robin developed a monobloc appliance geared at advancing the mandible in patients with glossoptosis syndrome, comprising of manifestations including severe mandibular retrognathia, adenoid facies and a high palatal vault. The appliance had pronounced lingual projections to facilitate retention along lingual surfaces of the mandibular and maxillary teeth, and included a palatal expansion screw in the palate to produce maxillary expansion. By virtue of forward posture, the appliance stimulated muscular activity. The overall treatment regime included conscious lip closure and appliance therapy, allied to physical and psychological support. The importance of muscular stimulation in the correction of malocclusion and dento-facial deformity was further emphasized by Alfred Rogers, a pupil of Angle's, who worked in Canada and advocated head and neck exercises in an effort to address malocclusion.[6,7] Rogers highlighted the role of facial muscles in the development and treatment of malocclusion. His theories have been exploited over the past 100 years.

Activators

A removable appliance was developed by Andresen in Norway in 1908 and subsequently popularized as the Andresen–Häupl appliance. The discovery was fortuitous: Andresen, who was a general dentist, fitted a vulvanite removable appliance in his daughter with the intention of retaining her post-orthodontic result. However, the appliance inadvertently involved 3–4 mm of forward activation, and night-time wear over a period of months resulted in sagittal occlusal change, prompting Andresen to explore the use of forward mandibular activation therapeutically.

Orthodontic Functional Appliances: Theory and Practice, First Edition. Padhraig Fleming and Robert Lee.

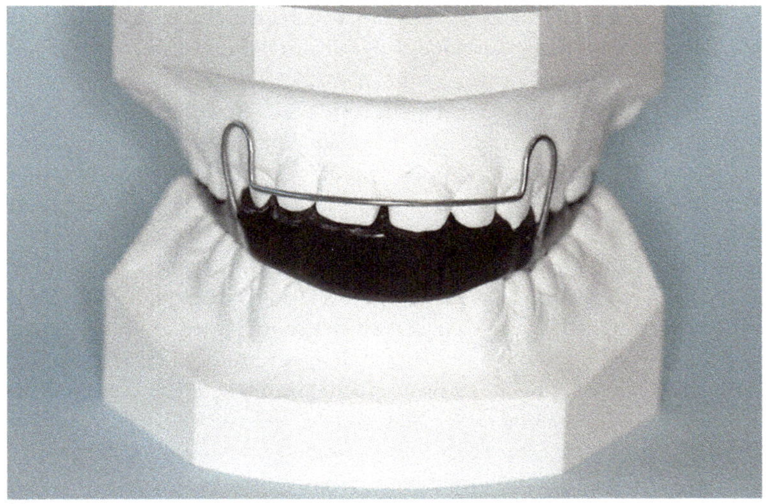

(a)

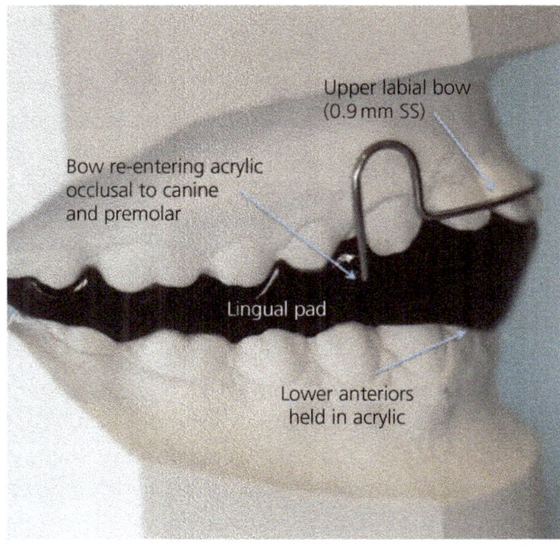

(b)

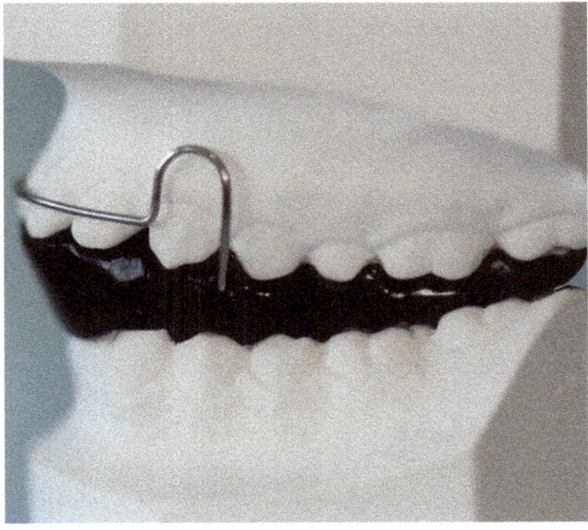

(c)

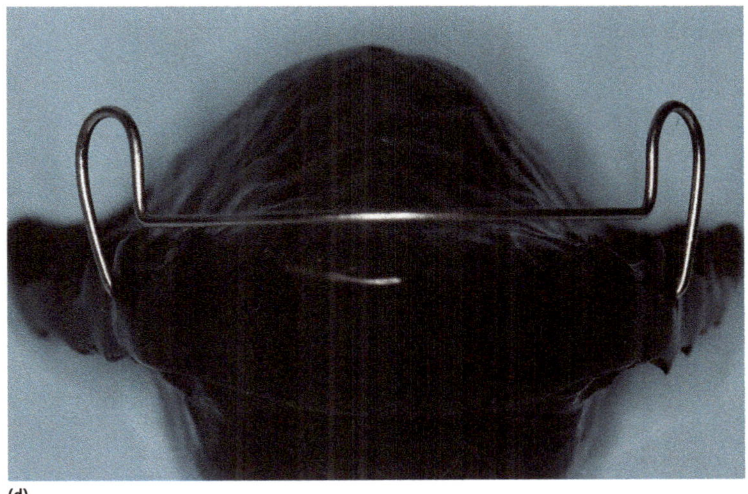

(d)

Figure 2.1 Andresen activator (a–d). Andresen believed that his passive appliance affected both the activity of the musculature and associated circulation, leading to an increase in biomechanical forces. The appliance involved little wirework, with early designs incorporating a coffin spring, although this is not now typical of the appliance. There is an upper labial arch, which can also involve loops to control the position of the maxillary canines. The labial bow is effectively passive and constructed from 0.9 mm spring hard stainless steel wire. The wire tagging enters the posterior blocks distal to the canines, elevated above the occlusal level of the contact points of the canines and premolars of the maxillary dentition. The tag ends of the labial bow should rest free of the maxillary dentition. The lower anterior teeth are held within the acrylic. Mandibular incisor proclination was common with this appliance, leading to lower anterior spacing. Fränkel, among other later developers, was critical of this and strove to limit forces to the lower anteriors to reduce proclination. Extensive functional trimming was typical of the Andresen in both the upper and lower regions of the posterior capping, but also the upper anterior palatal aspects of the appliance. This was designed to induce a 'bite thrust', as the patient continually bites into the appliance. Correct trimming of the posterior blocks should facilitate distal and transverse development of maxillary posteriors; directionally trimmed facets created at the chair-side permit the upper half of the posterior blocks to engage preferentially on the mesial aspects of the maxillary premolars and molars to encourage the desired tooth movement. The anterior palatal region of the appliance is trimmed on the fitting surfaces behind and along the anterior teeth. The space created allows posterior movement of the maxillary anteriors due to the unrestrained activity of the upper labial bow and soft tissues. Facets are present in the lower half of the posterior blocks only in the vertical plane, ensuring that they do not interfere with the vertical development of the mandibular posteriors. Judicious vertical trimming of the mandibular half of the blocks also prevents unwanted lingual tipping of the mandibular posterior teeth over the course of the functional phase.

The original Andresen activator was rigid, tooth-borne and loosely fitting. It was a bulky appliance, with acrylic blocks covering the palate and both arches. There were grooves to produce mesial tipping of lower teeth and distal tipping of upper posterior teeth. It was constructed to hold the mandible in a protrusive position, or to cause the mandible to occlude in a protrusive position. Essentially, patients cannot occlude in the normal retruded position, but rather into a more normal, forward position, with an associated reduction in the overjet and an improved position of the mandible. The appliance was loosely fitting based on the premise that it would activate the mandible to bite in a forward position, inducing muscular activation with these forces transmitted to the teeth and the tongue being stimulated by the appliance dropping against it. Conceptually, the patient would therefore intermittently bite in a more forward position, training the mandible to develop more normally. The tongue was also held in a further forward position due to the postural change with an increase in the airway dimension. Andresen also believed that the increased activity led to hypertrophy of the tongue muscles and improved the prospect of stability. The term 'activator' was therefore coined and subsequently many variants of this appliance have been introduced (Figure 2.1).

Initially, Andresen's design met with limited usage because it was removable. Andresen was also a proponent of extractions in orthodontics at a time when Angle was pre-eminent and his staunch advocacy of non-extraction approaches was in vogue. Moreover, while Angle propounded the treatment of malocclusion to an ideal state, Andresen suggested compromised goals in certain instances based on individual variation. Later, however, Andresen teamed up with a colleague in the University of Oslo, Karl Häupl, to further develop and popularize their approach, which became known as the 'Norwegian system'. The pair later published a book on functional jaw orthopaedics, which resulted in the system's widespread use. Some disagreement persisted regarding the appliance's mode of action and Selmer-Olsen[8] suggested that it was necessary to record the bite in a more open position, as the effects were due to stretching the underlying soft tissues rather than activating the mandible to bite forwards. Nevertheless, the activator endured due to a number of accepted advantages,[5] including the facility for early treatment in the deciduous and early or late mixed dentition due to its passive fit; the possibility of longer inter-appointment intervals; the requirement for night-only wear reducing the onus on compliance; and the ability to eliminate aberrant habits, including mouth breathing and tongue thrusting. It was, however, incapable of treating crowded malocclusions. Häupl, in particular, frowned on the use of fixed appliances in view of concerns relating to their safety, which stemmed from the work of Oppenheim alluding to iatrogenic damage attributed to fixed appliances.[9]

Bionator

The activator appliances are designed to be worn for as much time as possible, but their inherent bulk discourages their use during the day and also tends to encroach on the tongue space. The Bimler appliance[10] marked an attempt at streamlining, permitting daytime wear. The upper and lower components were connected by a wire, facilitating incremental activation. Similarly, the activator developed by Wilhelm Balters[11] had reduced bulk. It became known as the Bionator (Figure 2.2). Activators of reduced bulk have subsequently been referred to as Bionators.

The appliances were designed to facilitate correction of Class II malocclusion with mandibular retrognathia and were intended for part-time wear. It was a one-piece appliance with the upper component having a midline spring; midline expansion, however, was difficult. Clinically, they were found to be effective in correcting the occlusion consistently, subject to sufficient wear. Concepts of clinical trials with random allocation of patients and strict treatment protocols were not widespread until late in the twentieth century and there was therefore little agreement on the skeletal effects that this appliance achieved, other than a recognition of the occlusal changes that occurred until recent years. Nevertheless, these appliances have met with some use in both Europe and the United States.

Functional regulator

An elaborate functional appliance was developed in Zwickau in former East Germany by Dr Rolf Fränkel.[12] He exhibited records of patients achieving major occlusal changes and improvement of facial appearance with the use of a group of appliances that are referred to as functional regulators (FR). The first version of this appliance, the FR1, was used in Class II malocclusion with malaligned teeth; the FR2 (Figures 2.3 and 2.4) was used in patients with a large overjet or deep overbite; the FR3 for the correction of Class III malocclusion; and the FR4 for the correction of anterior open bite.

These appliances are unique in their construction as they are largely borne by the tissues and, therefore, are often referred to as tissue-borne appliances. Their objective is to alter soft tissue behaviour, chiefly the activity of the musculature, primarily the mentalis muscle of the lower jaw in Class II malocclusion and the cheek musculature, the buccinators, in Class II and Class III correction. Changes in the activity of the musculature are intended to produce normal functional activity and a more normal rest position of the lips, cheeks and tongue. Promotion of normal behaviour of these muscles in speech and facial expression with appropriate positioning of the mandible in all expressive and swallowing activities is inherent in the appliance design. It is not intended to correct the malocclusion by direct force on the dentition, but rather to induce tooth movement by alteration in soft tissue pressure. Expansion of the upper arch occurs due to the tongue pressure on the inside and elimination of buccal forces on the outside due to the addition of buccal shields, which are designed to remove the effects of the buccal musculature on the dentition. Similarly, movement of the upper incisor occurs due to the lower lip resting and acting labial to the teeth. Dr Frankel applied the concepts of Van der Klaauw, later made popular by Melvin Moss,[13] regarding functional cranial components. The objectives of functional therapy could, therefore, be described as the re-establishment of physiological space conditions by the placement of the appliance leading to correction of aberrant neuromuscular behaviour and pressures.

This appliance requires significant patient cooperation, technical skills during construction and design, and careful case selection.

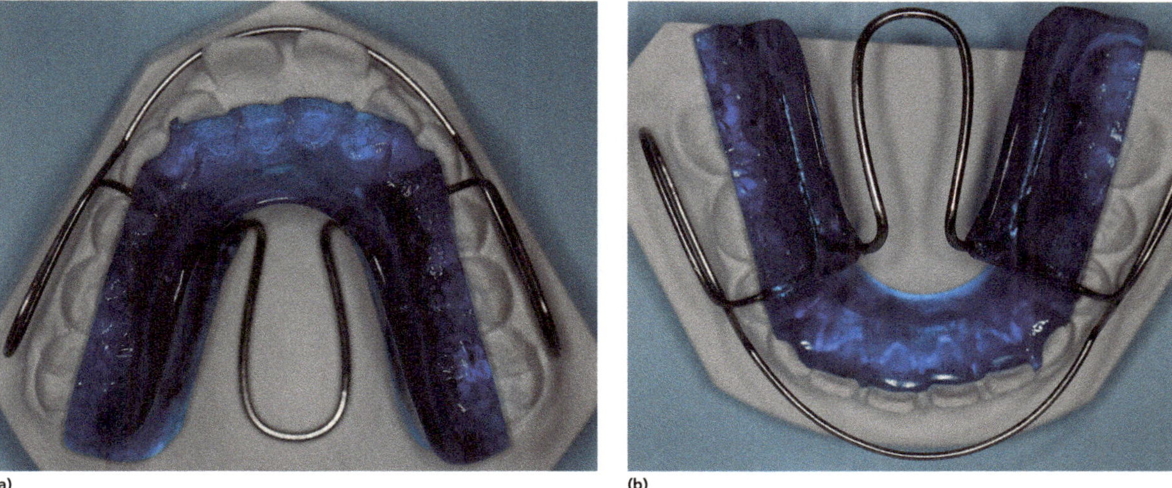

(a) (b)

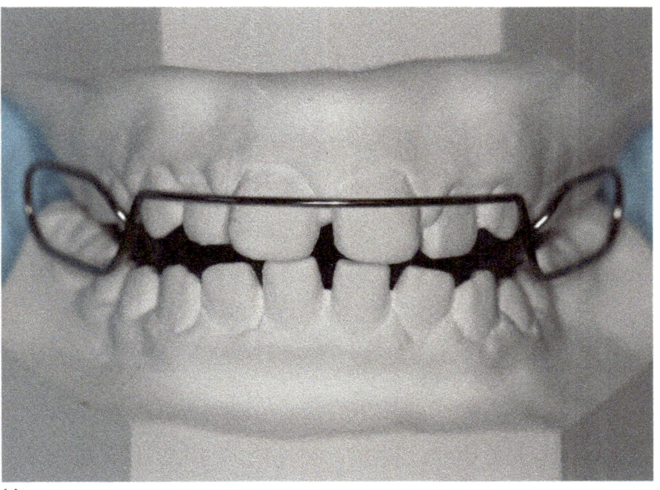

(c)

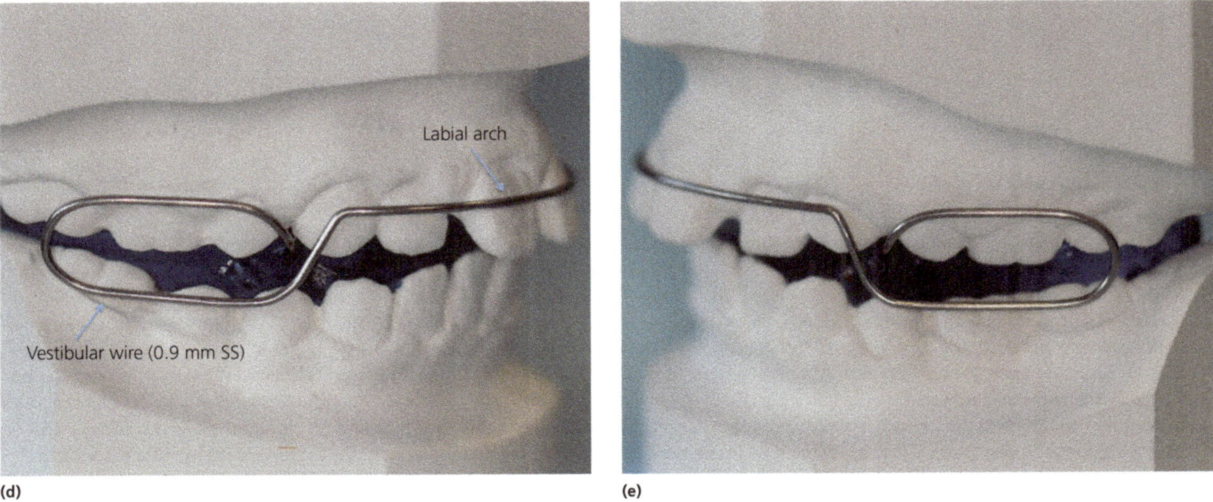

(d) (e)

Figure 2.2 Bionator (a–e). Balters believed in the centrality of normal soft tissue pattern and behaviour in the development of facial form and inter-maxillary relationships. As such, he emphasized the pivotal nature of the education of soft tissues, including improvement of lip seal and tongue posture and function, even publishing a paper on the 'self-healing' of malocclusion due to elimination of aberrant soft tissue patterns and behaviour. By advancing the mandible with the postured bite, Balters opined that dynamic space within the mouth was increased for functions including breathing and speech. The space for the tongue would also be increased with improved vascularization and lymphatic exchange. The appliance incorporates a vestibular and palatal arch and a resin body. The construction bite is normally taken with the incisors in an edge-to-edge relationship. The labial arch was initially suggested in an attempt to train the upper lip, promoting lip competence by introducing a stimulus for lip closure. Balters recommended prolonged wear of up to 20–22 hours daily, believing that the reduced bulk resulted in limited impairment of oral functions including speech, although removal was recommended for eating, oral hygiene, wind instruments and sport. The vestibular wire is fabricated from 0.9 mm spring hard stainless steel wire, with the palatal connector 1.2 mm in dimension. The vestibular wires should extend no further posteriorly than the mid-buccal groove of the maxillary first molars with separation of approximately 1 cm between upper and lower vestibular wires in the posterior region; it should also be clear of the teeth without encroaching on the buccal mucosa. There should be adequate clearance between the wire contouring labially and that in the vestibular region.

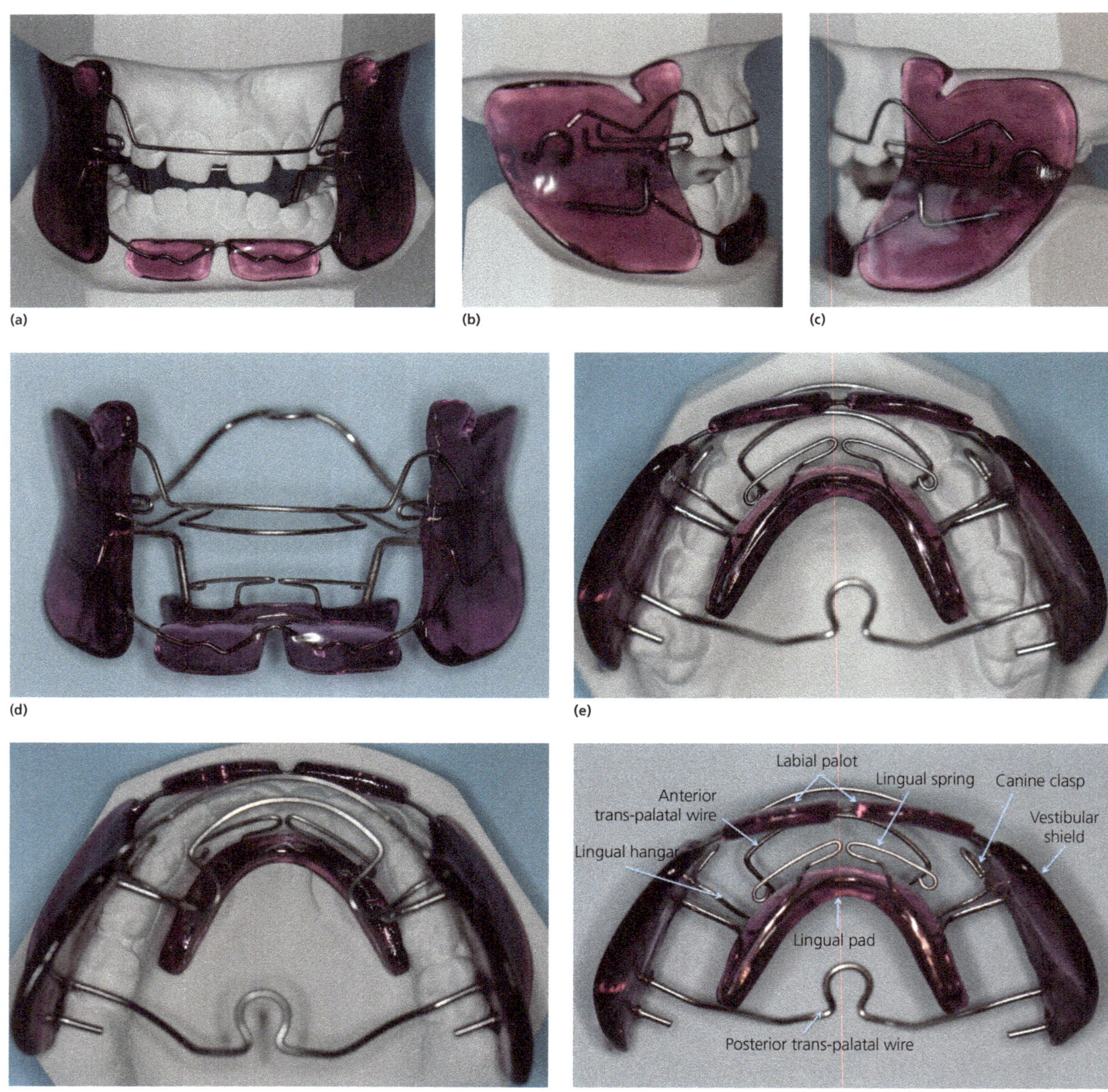

Figure 2.3 FR2 (a–g). Fränkel's appliances were based on his belief that the soft tissues were central to the development of malocclusion. He also aimed to restore normal muscle function with treatment. Consequently, the FR2 had vestibular shields to remove the influence of the buccal musculature on the dentition, allowing unopposed expansion due to the position and activity of the tongue. Moreover, by incorporating buccal shields Fränkel believed that more room was given to the tongue to allow tongue exercises to be undertaken. He also felt that this altered tongue behaviour would induce new bone in palatal growth sites, with minimal tipping of posterior teeth due to periosteal stretching. Moreover, the buccal shields and lower anterior palots were intended to induce traction on the periosteal layer, stimulating bone formation. The buccal shields are relieved 2.5 mm in the upper half and 0.5 mm in the lower half to facilitate expansion. Fränkel aimed to limit direct forces to the teeth from the wirework, with lower lingual shields designed to influence periodontal receptors and the mucosa, reflexly activating mandibular protractor muscles rather than allowing proclination of the mandibular incisors. He believed that forward mandibular posture was maintained by neuromuscular activity due to contraction of the extensor muscles rather than actively by the components of the appliance, suggesting that this would translate into less mandibular incisor proclination. The absence of occlusal rests on the lower dentition means that the vertical dimension is maintained by the height of the buccal shields. Consequently, while trimming of the shields may be undertaken in an effort to improve comfort and compliance, this may influence the vertical dimension and risk placing excessive forces from the lingual resting wires on the lower incisors causing further proclination, as these may contact the lower incisors in a more gingival position. Where excessive mandibular incisor proclination occurs, consideration may be given to removal of the lingual wires to allow the mandibular incisors to upright into a more stable position. The lingual pad is the heart of the appliance; it is carried by the lingual hangar and the lingual springs. The hangar is fabricated from 1.5 mm spring hard stainless steel with the lingual springs 0.7 mm in dimension; 0.9 mm spring hard stainless steel wires emerge from the buccal shields inferior to the teeth to carry the lower labial palots. Anteriorly the labial palots are relieved by 0.5 mm and they should not extend to the occlusal level of the lower incisors. The anterior labial bow is fabricated in 1 mm wire emerging from the buccal shields, rests gently against the maxillary incisors and is free of the canines. Recurved canine clasps are sited in the canine region and are not designed to engage with the canines. The anterior transpalatal wire is made in 0.9 mm spring hard stainless steel placed posterior to the cingulum of the maxillary incisors and features U-loops at its extremity that terminate in the buccal shields. The posterior transpalatal wire is made in 1.2 mm wire; it is recurved in the terminal aspect overlying the occlusal surfaces of the first molars.

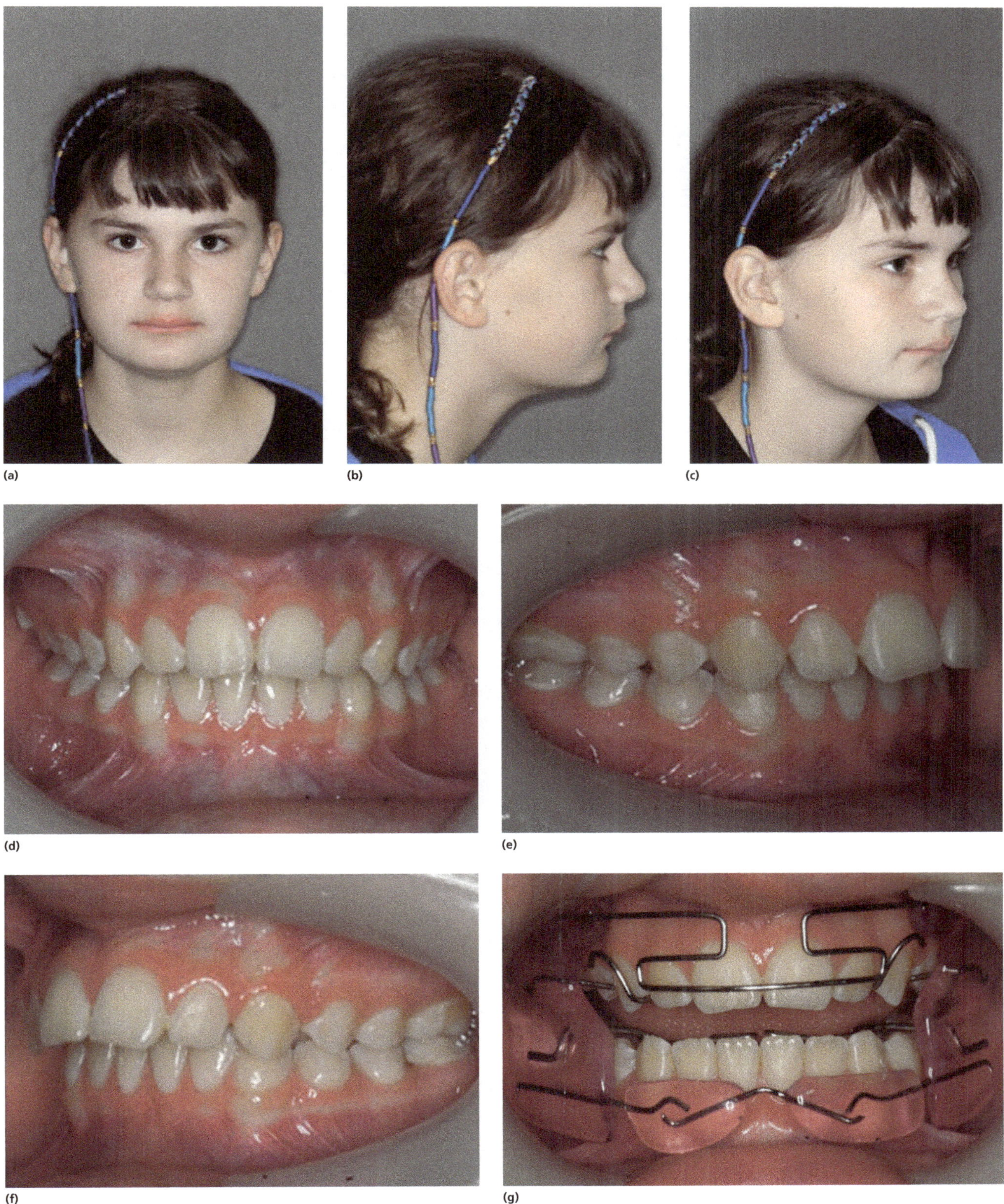

Figure 2.4 A 12-year-old female presented with a Class II division 1 incisor relationship in the early permanent dentition, with an increased overjet of 11 mm and Class II molar relationships bilaterally (a–f). There was a lower lip trap with a deep labio-mental groove, with the lower incisors upright on the lower dental base. An FR2 was fitted with lower labial palots and an upper labial bow (g). The lower palots were placed inferior to the lower incisors in the labial sulcus with the appliance fully engaged, inducing periosteal stretch. The appliance was worn for a period of 12 months resulting in full correction of the malocclusion with unfurling of the lower lip and a resultant advancement of the lower incisors; much of the overjet reduction was attributable to mandibular incisor proclination (h–p). The occlusion was detailed with fixed appliances thereafter over a period of 9 months (q–y).

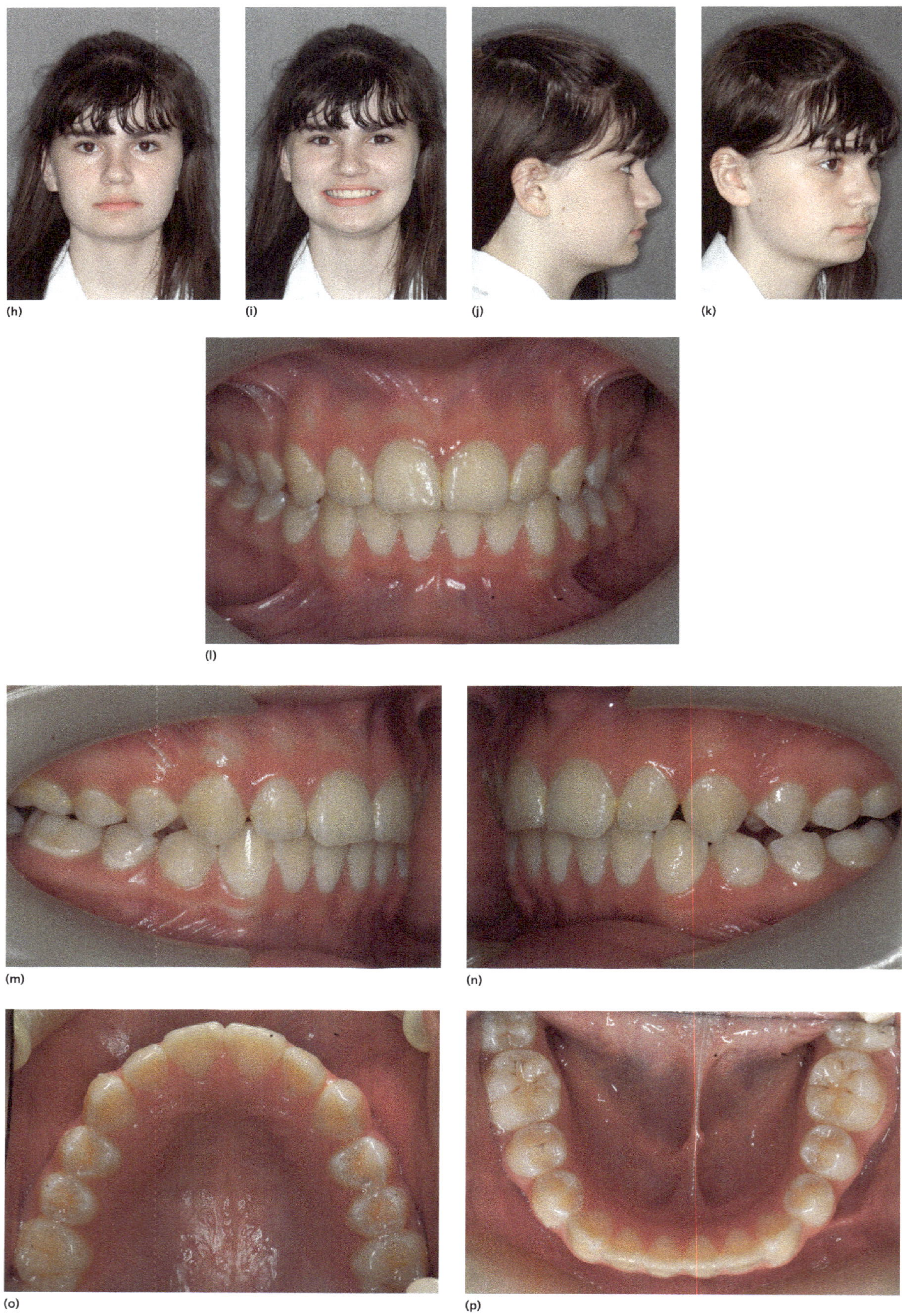

Figure 2.4 (*Continued*)

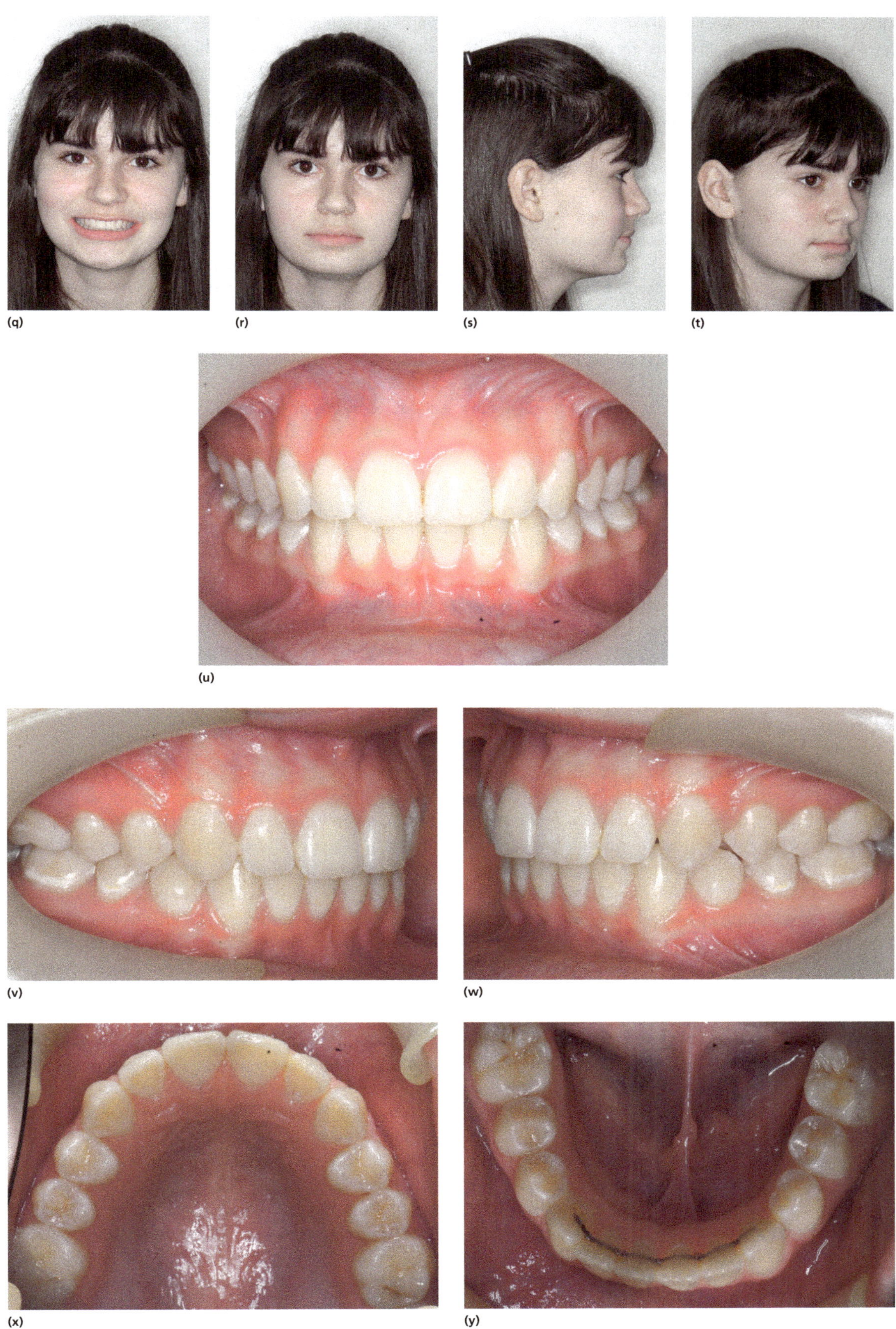

Figure 2.4 (*Continued*)

An advantage is that it can be applied prior to eruption of the permanent successors and in appropriate patients can produce quite dramatic changes in terms of overall facial appearance. The tenets on which the appliances are based are less accepted nowadays, however, and these appliances have largely been superseded, although they remain in usage. In the United Kingdom in particular, the tooth-borne Twin Block appliance has largely replaced both functional regulators and activators. However, in the United States, where early Class II treatment is more accepted and commonplace, activators remain in greater use, as they are less reliant on the presence of permanent teeth for retention. With respect to later treatment in the late mixed and early permanent dentition, fixed functional appliances, particularly the Herbst, have become increasingly popular in the United States over the past 20 years. It has also variously been recommended following fixed functional therapy in young adolescents that retention is provided by either an activator or a Bionator nocturnally until a fully established permanent dentition with occlusal intercuspation is achieved.

Twin Block

Subsequently, Clark[14] in Kirkaldy, Scotland developed an appliance system causing the mandible to posture forward in Class II, leading to correction similar in nature to the activators and Frankel appliances. This was a two-part appliance, which enabled the patient to wear it during eating. It is now known as the Clark Twin Block and is the most widely used appliance in the United Kingdom.[15] It is also being used to a limited extent elsewhere and has been the subject of a number of controlled clinical trials due to its effectiveness in producing occlusal correction in a fairly consistent manner.

The original appliance had shallow blocks with the upper and lower appliances set at 45 degrees to one another, a labial bow and a mechanism for the attachment of elastics from the lower appliances to a facebow to maintain a Class II effect during sleep. Clark[16] subsequently modified the design to increase the depth of the blocks, which are now set at approximately 70 degrees, and no longer advocates the use of a labial bow (see Chapter 5).

The primary limitations of the Twin Block are difficulties with retention in the mixed dentition and complexity in undertaking concurrent fixed appliance treatment with the removable Twin Block in place. Nevertheless, fixed variants have been developed to address the latter issue, while also removing the onus on compliance to achieve Class II correction.[17, 18]

Research reports on the Clark Twin Block[19, 20] show that the appliance has a limited effect in producing anterior posterior movement of the chin, with a consistent effect in leading to an increase in the vertical dimension of the face. Twin Block variants have been directed at reducing the bulk of the appliance and making it easier to wear, but the clinical effects have been impaired, often allowing the patient to avoid engaging the blocks with the mandible in the rest position.[21, 22]

Several attempts have been made to develop functional appliances that would not produce such an increase in the vertical dimension.[23, 24] These are recommended for concurrent use with headgear to limit vertical growth and posterior eruption. They therefore place an increasing onus on compliance, and definitive proof of the ability to restrain vertical maxillary growth remains lacking. Both the Bass Orthopaedic appliance and its successor the Bass Dynamax were introduced in an attempt to limit increases in the vertical dimension and to allow concurrent fixed appliance treatment, particularly in the lower arch.[25, 26] The Dynamax has a fixed lower element and a removable upper appliance with reduced bulk and a vertical wire extension to engage the fixed lower lingual arch. While less significant vertical changes have been reported with this appliance, it has also been shown to be less potent in terms of Class II correction compared to alternatives[27] and is technically demanding to make.[28]

Fixed functional appliances

These appliances have the advantage of requiring less patient compliance and also enabling the clinician to undertake concurrent fixed appliance therapy. As the patient cannot remove them, these appliances offer the advantage of 24-hour wear; this does mean that they are subject to the forces of mastication, with an associated heightened risk of fatigue and breakage.

Herbst

This appliance was introduced by Herbst[29] in 1905, although its development was not published until a later stage, and consisted of a fixed upper and lower splint mechanism with an interconnecting piston to force the mandible forward. It was initially used to modify growth and also in the management of temporomandibular joint disorders and the treatment of mandibular fractures. The use of the Herbst appliance has been popularized since the 1970s based on the work of Pancherz and co-workers in Germany.[30]

Pancherz[30] reported use of the Herbst in the mixed and early permanent dentition concurrent with fixed appliances. The effects of cast upper and lower splints in conjunction with fixed appliances were assessed via reports on a number of treated cases and the requirements for stability of the changes produced. Although the appliance is fairly robust, it is subject to breakage particularly in the piston mechanism and its attachments as the patient carries out antero-posterior and lateral excursions during mastication. Pancherz subsequently advocated use of the appliance in adults as a mechanism for disengaging the dentition and producing correction of the overjet and molar relationship. As the appliance design has not fundamentally changed, he has been able to report on the long-term effects and the relevance of long-term facial growth on treatment outcomes.[31] Nowadays, despite a lack of uptake over the first seven decades after its development, the Herbst is the most popular functional appliance in the United States and parts of Europe.[32]

Fixed mandibular advancement appliances

Various manufacturers have designed and marketed fixed functional appliances with the objective of reducing the bulk, allowing easier lateral excursions and insertion by the orthodontist without a requirement for laboratory construction. A host of such appliances have been produced over the past 20 years in particular.[33] This likely reflects a growing reliance on fixed appliance designs over the past three decades, particularly following the development of pre-adjusted Edgewise systems,[34] allied to an acceptance that functional appliances are largely incapable of producing significant skeletal change in the long term.

Fixed mandibular advancement appliances are particularly helpful in producing occlusal changes, but have yet to be shown to produce growth modification. Similar to the Herbst they are subject to breakage, but are effective in producing rapid changes in molar occlusion. Fixed functional appliances therefore have the facility to produce antero-posterior changes in the dentition, although the outcome is not devoid of the requirement for patient compliance. A range of these appliances have been developed and marketed in recent years (see Chapter 7).

Summary

It is clear that functional appliances have now been utilized as long as orthodontic practice has been undertaken. Their use has increased in Europe and the United Kingdom, particularly with the standard use of pre-adjusted Edgewise appliances, which are somewhat limited in the correction of antero-posterior discrepancies relative to precursors, including the Begg appliance. They are primarily used in adolescents with the objective of maximizing favourable growth changes. All functional appliances used in the correction of Class II malocclusion utilize forward and downward posture or the mandible to produce changes in the dentition involving tooth movement in the upper and lower arches to varying degrees.

References

1. Wahl N. Orthodontics in 3 millennia. Chapter 2: Entering the modern era. Am J Orthod Dentofacial Orthop. 2005; 127: 510–15.
2. Roux W. Der Kampf del Teile im Organismus. Leipzig: Engelmann; 1881.
3. Angle EH. The latest and best in orthodontic mechanism. Dental Cosmos 1928; 70: 1143–58.
4. Kingsley NH. A treatise on oral deformities. New York: D. Appleton; 1880.
5. Wahl N. Orthodontics in 3 millennia. Chapter 9: Functional appliances to midcentury. Am J Orthod Dentofacial Orthop. 2006; 129: 829–33.
6. Rogers AP. Making facial muscles our allies in treatment and retention. Dental Cosmos 1918; 64: 711–30.
7. Rogers A. Myofunctional treatment from a practical standpoint. Am J Orthod. 1940; 26: 1131–7.
8. Selmer-Olsen R. En kritisk betraktning over 'Det norske system'. Norske Tannlaegefor. Tidskrift. 1937; 47: 176–93.
9. Oppenheim A. The crisis in orthodontia. Int J Orthod. 1934; 20: 1201–13.
10. Bimler B. Hans Peter Bimler at age 85. Int J Orthod. 2002; 13: 19–20.
11. Balters W. Allgemeines zur Atmung und Atmungsstörung. Fortschr Kieferorthop. 1954; 15: 193–200.
12. Fränkel R. Funktiotnskieferorthopadie und der Mundvorhof als apparative Basis. Berlin: VEB Verlag Volk und Gesundheit; 1967.
13. Moss ML, Rankow RM. The role of the functional matrix in mandibular growth. Angle Ortho. 1968; 38: 95–103.
14. Clark WJ. The twin block traction technique. Eur J Orthod. 1982; 4: 129–38.
15. Chadwick SM, Banks P, Wright JL. The use of myofunctional appliances in the UK: A survey of British orthodontists. Dent Update. 1998; 25: 302–8.
16. Clark W. Design and management of Twin Blocks: Reflections after 30 years of clinical use. J Orthod. 2010; 37: 209–16.
17. Clark WJ. New horizons in orthodontics & dentofacial orthopedics: Fixed Twin Blocks & TransForce lingual appliances. Int J Orthod Milwaukee. 2011; 22: 35–40.
18. Read MJ, Deacon S, O'Brien K. A prospective cohort study of a clip-on fixed functional appliance. Am J Orthod Dentofacial Orthop. 2004; 125: 444–9.
19. Illing HM, Morris DO, Lee RT. A prospective evaluation of Bass, Bionator and Twin Block appliances. Part 1: Rhe hard tissues. Eur J Orthod. 1998; 20: 501–16.
20. Lund DI, Sandler PJ. The effects of Twin Blocks: A prospective controlled study. Am J Orthod Dentofacial Orthop. 1998; 113: 104–10.
21. Gill DS, Lee RT. Prospective clinical trial comparing the effects of conventional Twin-block and mini-block appliances. Part 1: Hard tissue changes. Am J Orthod Dentofacial Orthop. 2005; 127: 465–72.
22. Sharma AA, Lee RT. Prospective clinical trial comparing the effects of conventional Twin-block and mini-block appliances. Part 2: Soft tissue changes. Am J Orthod Dentofacial Orthop. 2005; 127: 473–82.
23. van Beek H. Combination headgear-activator. J Clin Orthod. 1984; 18: 185–9.
24. Teuscher U. A growth-related concept for skeletal class II treatment. Am J Orthod. 1978; 74: 258–75.
25. Bass NM. Dento-facial orthopaedics in the correction of class II malocclusion. Br J Orthod. 1982; 9: 3–31.
26. Bass NM. The Dynamax system: A new orthopaedic appliance and case report. J Orthod. 2006; 33: 78–89.
27. Lee RT, Kyi CS, Mack GJ. A controlled clinical trial of the effects of the Twin Block and Dynamax appliances on the hard and soft tissues. Eur J Orthod. 2007; 29: 272–82.

28. Thiruvenkatachari B, Sandler J, Murray A, Walsh T, O' Brien K. Comparison of Twin-block and Dynamax appliances for the treatment of Class II malocclusion in adolescents: A randomized controlled trial. Am J Orthod Dentofacial Orthop. 2010; 138: 144–e1.
29. Herbst E. Atlas und Grundriss der Zahnartztlichen Orthopadie. Munich: J.F. Lehmann; 1910.
30. Pancherz H. Treatment of Class II malocclusions by jumping the bite with the Herbst appliance: A cephalometric investigation. Am J Orthod. 1979; 76: 423–42.
31. Pancherz H. The Herbst appliance: Its biologic effects and clinical use. Am J Orthod. 1985; 87: 1–20.
32. Keim RG, Gottlieb EL, Nelson AH, Vogels DS. 2008 JCO study of orthodontic diagnosis and treatment procedures. Part 1: Results and trends. J Clin Orthod. 2008; 32: 625–41.
33. McSherry P, Bradley H. Class II correction-reducing patient compliance: A review of the available techniques. J Orthod. 2000; 27: 219–25.
34. Andrews LF. The straight-wire appliance, origin, controversy, commentary. J Clin Orthod. 1976; 10: 99–114.

CHAPTER 3

The role of genetics and environmental factors on the condyle in mandibular growth

Peter A. Mossey and Colin Larmour

The role of the condyle in mandibular growth remains an area of continued interest in the field of orthodontic science. Numerous studies over the years have been able to demonstrate the pattern of mandibular growth, and have provided information on the various sites of growth that contribute to the final mandibular form. The mandibular implant experiments of Björk, for example, have demonstrated that the condylar region is the main contributor to total ramus height, and a combination of resorption at the anterior border allied to apposition of the posterior border determines ramus width and body length.[1, 2]

The precise mechanisms involved are, however, less well defined. There are three principal mechanisms involved in the growth of the craniofacial skeleton:

- Primary cartilaginous growth at the spheno-occipital and spheno-ethmoiodal synchondroses and the nasal septum with the replacement of cartilage by bone are important primary growth centres under tight genetic control. Growth of the anterior cranial base, however, is complete by age 7 years with the fusion of the spheno-ethmoidal synchondrosis.[3]
- Sutural growth in which bones are united by connective tissue (synarthroses) is an important passive growth mechanism, subject to significant environmental influences, whereby there is bone deposition filling space created by a tension field. Sutural and endocondral sites have limited growth, and usually cease activity towards adulthood.
- Appositional and resorptive growth (bony remodelling) occurs on either the outer (periosteal) or inner (endosteal) surfaces of bone throughout life.

There are complex inter-relationships between these three mechanisms that remain incompletely understood. For example, growth of the upper facial skeleton and of the mandible occurs by entirely different mechanisms, yet growth of the maxilla and mandible needs to be closely correlated in three dimensions to ensure that occlusion is established.

Growth in the length of the mandible occurs primarily by resorption at the anterior border and deposition of bone along the posterior border of the ramus, and vertical growth is a result of upward and backward growth at the condyle, which rests against the articular fossa of the temporal bone at the cranial base, resulting in movement of the entire mandible downwards and forwards (see Figure 1.2).[4]

Controversy still exists as to whether mandibular growth is under strict genetic control or can be influenced by environmental stimuli. As a result, two philosophically distinct and somewhat conflicting schools of thought on the mechanism of mandibular growth have emerged. The classic view is that growth of the condylar cartilage is under genetic control and acts as a primary growth centre propelling the mandible downwards and forwards and thereby governing the overall size and shape of the mandible. The second view is that genetic control is mediated outside the skeletal system and that growth of bone and cartilage is controlled epigenetically (indirect genetic control) through response to a signal from other soft tissues. This view, put forward by Moss[5] as the functional matrix hypothesis (see Chapter 1), suggests that growth of the mandible occurs in response to functional needs and is mediated by the soft tissues investing the facial skeleton. As the mandible translates downwards and forwards in response to growth of the soft tissues, reactionary growth occurs at the mandibular condyle, increasing ramus length and maintaining the condyle/fossa articulation. Proffit[6] suggests that mandibular forward translation is influenced by the interlocking of the occlusion. As the maxilla remodels outwards and downwards, the occlusion maintains the downward and forward growth of the mandible in concert with the maxilla, thereby having its effect on the condyle.

This area continues to provoke much debate within orthodontics, because if environmental factors can make a significant impact then it should be possible to alter growth with appliances correcting any underlying disproportionate growth of the jaws. In a series of follow-up articles, Moss provides a less extreme view of the influence of genetics but continues to emphasize the major role of the functional matrix.[7–11]

Orthodontic Functional Appliances: Theory and Practice, First Edition. Padhraig Fleming and Robert Lee.

Genetic control of condylar growth

The future condyle develops from a condensation of alkaline phosphatase-positive cells that are continuous anteriorly with the mandibular periosteum.[12] This suggests that these cells are not truly mesenchymal in character, but have already differentiated into periosteum-like cells that may still be bipotent between osteogenic and chondrogenic lineages.[13] In the developing mandibular condylar cartilage (MCC), the bipotentiality of prechondroblastic cells is exemplified by their expression of both mRNA for osteogenic lineage markers, such as type I collagen, Runx2 and Osterix, and mRNA for Sox9, a marker for chondrogenic differentiation.[14] Notch1 and Twist, known as cell fate mediators in a variety of tissues, are both expressed largely in the prechondroblastic layer in the developing MCC[15, 16] and the expression levels of these factors may also play a role in the differentiation pathway. Experiments in secondary cartilage on the intra-membranous bones of the chick suggest that movement or articulation is necessary for diversion of the otherwise osteogenic precursors to chondrogenesis in the region of articulation between two bones.[17]

Notch proteins are cell surface receptors that mediate critical cellular functions through direct cell–cell contact. Interactions between Notch receptors and their ligands regulate cell fate decisions such as differentiation, proliferation and apoptosis in numerous tissues. Notch1 is localized primarily to the prechondroblastic (chondroprogenitor) layer of the MCC. Serrano et al.[18] analysed gene array data and demonstrated that the perichondrial layer of the MCC is rich in Notch receptors (Notch 3 and 4) and Notch ligands (Jagged and Delta) as well as various downstream facilitators of Notch signalling. Disruption of Notch signalling in MCC explants decreases proliferation and increases chondrocyte differentiation (as indicated by Sox9 expression), and helps explain the regulation of proliferation and differentiation in the MCC. Differences in gene expression between periosteal perichondrium and the underlying cartilage layers determine growth regulation and tissue regeneration in different zones of the MCC, and this unique bipotency is the characteristic that explains the growth response and response to mechanical stimulation, such as that during functional appliance therapy (Figure 3.1).

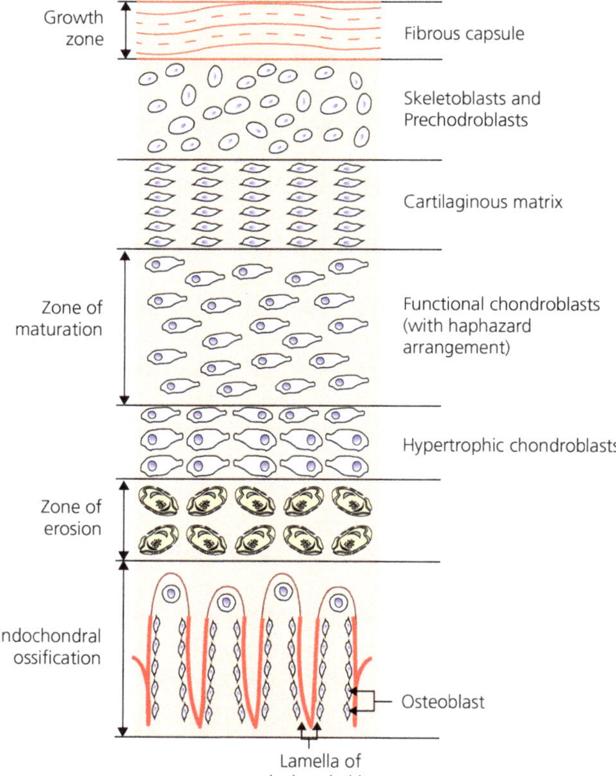

Figure 3.1 Arrangement of bone-producing cells within condylar growth sites. Specific differences relative to endochondral ossification in long bones include the haphazard arrangement of the cartilage-producing cells and the presence of a layer of dense fibrous connective tissue.

Evidence from animal experiments: Condylar injury, transplantation and growth factors

See Figure 3.2.

Condylar removal/injury

In animal experiments, Sarnat and Muchnic[19] found that condylectomy resulted in vertical facial growth deficiency in both growing and adult animals, in particular the maxillary and mandibular dento-alveolar regions. The fact that this was observed in both growing and adult monkeys indicated that the important factor was loss of integrity of the temporo-mandibular joint rather than loss of growth site. Spyropoulos and Tsolakis[20] demonstrated that following condylar injury and scarring, mandibular growth can be restored to normal by maintaining the mandible in a protrusive position with an intra-oral appliance; this suggests that following a functional disturbance, normal growth can be restored by overcoming the restriction and translating the mandible forwards in response to the soft tissue demands.

The effects of removing a cartilage on growth pattern are also informative. Fracture of the neck of the condyle results in the condylar head being retracted away from the glenoid fossa by the pull of the lateral pterygoid muscle. The condyle has effectively been removed and resorbs over a period of time. If the condyle was an important primary growth center, it would be expected that this injury would result in a severe impairment in mandibular growth if it occurred at a young age. However, two excellent Scandinavian studies[21, 22] appear to disprove this contention. Both studies demonstrated that the condyle tends to regenerate in the majority of children and that in the majority of cases (80%) there are no long-term adverse effects on mandibular growth. However, it has also been suggested that 20% of cases that have growth disturbances may result from intracapsular haemorrhage

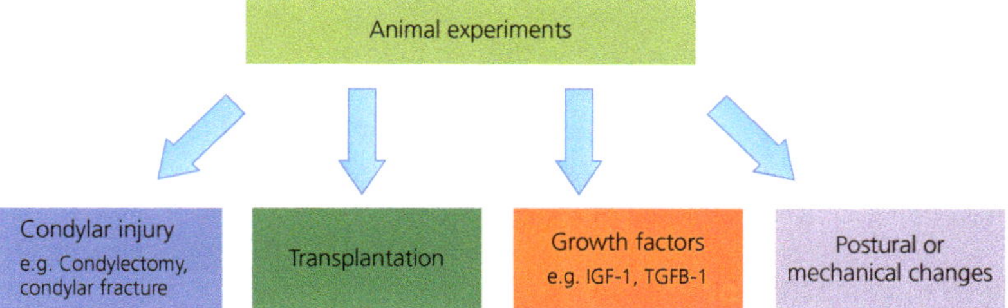

Figure 3.2 Experimental evidence for control of condylar growth.

and scar tissue formation.[23] This impeded mandibular translation is also seen in patients with ankylosis of the temporo-mandibular joints secondary to juvenile arthritis or infection.

Condylar transplantation experiments

Cartilage transplantation and culture growth experiments in rats[24–28] suggest that when the mandibular cartilage is transplanted or in tissue culture it appears to have little intrinsic growth potential. The effects of removing the condyle from its functional environment may be significant, since it is the cells of the proliferative zone that are responsible for the growth of the condylar cartilage. Experiments by Meikle have shown that the cells of the proliferative zone are multi-potential and can form either cartilage or bone depending on the environmental circumstances.[24]

Growth factor studies

Li et al.[29] suggest that growth factors can be produced locally by rat condylar cartilages. The growth factors IGF-1 (insulin-like growth factor) and TGF-B1 (transforming growth factor beta-1) appear to play an important role in the metabolism of condylar cartilages and probably growth. Other studies suggest that during puberty testosterone is important in local growth factor (IGF-1) production in the chondrocyte cell layers of the condylar cartilage.[30] In adults after completion of normal physiological growth, increased pituitary secretion may stimulate active sites of cartilage, producing the syndrome known as acromegaly. This particularly affects the extremities and the lower jaw, producing marked Class III malocclusion. That indicates that growth hormone can have an effect on the condylar cartilage.

The evidence supporting genetic control of condylar growth is therefore still inconclusive. The animal transplantation and growth experiments would suggest that the condylar cartilage has little inherent growth potential. However, the limitations of animal experiments have to be accepted, particularly since the proliferative zone of the cartilage is removed from its functional environment. The human trauma studies seem to support the argument that the condylar cartilage is not an important primary growth centre. Nevertheless, the recent work looking at growth factors suggests that there may be some degree of intrinsic growth potential within the condyle and therefore that it may exert genetic control on mandibular growth.[29, 30]

Achondroplasia is a rare genetic condition in humans and its effects on cartilaginous growth in the long bones contrasted with that in the cranial base and craniofacial complex are interesting. In addition to short limbs, the cranial base does not lengthen normally because of the deficient growth at the synchondrosis. The maxilla therefore is not translated forwards to the normal extent and a relative mid-face deficiency occurs. There is no apparent effect on mandibular growth, however, and these patients therefore tend to have relative mandibular prognathism, which further emphasizes the distinction between the genetic control of epiphyseal and that of condylar cartilages.[31]

Response of the condyle to postural or mechanical changes

Animal experiments provide evidence of alteration of the condylar cartilage response to changes in habitual position and/or movements of the mandible.

Effects on the glenoid fossa

In experiments where the mandible functions in a protruded posture, fibrocartilage thickening is noted on the articular eminence; however, the fibrocartilage layer is diminished or eliminated altogether in experiments in which the mandible is retruded (Class III traction) or restricted in movement. In the glenoid fossa region, new bone formation is noted in association with a protrusive repositioning of the lower jaw, while increased resorption of bone accompanies retrusion. Therefore, the position of the condyle rather than function or movement seems to be the crucial factor eliciting the response. These changes appear to be transient, however, and the resultant alterations in glenoid fossa morphology are restored to their initial states by resumption of 'normal' mandibular position and function.

Effect of immobilization of the mandible

Rubak et al.[32] have shown that joint motion is important for the maintenance of the chondrocytic phenotype in periosteal grafts. Hall[33] demonstrated that *in vivo* immobilization produced by paralysis caused the secondary cartilage of the condyle to be transformed into a bone-like tissue. In his study, the chondrocytes became smaller and came to resemble osteoblasts, and the matrix began to undergo calcification. These changes are similar to those noted on the articular eminence in Class III and 'protrusive fixation' animals. It is reasonable to assume therefore that in the human clinical situation the type of tissue formed (bone, cartilage or an intermediate tissue) and its route of formation are contingent on some aspect of the biomechanical environment in different parts of the joint.

Condylar growth during application of mechanical forces

Animal culture experiments[34] reveal differences in the response to continuous versus intermittent compressive forces. Continuous compressive force inhibits condylar growth even if it is relatively small in magnitude, whereas intermittent compressive force, while reducing the growth rate, permits condylar cartilage to grow *in vitro* even when the forces are of a considerably greater magnitude. In both instances there is reactivation of growth on removal of the forces and catch-up growth is also observed until a new balance has been achieved.

Functional/biochemical interface

It has been suggested[35] that the condylar cartilage functions mainly as a growth cartilage during the foetal and neonatal stages. Subsequently, as the articular function of the condyle increases, the growth activity decreases. Paulsen et al.[36] have recently carried out a scanning electron microscope analysis of cartilage characteristics and bone remodelling activity in autopsy samples of condyles from 20 individuals, ranging in age from 18 to 35 years. Quantitative and qualitative assessment of the turnover activity in the cartilage and bone suggests that although the growth activity decreases, some growth activity in the condyle was evident up to 30 years of age, and in acromegaly the condyle is responsive up to 37 years of age.

Other investigators provide evidence of the role of functional factors in subsequent growth, maturation and functional adaptation of the condylar cartilage. Kantomaa and Hall[37] investigated the importance of cyclic adenosine-monophosphate (cAMP) and calcium ions (Ca++) in mandibular condylar growth and adaptation. They reported that the cells in the proliferative zone of the condylar cartilage are undifferentiated mesenchymal cells or prechondroblasts, which later mature and hypertrophy. Function affects the maturing process and is mediated by cAMP and Ca++. An increase in the levels of cAMP and Ca++ accelerates the differentiation of mesenchymal cells and their maturation to hypertrophic cells. Function appears to favour differentiation of the prechondroblasts into chondroblasts (with condylar growth), whereas a lack of function favours differentiation into osteoblasts and conversion of the condylar cartilage to bone.

This difference in susceptibility to various biomechanical forces might be ascribed to the different localization of the cells. The prechondroblasts, which respond to the continuous forces, are situated near the surface of the condylar cartilage, while the functional chondroblasts, which produce the cartilage matrix, lie deeper. Since the nutritional supply for the condylar cartilage cells is produced by diffusion, it is conceivable that the pumping or blockading effect on diffusion by intermittent forces has a differential effect on the metabolic activity of the functional chondroblasts. Moreover, there is increasing evidence that membrane-bound adenylate-cyclase in a complex interplay with calcium ions and prostaglandins is a mediator in translation of the biomechanical stimuli into cellular reactions.

Epiphyseal growth rates are also sensitive to hormone and vitamin deficiency.[38] Although there is some recent evidence that the mandibular condyle is sensitive to testosterone, it would appear that it is also sensitive to mechanical pressure stimuli.[30] The pressure effects may be due to a unique proteoglycan (versican) in the condylar cartilage, which seems to be involved in the control of cell proliferation and differentiation.[39]

Environmental influences through functional appliance therapy

Effect of orthopaedic forces

The small continuous compressive force applied *in vitro* corresponds to continuous *in vivo* pressure exerted on the condyle by the perichondreal envelope. The functional activity of the mandibular joint *in vivo* is thought to generate small intermittent forces to simulate those already outlined. The insertion of an intra-oral or extra-oral appliance to protrude the mandible and therefore reduce the intermittent forces on the condyle results in an increase in activity in the proliferative zone of the cartilage, followed by a period of catch-up growth of the condylar cartilage, which continues until a new balance is achieved.

There are few clinical studies in the literature examining the influence on compressive forces in matrix synthesis in the condylar cartilage *in vivo*, but Petrovic et al. produced an overload on the condylar cartilage in rats with a chin cup and observed an inhibition in growth.[13] Petrovic et al.[40–42] have reported that the fitting of appropriate orthopaedic appliances that maintained the rat mandible in a forward postural position increased not only the condylar growth rate, but also the absolute size of the mandible. The mandible was 5–15% longer than that of the control animals. They also reported that no genetically predetermined final length of the mandible could be detected. McNamara[43, 44] has also carried out functional protrusive experiments using young adult rhesus monkeys and reported a consistent increase in the amount of condylar growth compared with the control animals.

Limitations of animal experiments

McNamara[45] recognized the limitations of animal experiments and carried out clinical trials to evaluate the treatment effects of functional appliances on mandibular and maxillary growth. The clinical trials using the functional regulator appliance suggested that the effects on mandibular growth in human subjects were much more modest (approximately 1–2 mm of extra growth). McNamara concluded that the results were characterized by unpredictability and that the amount achieved may be statistically but not clinically significant. Pancherz and Hansen[46] confirmed these findings with the Herbst fixed functional appliance and also demonstrated the short-term nature of any extra growth, with partial relapse over the following year. More recently, long-term radiographic studies have demonstrated that the Herbst appliance can increase condylar growth by 2–3 mm during the treatment period, again with a return to normal growth post treatment.[47, 48] These findings have been echoed more recently in randomized clinical studies. Apart from the difficulties of extrapolation of animal experiments to the human situation because of the differences in growth rates and physiological response to orthopaedic forces, the degree and duration of protrusion in these experiments would preclude their use in the human clinical context. The animal experiments also showed that relapse would occur if the appliance were removed before growth was completed.

Overall control of mandibular growth

Gene–environment interaction

Studies assessing the effects of functional disturbances and of orthopaedic forces confirm that the environment can influence mandibular growth and provide support for the functional matrix argument.[5] However, the consistent overall pattern of craniofacial growth with racial and familial similarities irrespective of environment or function is a strong indicator of overall genetic control. This is very apparent in cases where there is an obvious skeletal disproportion such as severe mandibular prognathism, for example familial Class III, where the inherent growth potential has overcome the capacity of the complex biomechanical feedback mechanism, of which the functional matrix is a part, to compensate.

Growth modification due to functional effects

Kantomaa and Hall[37] have applied their theory to explain the influence that function might have on mandibular cartilage differentiation and therefore mandibular form. When the mandible is rotated down and back, as for example in mouth breathing and digit sucking, the anterior aspect of the condyle has less functional stimulus, which results in less cartilage proliferation, more bone formation and ultimately less growth. This can then result in a more downward and backward mandibular growth rotation as development proceeds.

Conversely, experimental and clinical studies of functional orthopaedic appliances reveal that there is no doubt that the displacement of the condyle downwards and forwards out of the glenoid fossa results in an increased proliferation of the condylar cartilage while there is still growth potential in the cartilage.[43–45] This has been likened to the 'suture-like' infill growth mechanism, which operates in a tension field. However, clinical studies suggest that the mandible will revert to its inherent growth pattern once the appliance is removed. There is no overall increase in mandibular size relative to that occurring with normal growth. In other words, although a temporary acceleration of growth is achieved, it is not possible to stimulate growth to produce an ultimate increase in mandibular ramus or body length beyond that which is genetically predetermined.

Hence there is a rational reconciliation between the genetic and environmental views. The functional matrix theory does not preclude the influence of genotype on craniofacial growth and form and there is evidence that growth can be influenced by environmental factors. This is consistent with the epidemiological, experimental and therapeutic evidence. The reconciliation can be rationalized in the context of functional appliance therapy by the realization that the mandibular growth can be accelerated up to, but not beyond, a predetermined growth potential.

Relapse

If there are restraining forces on the osteogenic tissues, the normal growth and development can be retarded, as in condylar injury with scarring. Conversely, the removal of restraint can allow restoration of normal growth potential and also the direction can be modified to some extent, as for example in the use of a functional appliance following condylar injury.[20] This is referred to as 'optimizing' the functional matrix and results in secondary effects on bone growth. The extent to which the soft tissue matrix can be manipulated is, however, very limited and dependent on the characteristics of the individual. Bone movement to the extent that there is conflict with the investing soft tissue matrix will tend to relapse. Proffit[6] in his 'envelope of discrepancy' suggests that surgical advancement of the mandible greater then 12 mm will encroach on the soft tissues and tend to relapse. However, accurate parameters, which enable prediction of the degree to which bones or the dentoalveolar complex can be moved without violate the soft tissues, have not been clearly defined. Due to the spectrum of biological variation involving skeletal, soft tissue and growth factors, such prediction in an individual case is extremely difficult.

Summary

The condylar cartilage, unlike primary epiphyseal cartilage, appears to possess limited intrinsic growth potential. During post-natal development of the condyle, local and general growth factors modulate and preserve a complex interaction with biomechanical factors to influence the intrinsic proliferation and differentiation rates of the condylar cartilage. Therefore, while intrinsic genetic factors provide the potentiality of growth, its expression can only occur through the operation of extrinsic (functional) factors provided by the matrices.

Mechanical stimuli from the functional environment such as functional appliances are necessary to maintain the normal condylar growth pattern and can be used to optimize the expression of the morphogenetic potential for growth that resides in the condylar cartilage and can therefore influence the ultimate condylar shape. However, they cannot increase the absolute size of the mandible and if 'growth' beyond a physiological equilibrium is induced it will be condemned to relapse. Hence the early assertion of Sarnat and Robinson[49] that the condyle is unique and acts as the 'pacemaker and organizer of mandibular growth' seems to be a reasonable description of its role.

References

1. Björk A. Variations in the growth pattern of the human mandible: Longitudinal radiographic study by the implant method. J Dent Res. 1963; 42: 400–11.
2. Björk A, Skieller V. Normal and abnormal growth of the mandible: A synthesis of longitudinal cephalometric implant studies over a period of 25 years. Eur J Orthod. 1983; 5: 1–46.
3. Goose DH, Appleton J. Human dentofacial growth. Oxford: Pergamon Press; 1982.
4. Enlow DH. Facial growth, 3rd ed. Philadelphia, PA: WB Saunders; 1990.
5. Moss ML, Salentijn L. The primary role of functional matrices in facial growth. Am J Orthod. 1969; 55: 566–77.
6. Proffit WR, Fields HW, Sarver DM. Contemporary orthodontics. Oxford: Elsevier Health Sciences; 2014.
7. Moss ML. The functional matrix hypothesis revisited: 4. The epigenetic antithesis and the resolving synthesis. Am J Orthod Dentofacial Orthop. 1997; 112: 410–17.
8. Moss ML. The functional matrix theory revisited: The role of mechanotransduction. Am J Orthod Dentofacial Orthop. 1997; 112: 8–11.
9. Moss ML. The functional matrix theory revisited: The role of an osseous connected cellular network. Am J Orthod Dentofacial Orthop. 1997; 112: 221–6.
10. Moss ML. The functional matrix theory revisited: The genomic thesis. Am J Orthod Dentofacial Orthop. 1997; 112: 338–42.
11. Moss ML. The functional matrix theory revisited: The epigenetic antithesis and the resolving synthesis. Am J Orthod Dentofacial Orthop. 1997; 112: 410–17.
12. Shibata S, Fukada K, Suzuki S, Yamashita Y. Immunohistochemistry of collagen types II and X, and enzyme-histochemistry of alkaline phosphatase in the developing condylar cartilage of the fetal mouse mandible. J Anat. 1997; 191: 561–70.
13. Petrovic AP, Stutzmann J, Oudet CL. Control processes in post natal growth of the condylar cartilage in mandible. In: McNamara JA Jr ed., Determinants of mandibular form and growth. Craniofacial Growth Series, vol. 4. Ann Arbor, MI: Center for Human Growth and Development, University of Michigan; 1975: 101–54.
14. Shibata S, Suda N, Suzuki S, Fukuoka H, Yamashita Y. An in situ hybridization study of Runx2, Osterix, and Sox9 at the onset of condylar cartilage formation in fetal mouse mandible. J Anat. 2006; 208: 169–77.
15. Capps C, So S, Hinton R. Cell fate mediators in mandibular condylar cartilage. J Dent Res. 2007; Abstract 1233.
16. So S, Serrano M, Hinton RJ. Notch signaling in mandibular condylar cartilage. J Dent Res. 2007; Abstract 3010.
17. Buxton PG, Hall B, Archer CW, Francis-West P. Secondary chondrocyte-derived Ihh stimulates proliferation of periosteal cells during chick development. Development. 2003; 130: 4729–39.
18. Serrano MJ, So S, Hinton RJ. Roles of notch signalling in mandibular condylar cartilage. Arch Oral Biol. 2014; 59: 735–40.
19. Sarnat BG, Muchnic H. Facial skeletal changes after mandibular condylectomy in growing and adult monkeys. Am J Orthod. 1971; 60: 33–45.
20. Spyropoulos MN, Tsolakis AI. Altered mandibular function and prevention of skeletal asymmetries after unilateral condylectomy in rats. Eur J Orthod. 1997; 19: 211–18.
21. Gilhuus-Moe O. Fractures of the mandibular condyle in the growth period: Histologic and autoradiographic observations in the contralateral, nontraumatized condyle. Acta Odontol Scand. 1971; 29: 53–63.
22. Lund K. Mandibular growth and remodelling process after mandibular fractures. Acta Odont Scan. 1974; 32: Suppl 64.
23. Sahm G, Witt E. Long term results after childhood condylar fracture: A CT study. Eur J Orthod. 1990; 11: 154–60.
24. Meikle MC. In vivo transplantation of the mandibular joint of the rat: An autoradiographic investigation into cellular changes at the condyles. Arch Oral Biol. 1973; 18: 1011–20.
25. Meikle MC. The role of the condyle in the postnatal growth of the mandible. Am J Orthod. 1973; 64: 50–62.
26. Copray JC, Dibbets JM, Kantomaa T. The role of condylar cartilage in the development of the temporomandibular joint. Angle Orthod. 1988; 58: 369–80.
27. Copray JC. Growth of the nasal septal cartilage of the rat in vitro. J Anat. 1986; 144: 99–111.
28. Peltomaki T, Kylamarkula S, Vinkka-Puhakka H. Tissue separating capacity of growth cartilages. Eur J Orthod. 1997; 19: 473–81.
29. Li XB, Zhou Z, Luo SJ. Expressions of IGF-1 and TGF-beta 1 in the condylar cartilages of rapidly growing rats. Chinese J Dent Res. 1998; 1: 52–6.
30. Maor G, Segev Y, Philip M. Testosterone stimulates insulin-like growth factor 1 and insulin-like growth factor-1-receptor gene expression in the mandibular condyle: A model of endochondrial ossification. Endocrinology 1998; 140: 1901–10.
31. Brewer AK, Johnson DR, Moore WJ. Further studies on skull growth in achondroplasic (cn) mice. J Embryol Exp Morphol. 1977; 39: 59–70.
32. Rubak JM, Poussa M, Ritsila V. Effects of joint motion on the repair of reticular cartilage with free periostiografts. Acta Orthop Scand. 1982; 53: 187–91.
33. Hall RK. Injuries of the face and jaws in children. Int J Oral Surg. 1972; 1: 65–75.
34. Ehrlich J, Bab I, Yaff A, Sela J. Calcification pattern of rat condylar cartilage after induced unilateral malocclusion. J Oral Path. 1982; 11: 366–73.
35. Berraquero R. The role of the condylar cartilage in mandibular growth: A study in thanatophoric dysplasia. Am J Orthod Dentofacial Orthop. 1992; 102: 220–26.
36. Paulsen HU, Thomsen JS, Hougen HP, Mosekilde L. A histomorphometric and scanning electron microscopy study of human condylar cartilage and bone tissue changes in relation to age. Clin Orthod Res. 1997; 2: 67–78.
37. Kantomaa T, Hall BK. The importance of cAMP and Ca++ in mandibular condyle growth and adaptation. Am J Orthod. 1991; 99: 418–22.

38. Yamashiro T, Takano-Yamamoto T. Differential responses of the mandibular condyle and femur to oestrogen deficiency in young rats. Arch Oral Biol. 1998; 43: 191–5.
39. Roth S, Muller K, Fischer DC, Dannhauer KH. Specific properties of the extracellular chondroitin sulphate proteoglycans in the mandibular condylar growth centre in pigs. Arch Oral Biol. 1997; 42: 63–76.
40. Petrovic A. Control of postnatal growth of secondary cartilages of the mandible by mechanisms regulating occlusion: Cybernetic model. Trans Eur Orth Soc. 1974; 50: 69–75.
41. Petrovic A, Stutzmann J, Gasson N. The final length of the mandible: Is it genetically determined? In: Carlson DS, ed., Craniofacial biology. Cranofacial Growth Series, vol. 10. Ann Arbor, MI: Center for Human Growth and Development, University of Michigan; 1981.
42. Petrovic A, Stutzmann J. Further investigations into the functioning of the 'comparator' of the servosystem (respective positions of the upper and lower dental arches) in the control of the condylar cartilage growth rate and the lengthening of the jaw. In: McNamara JA Jr, ed., The biology of occlusal development. Cranofacial Growth Series, vol. 7. Ann Arbor, MI: Center for Human Growth and Development, University of Michigan; 1977.
43. McNamara JA, Connelly TG, McBride MC. Histological studies of tempromandibular joint adaptations. In: McNamara JA Jr, ed., Determinants of mandibular form and growth. Cranofacial Growth Series, vol. 4. Ann Arbor, MI: Center for Human Growth and Development, University of Michigan; 1975.
44. McNamara JA, Hinton RJ, Hoffman DL. Histological analysis of tempromandibular joint adaptation to protrusive function in young adult rhesus monkeys (Macaca mulatta). Am J Orthod. 1982; 82: 288–98.
45. McNamara JA Jr. Dentofacial adaptations in adult patients following functional regulator therapy. Am J Orthod. 1984; 85: 57–71.
46. Pancherz H, Hansen K. Occlusal changes during and after Herbst treatment: A cephalometric investigation. Eur J Orthod. 1986; 8: 215–28.
47. Pancherz H, Ruf S, Kohlhas P. 'Effective condylar growth' and chin position changes in Herbst treatment: A cephalometric roentgenographic long term study. Am J Orthod Dentofac Orthop. 1998; 114: 437–46.
48. Croft RS, Buschang PH, English JD, Meyer R. A cephalometric and tomographic evaluation of Herbst treatment in the mixed dentition. Am J Orthod Dentofac Orthop. 1999; 116: 435–43.
49. Sarnat BG, Robinson IB. Surgery of the mandible: Some clinical and experimental considerations. Plast Recons Surg. 1956; 17: 25–57.

CHAPTER 4

Functional appliance therapy: Indications and case selection

While functional appliance therapy has met with significant usage in Europe for decades, alternative forms of Class II correction were preferred in the United States until relatively recently. Geographical trends regarding choice of orthodontic treatment modality are not unique to functional appliances, with great variation in the uptake of standard edge-wise, pre-adjusted edge-wise and Begg appliances among others over the years. Often these patterns are dictated by the ideas and concepts of gurus; the pioneers of functional appliances primarily came from Europe, a factor likely to have increased their popularity in this region. In recent years this pattern has altered somewhat, with a majority of US practitioners utilizing functional appliances by 2008.[1] However, differences remain with respect to the specific choice of functional appliance in most common usage: fixed variants are popular in the United States, while removable functional appliances predominate in the United Kingdom.

Similarly, the specific indications for the use of functional appliances are varied. As with many orthodontic treatment planning decisions, including use of extractions,[2,3] the selection of the optimal approach to Class II correction involves a degree of individual preference. Indeed, there is evidence to suggest that varying modes of Class II correction have similar success rates and introduce broadly similar patterns of occlusal and facial change.[4] Nevertheless, there are a number of accepted indications for successful functional appliance therapy, as well as indications for a particular appliance or modification.

Age

Functional appliance therapy is typically undertaken in a growing Class II patient, ideally during the period of maximal pre-pubertal growth. The importance of timing reflects the ability of a functional appliance to modify mandibular growth, at least on a temporary basis. This growth modification effect is sufficient to address significant Class II dental relationships and has been shown to produce skeletal changes in the short term, the majority of which appear to diminish by skeletal maturity.

Prediction of the peak timing of mandibular growth has proven complex, with limited correlation between chronological age and rate of growth. However, arbitrarily chronological ages of 10 to 13 years in females and 11 to 14 years in males are typically regarded as conducive to successful functional appliance therapy.

Other practical approaches to predicting the maximal rate of mandibular growth include:

- Standing height measurements: Sullivan[5] adapted a technique based on standard growth velocity charts (Tanner[6]) by recording standing height at four-monthly intervals from 9 years of age. The accuracy of this technique has been found to be acceptable, although less so in females than in males.[6] However, Tanner's data is slightly outmoded; in view of secular trends, expected changes in contemporary society may be gauged more accurately using updated growth charts.[7]
- Hand–wrist radiographs: Hand–wrist radiographs were routinely used as an adjunct to facilitate identification of peak mandibular growth rates internationally. However, limited correlation between skeletal age and peak mandibular velocity has been demonstrated.[8,9] Consequently, their usage has declined in recent years due to concerns pertaining to limited diagnostic yield allied to the requirement for additional ionizing radiation.
- Cervical vertebral maturation (CVM): The CVM technique involves assessment of the appearance of the cervical vertebrae on a lateral radiographic view. It has been used to assess skeletal maturation and has gained wider acceptance following update[10] and further simplification, and has the advantage of being apparent on the standard lateral cephalometric radiograph.[11] It has been suggested that the peak rate of mandibular growth occurs within 12 months of the attainment of cervical vertebral maturation stage II, characterized by concavities on the lower border of C2 and C3. At this juncture the vertebral bodies of C3 and C4 may be either trapezoid or rectangular horizontal in shape. By maturation stage III, concavities are present on the lower borders of C2, C3 and C4. The bodies of both C3 and C4 are rectangular horizontal in

Orthodontic Functional Appliances: Theory and Practice, First Edition. Padhraig Fleming and Robert Lee.

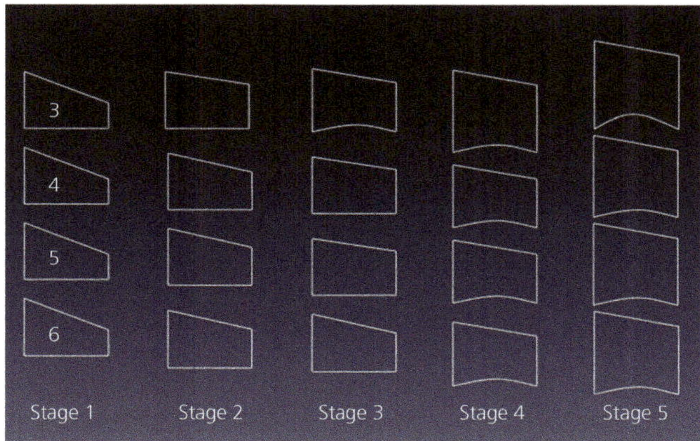

Figure 4.1 Cervical vertebral maturation (CVM) technique.

shape (Figure 4.1). Typically, the peak rate of mandibular growth has occurred 1 or 2 years prior to this stage. The reproducibility of the technique in terms of both inter-rater and intra-rater agreement has been questioned,[12] although some researchers have demonstrated high levels of agreement.[13]

The theoretical advantage of timing functional treatment with a period of maximal growth has been borne out in prospective studies. However, significant debate and indeed controversy have surrounded the relative merits of 'early' functional appliance therapy commenced prior to the pre-pubertal growth spurt in an attempt to harness growth potential at an earlier juncture. Results from these studies have indicated that early treatment, which usually involves two phases often combined with a prolonged retention phase, is no more effective and indeed is less efficient than treatment postponed until the pre-pubertal growth spurt.[14] There is also no evidence to suggest that earlier intervention will induce a meaningful difference in the skeletal pattern in the longer term.[15]

While there is limited prospective research on the relative merits of treating patients with a functional appliance at or after the period of maximal growth,[16] a randomized controlled trial specifically directed at answering this question would likely be unethical given the risk of depriving patients treated at a more advanced age of the benefits of what is considered the most timely treatment. Comparing the effects of appliances at different time periods, the Bass appliance was found to be more effective in boys treated during the period of peak height velocity, rather than before.[17, 18] Similarly, condylar growth has been reported to be increased in patients treated at the peak of condylar growth with a Herbst appliance,[19] being twice the rate of that in patients treated 3 years before or after this peak period. Similar findings were observed in a further retrospective investigation[20] with forward projection of Pogonion of 2.5–2.6 mm being reported; changes were slightly more marked in the group undergoing active treatment during the growth spurt. In a further retrospective study, Konik et al.[21] compared 22 patients undergoing early Herbst treatment and 21 patients having later treatment, with assessment of growth potential using hand–wrist radiographs. The group having treatment before the growth spurt experienced 3.1 mm of forward movement of Pogonion, while the group treated after this period had just 2.4 mm of forward projection despite undergoing active treatment for a longer period.

The use of functional appliances in non-growing adults, including the Herbst appliance, has been championed by a German research group.[22] The authors reported molar correction of over 4 mm; 22% of this change was attributed to skeletal effects. Moreover, 13% of the overjet decrease was related to skeletal modification. The authors therefore advocate the use of fixed functional appliances as a less invasive alternative to orthognathic surgery in adult skeletal II patients with relatively mild skeletal discrepancy. The reported skeletal changes include significant condylar and glenoid fossa remodelling based on both magnetic resonance imaging (MRI) and cephalometric radiographs. While these results are encouraging, the ability to modify skeletal pattern in adults without resort to surgical correction is limited and appears to produce changes almost identical to orthodontic camouflage. This treatment approach has met with limited application; with the exception of usage in sleep disordered breathing, functional appliances are therefore typically reserved for children and young adolescents.

Growth pattern

Just as predicting the timing of growth changes has proven complex, the ability to predict the pattern, direction and magnitude of facial growth remains limited. A significant amount of research has been dedicated to facilitating prediction:

- Cross-sectional and longitudinal growth studies: These analyses, particularly large growth studies undertaken in North America including the Bolton Brush,[23] Michigan[24] and Burlington[25] growth studies, have provided invaluable normative data in orthodontics. Studies based on these resources typically contain a mixture of age ranges, genders, occlusal and skeletal relationships and ethnic groups. Furthermore, mean changes are usually presented that fail to account for individual variation. Templates derived from these growth studies[26, 27] are used to forecast average changes, but have not proven sufficiently accurate to lead to reliable prediction on an individual basis. Additionally, earlier achievement of skeletal maturation and greater growth increments in present-day advanced societies will be reflected in facial growth as well as general stature and body mass.
- Longitudinal method: Serial cephalometric films can be superimposed on potentially stable structures[28] to establish the pattern of growth, which may be indicative of the likely direction of growth. However, the relationship between past and future growth has been shown to be surprisingly weak.[29]

- Metric approach: Björk[28] suggested that measurements from a single cephalometric view could be used to predict the future growth pattern. Once again, this method has not been proven to be effective.
- Structural method: Björk[28] also identified seven allied morphological features that he believed to be indicative of forward or backward growth rotations. These signs included inclination of the condylar head, curvature of the inferior dental canal, shape of the mandibular lower border, inclination of the symphysis, inter-molar angle, inter-incisal angle and lower anterior face height. It has been suggested that the presence of a greater number of these features would lead to greater predictive accuracy. However, Ari-Vivo and Wisth[29] concluded that the likely growth pattern could only be forecast in the presence of extreme rotations; more subtle variations could not be identified. Limitations of this approach have also been exposed in further studies.[30, 31] In a retrospective study, no relationship was found between the morphology of the lower border of the mandible and skeletal and dental improvements with Twin Block treatment.[32] The degree of concavity or convexity of the lower mandibular border, which Björk regarded as a structural sign indicative of mandibular growth pattern, was shown to have no relationship with treatment outcome.

Typically, however, it is believed that individuals with apparent posterior growth rotations are likely to respond less favourably to functional appliance therapy than those with anterior growth rotations, the latter being characterized by an increased overbite, reduced lower anterior facial height and decreased Frankfurt–mandibular planes angle. However, our ability to predict growth pattern and hence response to growth modification treatment remains limited. In the future, application of three-dimensional imaging modalities including cone-beam computed tomography may permit more detailed morphological and volumetric assessment of mandibular size and shape[33] and the outcome of growth modification treatment.

Vertical skeletal pattern

The relationship between pre-treatment skeletal pattern and occlusion in terms of the outcome of functional appliance treatment has been considered in both prospective and retrospective studies. In particular, skeletal dimensions, including overall mandibular length, ramus height, ratio of posterior to anterior facial height, cranial base length and occlusal predictors, chiefly overbite depth, have variously been linked to successful therapy.[34, 35] However, these associations have not been uniformly confirmed.

Functional appliances are typically indicated in the presence of average to reduced lower anterior facial height. While a number of the larger trials focusing on early treatment did not report vertical skeletal changes,[15, 36] facial height is known to increase during functional therapy due to a combination of accelerated growth and the orientation of the occlusal plane, with the latter being tipped interiorly and anteriorly. Illing et al.[37] reported an increase of 4.2 mm in lower anterior facial height during Twin Block therapy in a pre-adolescent group. Minor increases in the maxillary–mandibular planes angle (MMPA) are also typical, with Yaqoob et al.[38] alluding to changes of less than 0.65 degrees. The lack of significant change in the angular relationship is likely to reflect corresponding, albeit slightly smaller, increases in posterior facial height during therapy due to increases in condylar length and posterior eruption.

However, research has often failed to confirm the importance of vertical skeletal pattern to either occlusal or skeletal changes. The failure consistently to show a negative correlation is likely to be due to selection bias, with clinicians typically avoiding functional appliances in high-angle cases on clinical grounds; consequently, this may obscure a likely relationship by omitting subjects with significant increases in vertical dimension.[39, 40] Similar findings have also been reported in prospective studies.[41–43] In the study by Fleming et al.[40] involving the Twin Block, the mean MMPA of participants at the outset was slightly reduced (25.2 degrees), likely reflecting operator preferences and convictions given the retrospective design. Significant vertical excess is likely to have been managed without recourse to the Twin Block in many cases due to concerns about further increasing the vertical dimension. Consequently, pronounced vertical increase is likely to have been absent in this sample, making identification of significant relationships less likely. Assessment of the influence of vertical discrepancy on the outcome of Twin Block therapy would therefore necessitate prospective follow-up irrespective of vertical skeletal pattern.

Franchi and Baccetti,[42] based on a prospective study, have suggested that mandibular shape, specifically Co-Go-Me angulation, was predictive of both hard and soft tissue responses to headgear and Herbst appliance therapy. The authors observed that obtuse angles (in excess of 123 degrees) were less likely to undergo favourable treatment-related changes. This measurement provided an estimation of the skeletal discrepancy in both vertical and sagittal directions. In a more recent retrospective study with a shorter period of follow-up, however, this relationship could not be confirmed, with no association or threshold values observed.[40]

Antero-posterior skeletal pattern

The amount of change in the antero-posterior (A-P) projection of the mandible has been shown to be positively correlated with the extent of the initial inter-maxillary skeletal discrepancy[40] and SNB value in isolation,[41] with lower SNB values likely to increase more significantly during treatment than higher values. This finding may reflect the requirement for a greater degree of skeletal change in those with more significant skeletal discrepancy. The majority of studies have demonstrated forward movement of Pogonion of approximately 1–3 mm during appliance therapy. Baccetti et al.[43] reported 2.7 mm of relative forward movement of Pogonion in their prospective study involving two-phased treatment commenced with bonded Herbst appliance treatment. Similarly, in a meta-analysis Harrison et al.[44] reported a mean improvement in ANB value of 1.35 degrees with functional therapy during early treatment verses an untreated control; in adolescents the mean difference between treated and untreated groups increased to 2.27 degrees.

Transverse skeletal abnormality

Most functional appliances are capable of a degree of transverse correction. Fixed variants, such as the Herbst appliance, may incorporate rapid palatal expansion. Removable variants typically rely on midline expansion screws or springs (e.g. coffin spring) to achieve transverse improvement through tipping movements. With midline screws transverse expansion is usually started early in treatment and proceeds at a rate of 0.2–0.5 mm per week, with one or two turns of the expansion screw recommended on a weekly basis (Figure 4.2).

Expansion may be required to address both pre-existing crossbites and crossbites arising secondary to sagittal correction as a wider part of the lower arch moves forward in concert with Class II improvement. Certain removable functional appliances, particularly one-piece appliances involving acrylic coverage of the incisor teeth, do not permit transverse correction. Consequently, these appliances may be preceded by a preliminary expansion phase, usually with a removable appliance.

Rarely, functional appliances are indicated in the management of developing asymmetries that may be the result of trauma or craniofacial abnormalities, for example hemifacial microsomia. Typically, hybrid-type appliances may be used to advance the mandible on the side displaying deficient growth, while permitting eruption of posterior teeth on the same side to encourage levelling of associated occlusal canting, primarily by encouraging dento-alveolar changes (Figure 4.3).[45]

Occlusal features

Occlusal features including increased overjet and overbite have been linked to the success of appliance therapy in research studies. However, this pattern may merely reflect the extent of the presenting problem, with the aim of treatment being to reduce the overjet fully irrespective of the initial value. Arbitrarily, in Class II division 1 incisor relationships, functional appliances are typically considered with overjet in excess of 7 mm. In the presence of more limited overjet, functional appliances are often regarded as unnecessary, unduly complicating and potentially prolonging treatment. Nevertheless, the use of functional appliances is not restricted to Class II division 1, with successful usage in conjunction with Class II division 2 incisor relationships also common, particularly where correction of the molar relationship is required.[46] To facilitate this, simultaneous or prior decompensation of retroclined maxillary incisors may be undertaken, either with fixed appliances or with active components inherent in the functional design.

The possibility of improved success rates in the presence of an increased overbite[41] may relate to the likely co-existence of increased overbite with reduced lower anterior facial height and associated muscle pattern and soft tissue behaviour. The use of a functional appliance in these cases may, therefore, by a combination of forward mandibular posture and disclusion, allow the full and timely expression of mandibular growth to facilitate occlusal and skeletal correction. Moreover, with respect to the use of the Twin Block, with increased overbite sufficiently thick blocks (6–7 mm) can be incorporated without increasing the vertical opening in the incisor region excessively, enhancing patient comfort.

While most prospective studies have alluded to a ratio of dental to skeletal correction contributing to overjet correction of roughly 2:1, efforts are often made to maximize the proportion of skeletal change while limiting dento-alveolar correction. Consequently, modifications may be made to functional appliances to limit maxillary incisor retroclination or lower incisor proclination by, for example, including torquing spurs to the maxillary incisors or lower incisor capping. There is, however, limited evidence of a significant effect related to these modifications. Indeed, in certain cases it may be appropriate to maximize incisor movement intentionally in order to address pre-existing dental discrepancy (Figure 4.4).

Soft tissues

While the association between facial form and function is established, the causal link is less clear. It is suggested that a genetically determined facial skeletal morphology may influence the morphology and strength of the facial musculature; however, it is also conceivable that a strong musculature may in itself influence facial form.[47, 48]

Alteration in the development of the orofacial musculature has been shown to introduce significant changes in the shape of the mandible in animal studies.[49–52] Moreover, in humans increased bite forces are typical of reduced lower anterior facial height, while the reverse is true with increased lower facial height. In individuals with reduced lower face height, higher levels of Type II fibres are found than in those with normal facial dimensions, while high-angle individuals have a decreased number and size of Type II fibres.[53] However, it is believed that the orofacial musculature may have some limited degree of adaptive capacity, and that therefore it may possibly be susceptible to fibre-type switch in response to functional stimuli such as postural changes introduced by functional appliances,[54] with resultant alteration in contractile capacity.[55]

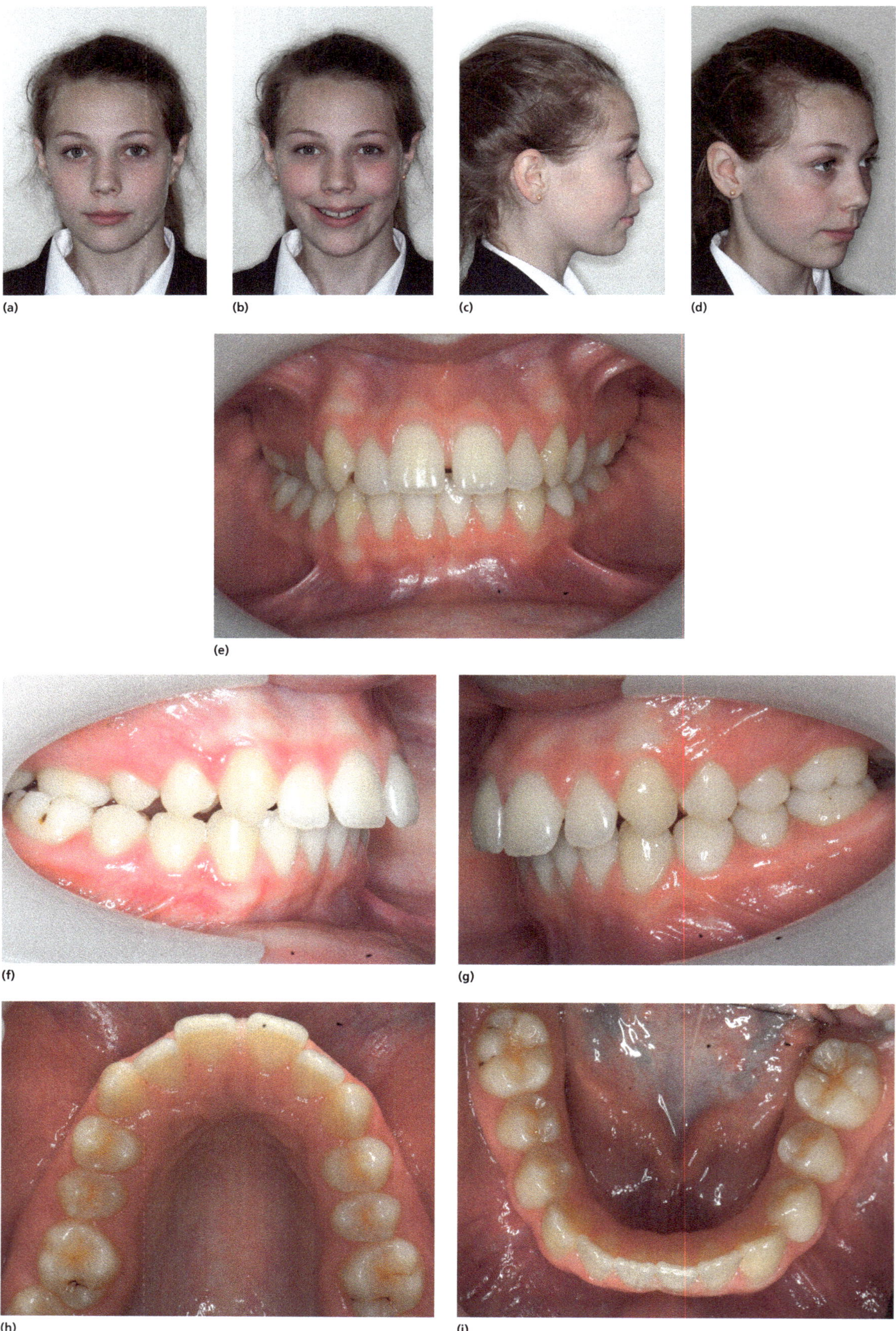

Figure 4.2 This 12-year-old female presented with a Class II division 1 incisor relationship on a skeletal II pattern. The malocclusion was complicated by a combination of increased overjet of 8 mm, upper and lower anterior malalignment and a unilateral posterior crossbite with displacement to the right side (a–i). She was treated with a modified Twin Block appliance for a period of 9 months to address the Class II element. The transverse issue was partially addressed during the functional phase with upper arch expansion (j–l). However, a crossbite tendency remained. This was resolved during the subsequent fixed phase (m–o). Total time for active treatment was 20 months. An upper Hawley retainer in conjunction with upper and lower bonded retainers was placed to retain the result (p–x).

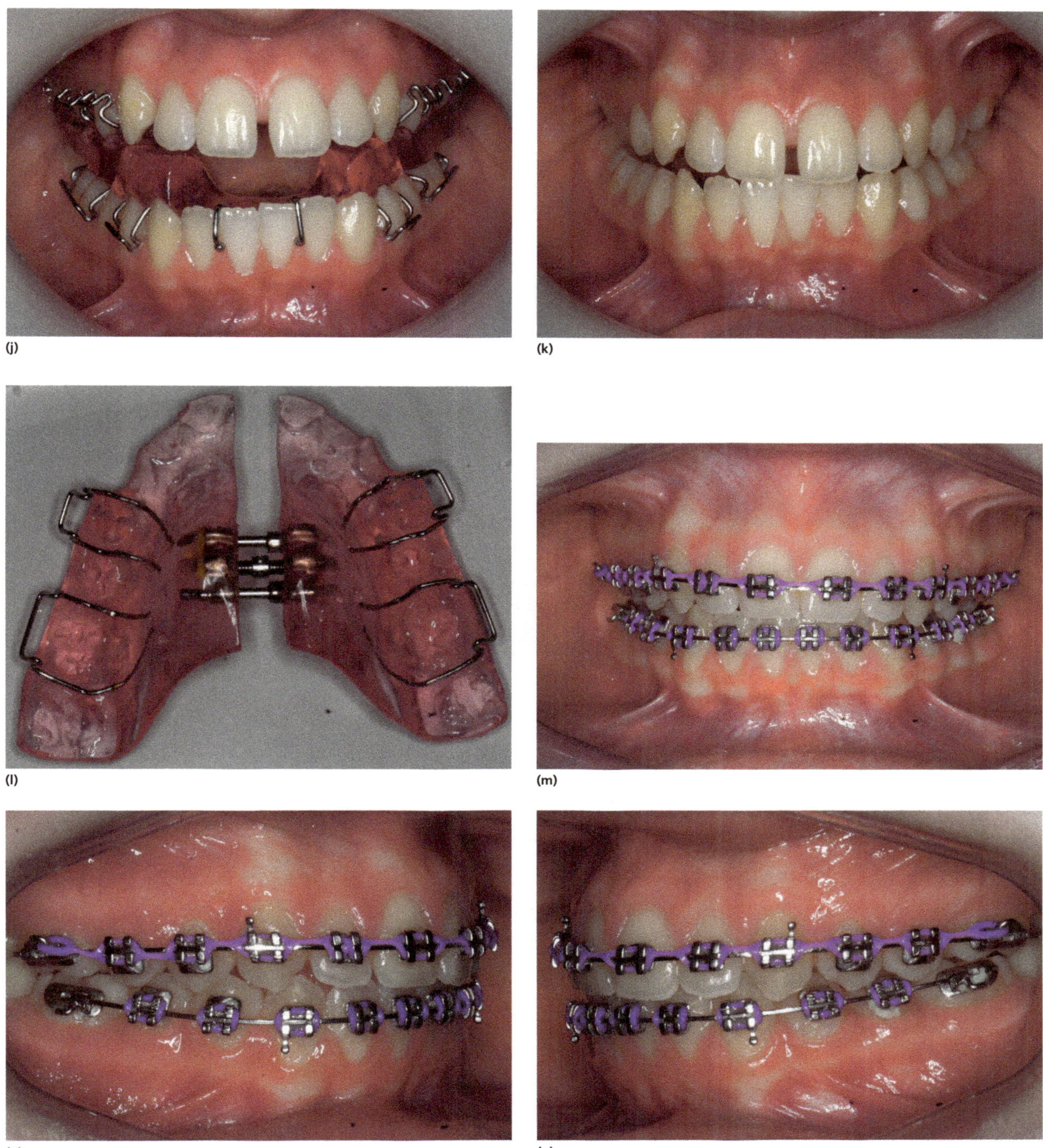

(j) (k) (l) (m) (n) (o)

Figure 4.2 (*Continued*)

Early use of myofunctional treatment in an effort to alleviate aberrant neuromuscular behaviour has received some attention, particularly in Europe. This treatment is based on the premise that malocclusion may be related to muscular behaviour and oral function. Van Dyck et al.,[56] in a pilot study comprising 22 children aged between 7 and 11 years, reported a marginal improvement in tongue elevation and posture with an associated increase in the prevalence of complete overbite. No improvements in speech or transverse changes were noted. The impact of functional appliances on bite force also appears to be equivocal.[57] A reduction in force levels in both the molar and incisor regions after 9 months of Andreasen treatment has been shown. These results were confirmed in a further analysis involving a Schwarz activator,[58] although the latter also highlighted a link between lower initial bite forces and enhanced dental and skeletal responses to appliance therapy. The authors

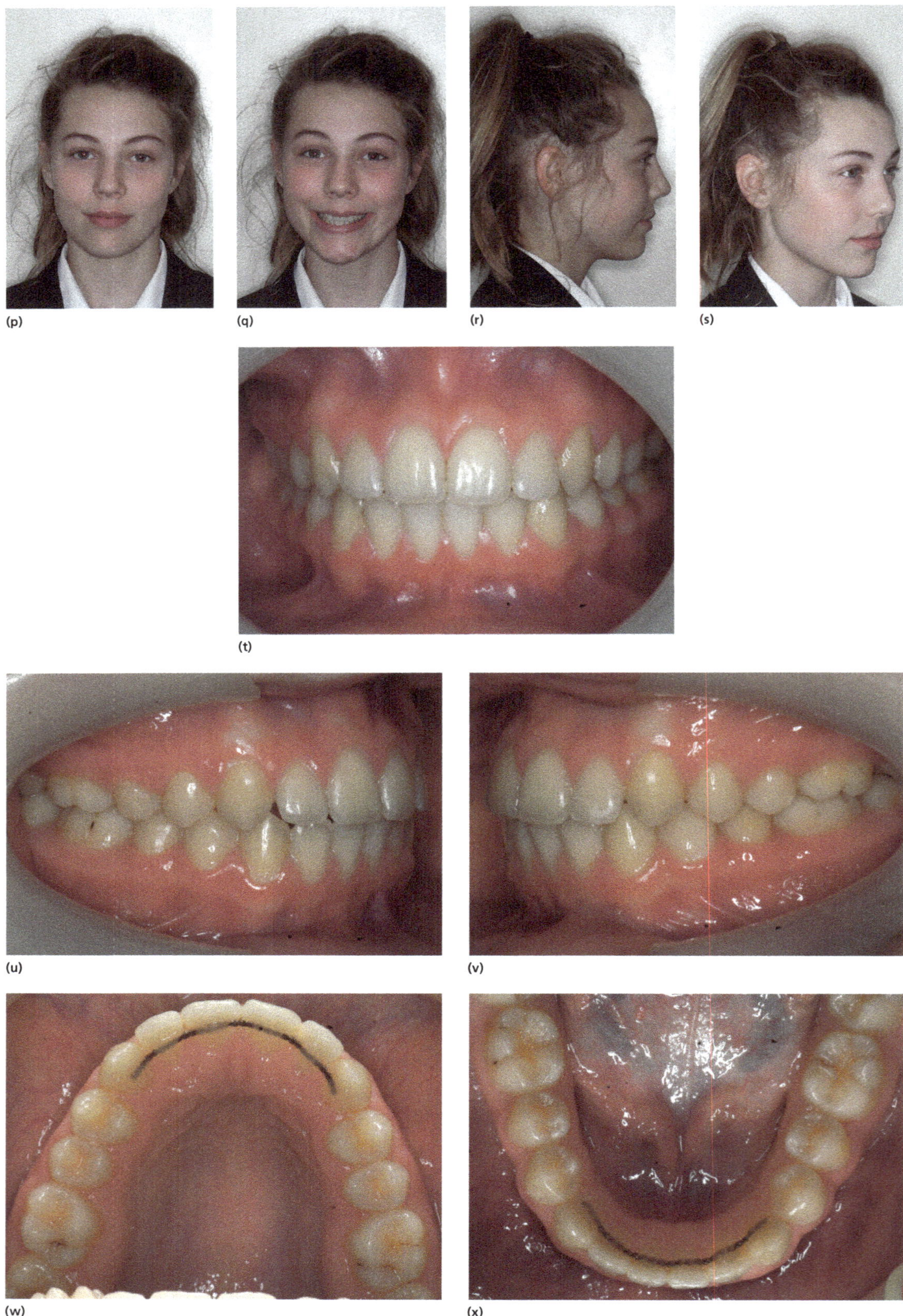

Figure 4.2 (*Continued*)

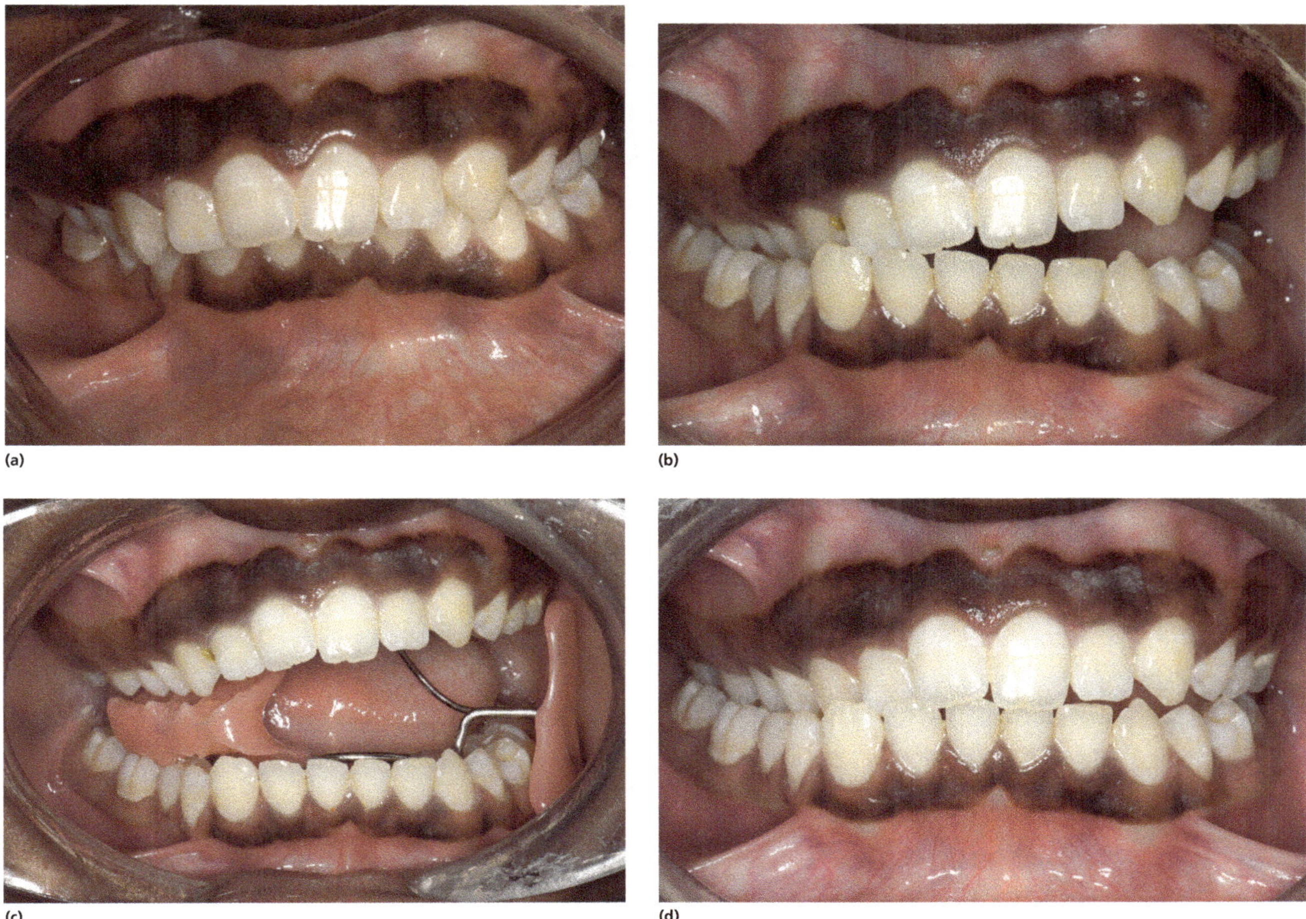

Figure 4.3 This 12-year-old male presented with a significant skeletal II discrepancy and mandibular asymmetry related to traumatic injury to the left condyle in infancy (a). This had resulted in a significant maxillary cant; mouth opening was also restricted (See Chapter 11). He was treated with mandibular distraction to address the skeletal II discrepancy and asymmetry in adolescence, resulting in increase in the ramal height on the left side and leading to a significant open bite on that side (b). A hybrid functional appliance with occlusal coverage on the right side only was fitted to maintain Class II correction while promoting vertical development of the left maxillary dentition (c, d). Fixed appliances were subsequently placed to settle the buccal occlusion.

attributed this differential effect to greater anchorage resisting forward mandibular displacement with thicker, stronger musculature. Conversely, weaker muscles may offer greater capacity for growth stimulation. In a 12-month follow-up of this sample, however, more dento-alveolar relapse was found in the subset with lower initial bite forces.[59] These conflicting data, allied to the methodological difficulties in measuring bite forces and masticatory muscle activity, mean that the role of orofacial musculature in both the indications for and indeed the response to functional appliance therapy remains speculative.

Individuals with increased vertical dimensions are believed to exhibit more obliquely oriented jaw muscles, leading to a more vertical direction of facial growth. With reduced lower facial height, muscle pattern may be more vertical; contractile effects may therefore act to limit increases in the vertical dimension, favouring an anterior rather than posterior growth rotation. This characteristic muscular pattern and behaviour may have an impact on the effectiveness of functional appliance therapy in high-angle patients, as functional appliances are reliant on forward mandibular posture, with associated alteration in muscle fibre orientation and muscle contraction required to introduce skeletal and dental effects.

Compliance

Functional appliance therapy is associated with some impairment of oral health–related quality of life during treatment. Indeed, in a prospective investigation, a similar level of impairment as that arising with headgear treatment was noted.[60] There is, therefore, a premium on compliance to achieve optimal outcomes. As functional appliances are mainly used in adolescence, varying degrees of compliance are to be expected from juveniles who are not necessarily compliant with operators, or may not entirely understand the necessity or potential benefit of treatment. Treatment may therefore be motivated externally by parents, peers or clinicians. The use of a fixed functional appliance that is not removable for adjustment might be expected to

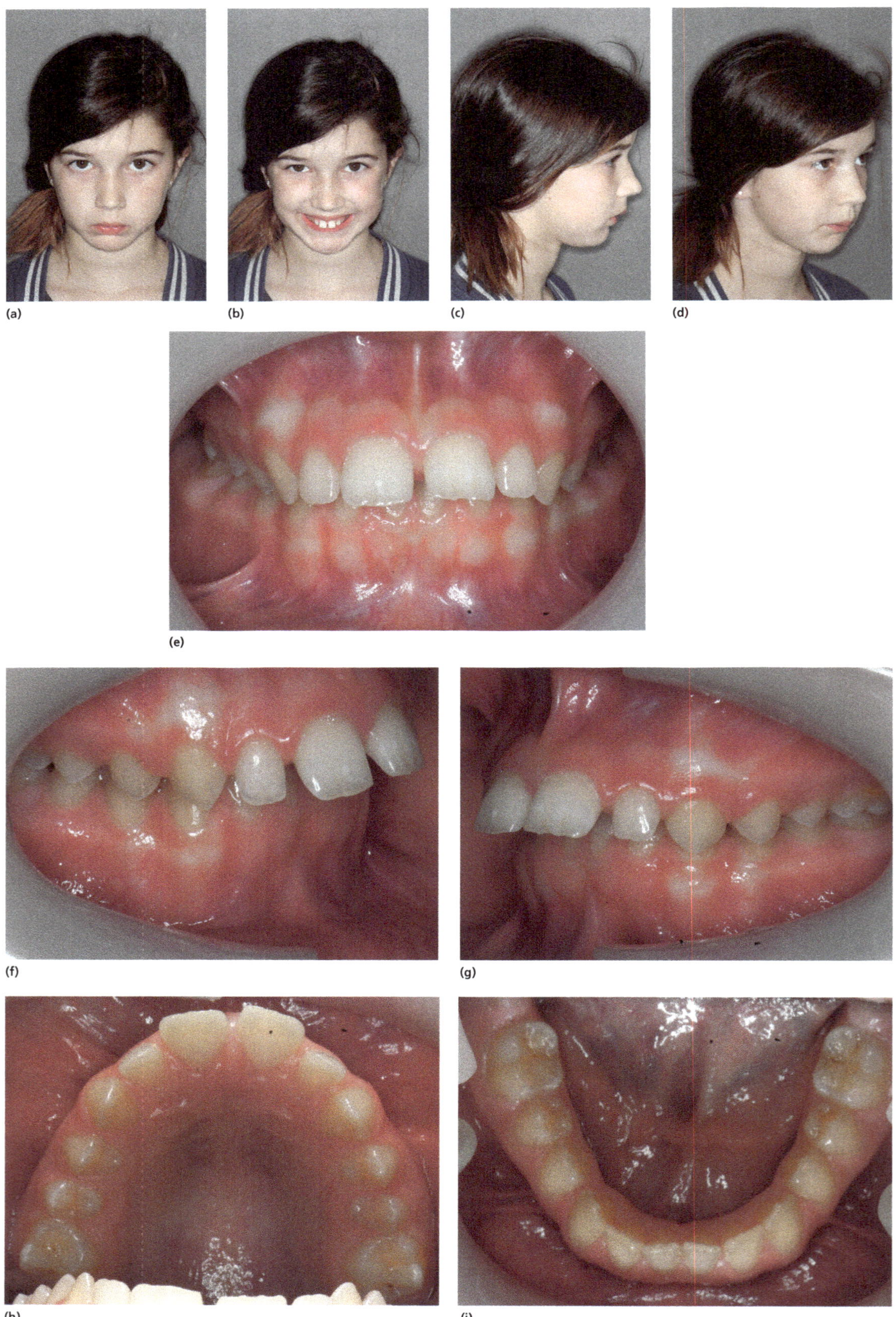

Figure 4.4 This 11-year-old female presented with an increased overjet of 12 mm. The molar relationships were Class II bilaterally. The maxillary incisors were spaced and proclined at 125 degrees to the maxillary plane with a lower lip trap. In this instance a modified Twin Block was fitted to address the Class II dental and skeletal relationships. An upper labial bow was incorporated to promote uprighting of the maxillary incisors. The labial bow was activated with the acrylic palatal to the incisors trimmed (j, k). The overjet was addressed with a combination of skeletal and dento-alveolar changes.

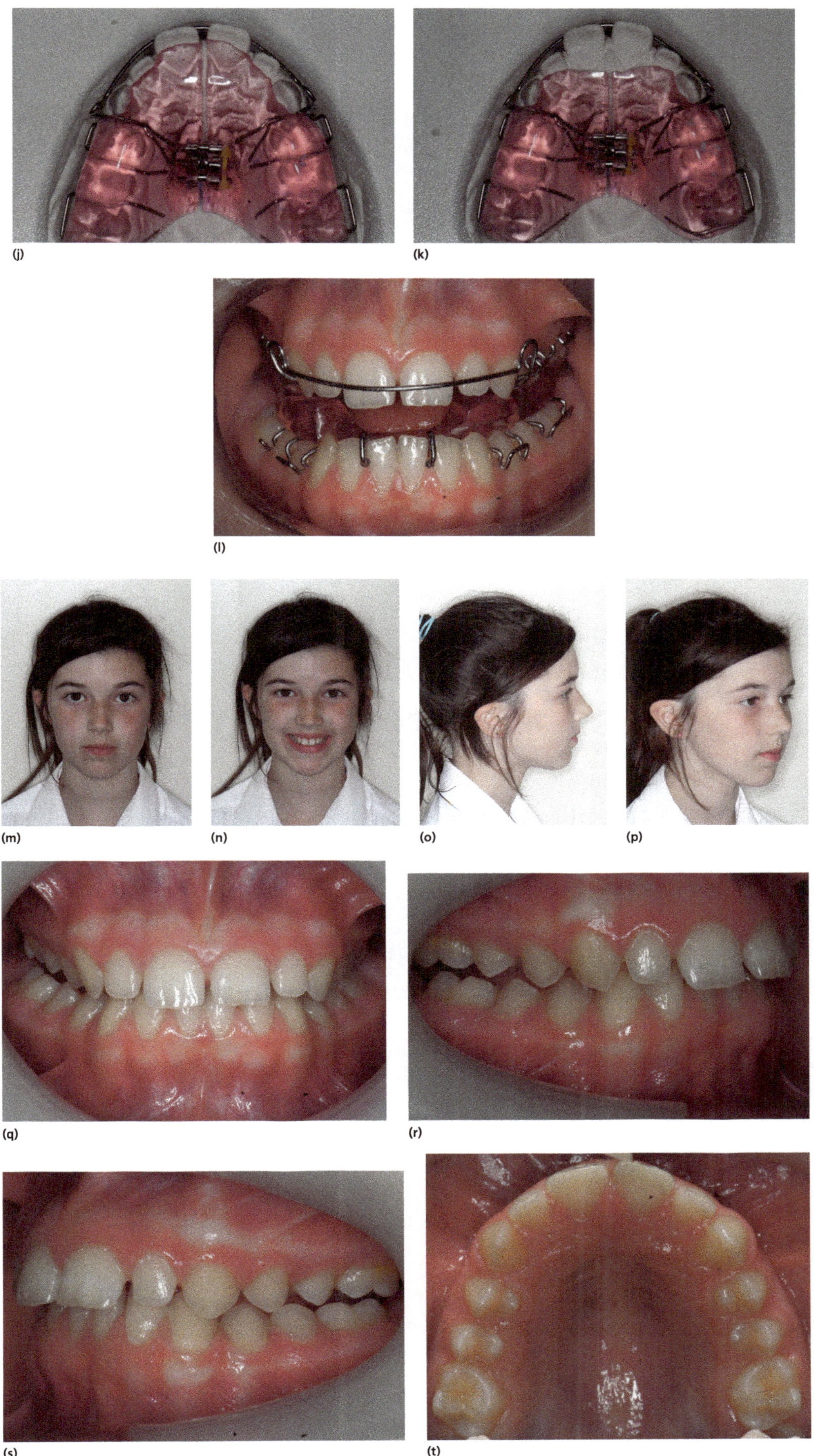

Figure 4.4 (*Continued*)

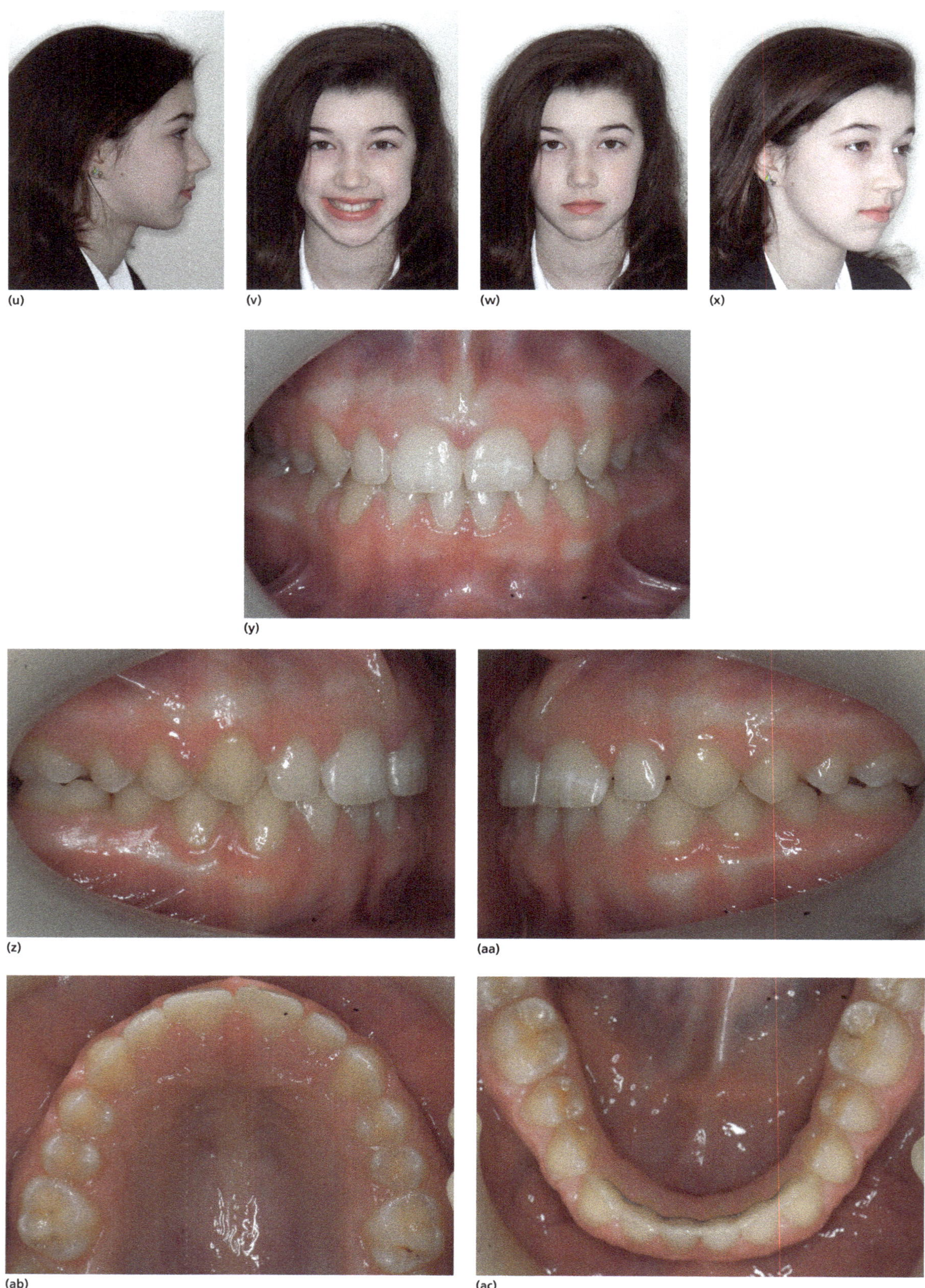

Figure 4.4 *(Continued)*

be associated with improved compliance, particularly if the duration of wear is reduced relative to removable variants. Appliances that can be removed by the patient may be worn intermittently and sporadically and thus the duration of overall treatment necessary to address the malocclusion is likely to be increased.

A randomized controlled trial comparing treatment with the Herbst appliance and the Twin Block alluded to a failure rate with fixed functional appliances of up to 13%.[61] However, the removable functional appliance used in this study was associated with a longer period of active treatment, with a mean duration of 11.2 months, while the mean treatment time with the Herbst appliance was 5.81 months. Moreover, one-third of subjects undergoing treatment with the Twin Block failed to complete the treatment. In a similar design, Read et al.[62] reported on the use of a fixed Twin Block design and reported a mean treatment duration of 5.1 months and a non-compliance rate of 6%.

Estimation of the wear of removable appliances is complex. Sahm et al.[63] incorporated a micro-electronic monitoring device in a Bionator and demonstrated wear in the region of 50–60% of the level requested by the orthodontist. Moreover, Tulloch et al.[36] found no relationship between reported compliance and the treatment response. Compliance was gauged by patients' reports of appliance wear and clinicians' subjective assessment of compliance. Similarly, in a recent analysis of the duration of wear of Hawley retainers and functional appliances, patterns of wear were found to be inconsistent and to vary between individuals, with median daily wear of 7 hours over an observation period of up to 18 months.[64] Retainer wear was found to be more diligent among females and in those paying for treatment. In a prospective analysis focusing on removable functional appliances, Tsomos et al.[65] reported wear for less than 9 hours per day despite 14 hours being prescribed during the active treatment phase. However, when instructed to wear the appliance 8 hours daily during the retention phase, this was exceeded with mean measured wear of 9 hours. Younger patients were found to comply better, although no association with gender was found. During functional appliance therapy, active involvement of patients and demonstration of progress during treatment, by, for example, highlighting changes in overjet, has been recommended as a motivational tool.[66]

Indications for specific appliances

While geographical trends and individual preferences heavily influence appliance design, the selection of functional appliance and specific design modifications is typically tailored to the presenting skeletal imbalance and malocclusion. High-angle cases with increased lower anterior facial height and often reduced overbite usually lend themselves to appliances geared to restricting posterior vertical maxillary growth likely to accentuate an underlying posterior growth rotation and a tendency to an increase in lower anterior facial height (Figures 4.5 and 4.6). This 'activator effect' can be limited by the use of high-pull orthopaedic headgear directed through the centre of resistance of the maxilla, estimated to lie between the roots of the maxillary premolars. Appliances such as the van Beek and Teuscher appliances are used exclusively with headgear in an attempt to produce these effects. The relative merits of these appliances have been assessed in retrospective studies; many of these studies have lacked either untreated or positive controls. In a comparison of subjects treated with the van Beek appliance and those treated with either the Herbst appliance or activator in isolation, similar levels of occlusal and facial change have been reported. However, maxillary protrusion was reduced with the van Beek–headgear combination, while greater mandibular projection was observed in the other group, most likely reflecting the effects of the adjunctive headgear. This study, however, lacked baseline matching of participants and may well have involved assessment of vertical growing individuals (with a mean MMPA of 39 degrees) in the activator group. In a retrospective comparison of a headgear–activator group and an untreated growing control, occlusal correction in the activator group was accompanied by a mean increase of 3.9 mm in lower anterior face height; the corresponding increase in the control group was just 1.3 mm.[67] In a controlled clinical trial comparing Twin Block therapy with and without the supplementary use of headgear, it was found that the main effect of the headgear was to increase the amount of upper incisor retraction rather than producing the intended control of vertical anterior face height.[68]

Modifications can also be made to more versatile appliances, for instance Twin Block, Bionator[69] or Herbst, to limit vertical increases. In particular, a high-angle variants of the Twin Block have been advocated, with posterior capping to prevent eruption of terminal molars and torquing spurs to maintain optimal palatal root torque to the maxillary incisors. These can also be adapted with the addition of headgear tubes to facilitate headgear-mediated vertical control. The effect of this technique has been demonstrated in prospective research,[70] with the ratio of lower face height to total anterior facial height increasing significantly less with the use of the modifications, although a slightly larger increase in total anterior face height (6.2 mm vs 4.9 mm) was also observed in this group.

Orthodontic mechanics have limited ability to control vertical facial growth and resultant increases in the vertical facial dimension.[71] However, the presence of significant skeletal discrepancy or indeed the existence of an increased vertical dimension may indicate an alternative treatment approach to Class II correction without recourse to functional appliances. In particular, consideration can be given to treatment involving extractions, or with Class II correction mediated by extra-oral traction to limit increases in the vertical dimension while facilitating sagittal correction of the malocclusion.

In the presence of reduced lower anterior facial height and increased overbite, eruption of the buccal segments and restraint of incisor eruption is considered favourable. A variety of appliances can be used to achieve this, including median opening activators, Twin Block and fixed functional appliances (Figure 4.7). The median opening activator incorporates acrylic capping in the lower incisor region, acting both to posture the mandible anteriorly and to limit eruption of the mandibular incisors (Figure 4.8). In the presence of an increased curve of Spee, significant opening is created in the posterior regions,

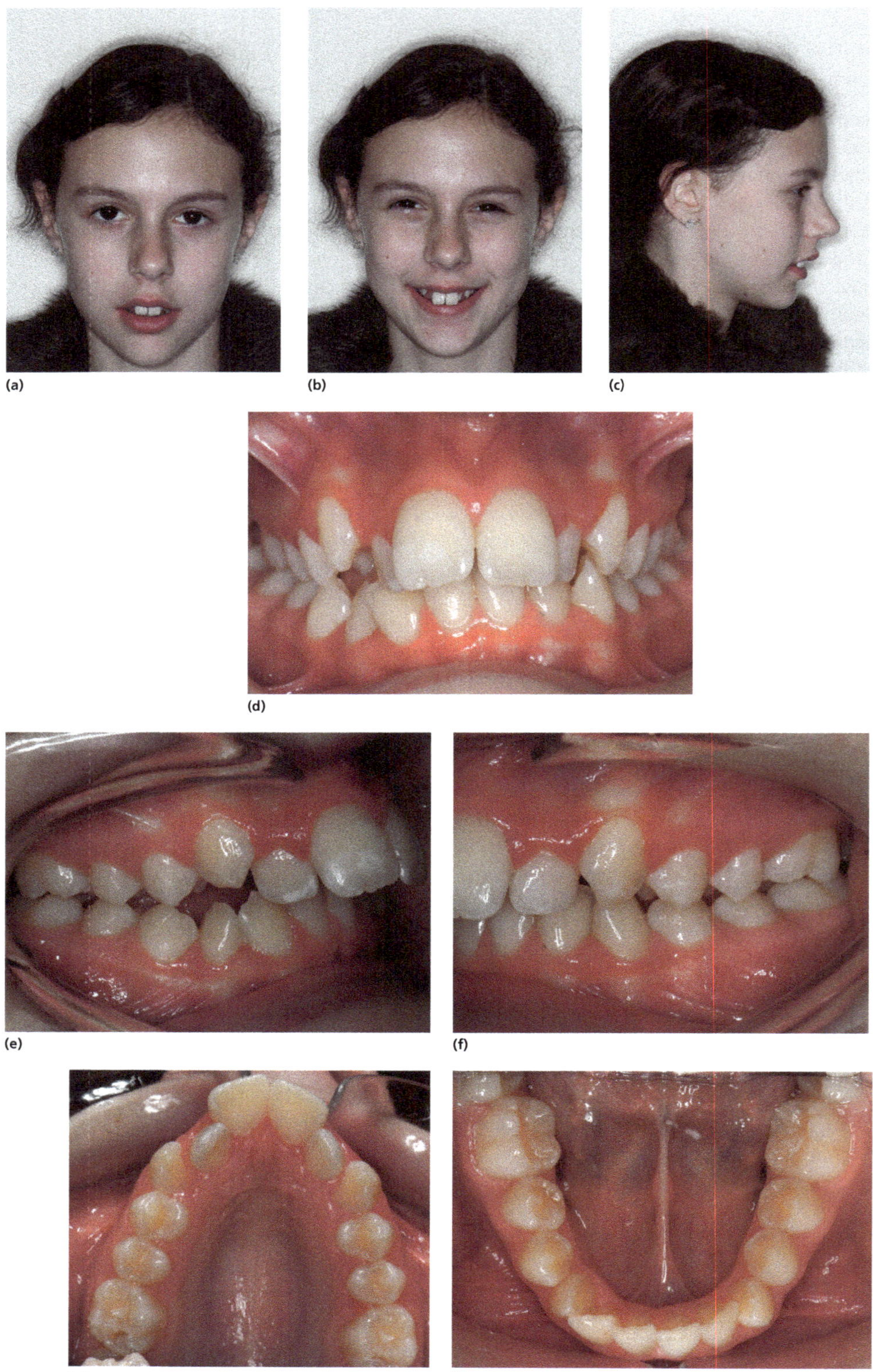

Figure 4.5 This 12-year-old female was referred by her orthodontic specialist in relation to her increased overjet. Extra-orally she had a moderate skeletal II pattern with increased lower anterior facial height and FMPA. The lips were incompetent, with 6 mm of incisal display at rest and 3 mm of gingival exposure on smiling. There was crowding in both arches and an overjet of 12 mm (a–h). The aims of treatment included improvement in the skeletal II discrepancy and correction of the incisor relationship. However, significant further increase in the vertical dimension would be undesirable facially, risking further lip incompetence, and from an occlusal standpoint, as reduction in the overbite was not required. While a Twin Block may have been considered in this case, it may have risked further increase in the vertical dimension, necessitating vertical control possibly with headgear. Notwithstanding headgear use, further vertical increase would have been difficult to avoid. Consequently, a Dynamax appliance was used in this case in conjunction with orthopaedic headgear (i, j). Limitation of increases in lower anterior face height may be facilitated by restraint of vertical maxillary growth; supplementary use of orthopaedic headgear and use of specific functional appliances, e.g. Teuscher, van Beek, Dynamax, have been proposed to achieve this. The Dynamax was used in isolation for 9 months in this case before committing to extraction of four second premolar units to facilitate relief of crowding and arch alignment. The functional appliance was maintained while initial alignment was achieved with fixed appliances, eliminating the need for the interim stabilization phase required with many removable functional appliances (k–n). Fixed appliances were subsequently used for 18 months to align the arches (o–q), closing the extraction spaces and resulting in solid buccal segment interdigitation favouring stable Class II correction. The final result is shown in r–y.

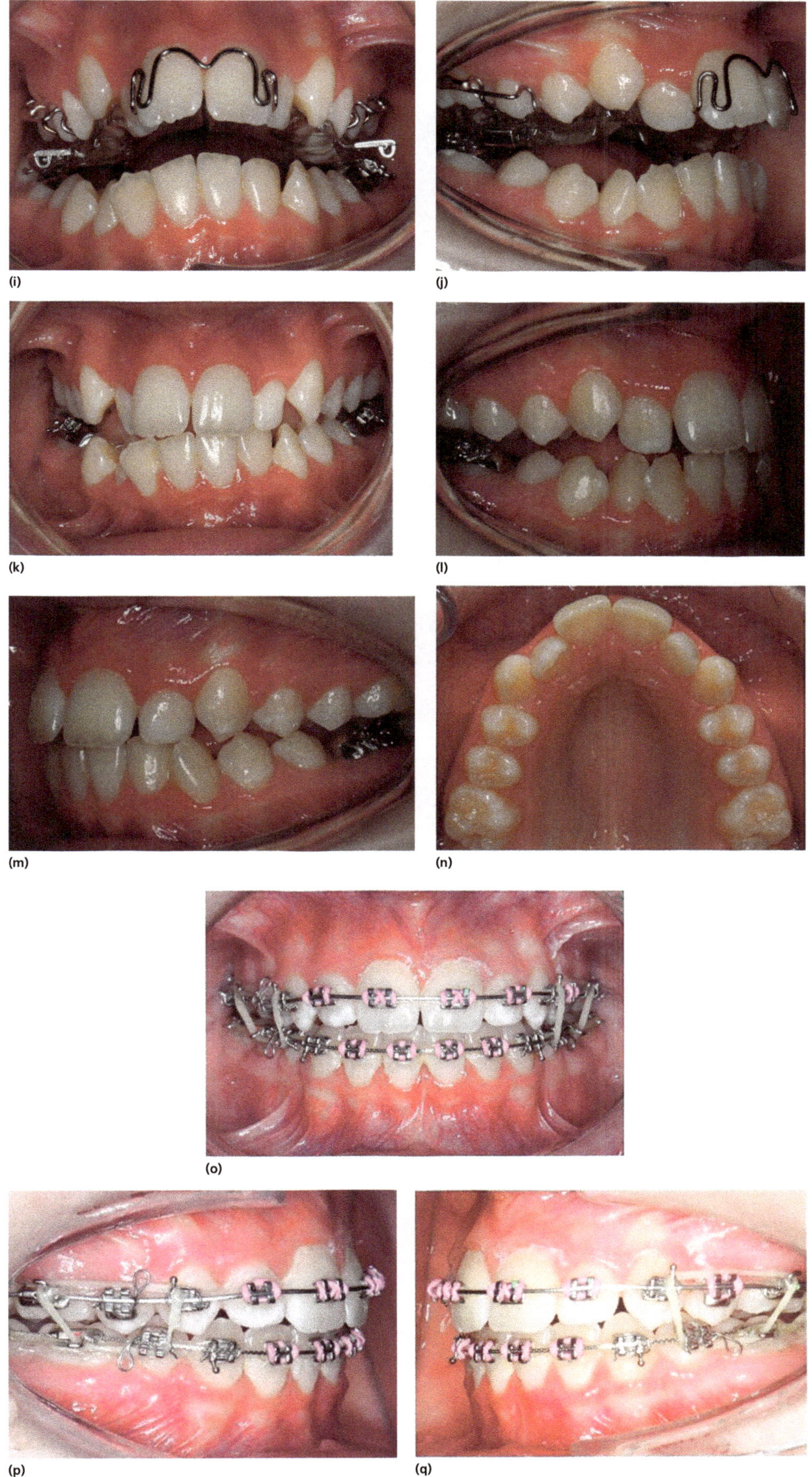

Figure 4.5 (*Continued*)

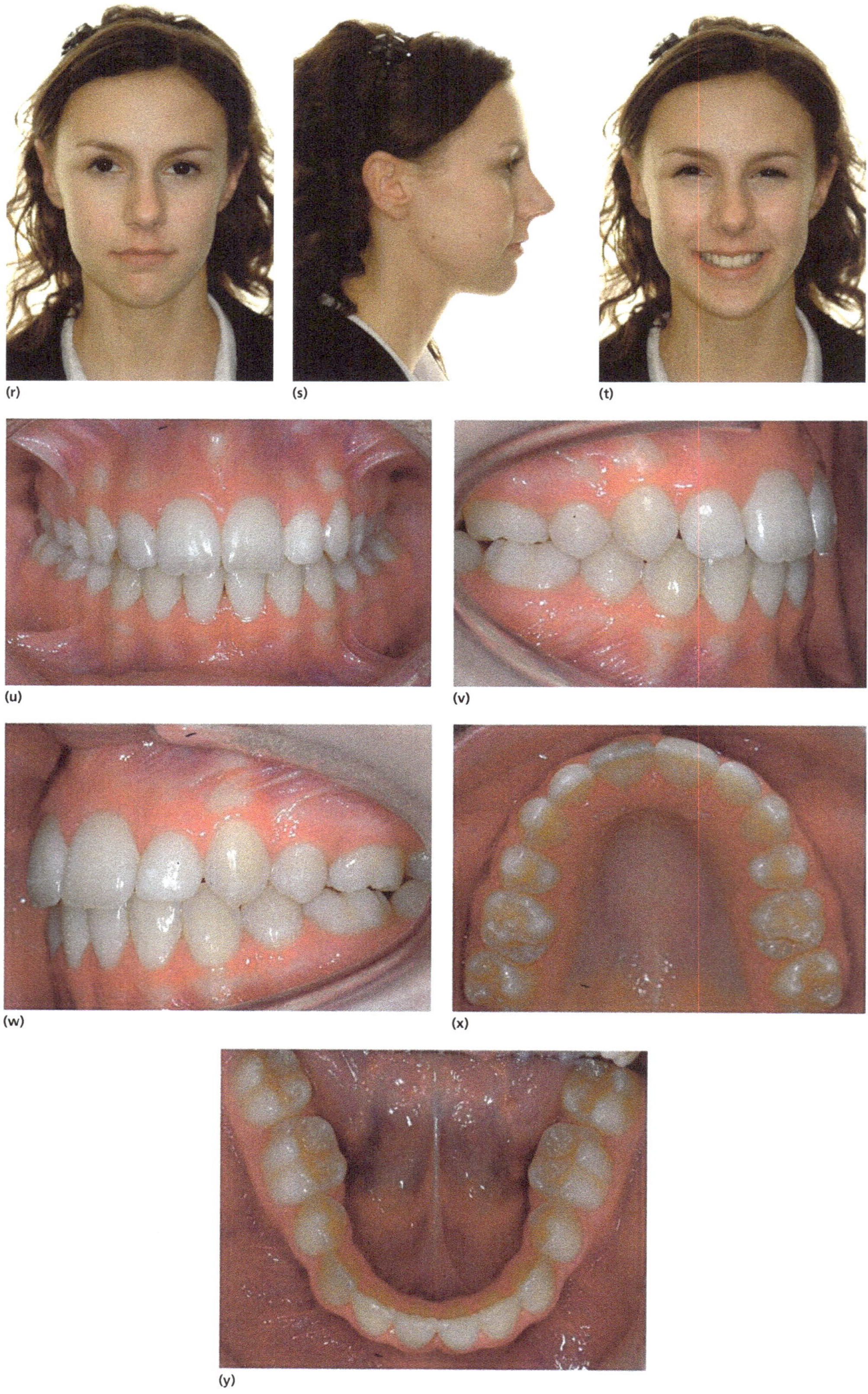

Figure 4.5 (*Continued*)

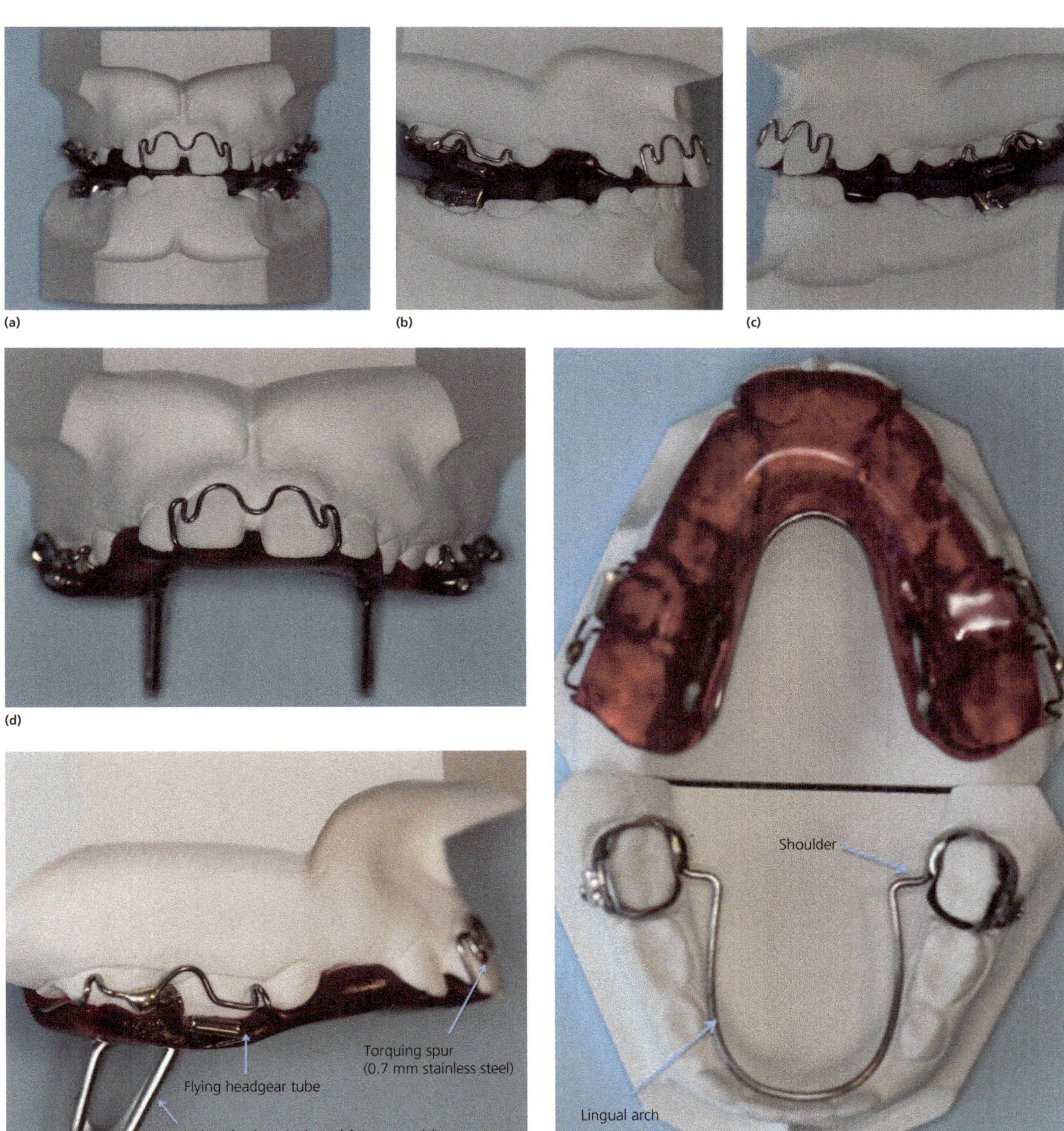

Figure 4.6 The Dynamax appliance (a–f) incorporates a modified lower lingual arch with lingual shoulders or steps designed to accommodate vertical projections from the upper component to maintain forward mandibular posture following an initial 3–4 mm of advancement by encouraging an avoidance reflex. The vertical projections are activated incrementally by approximately 2 mm on a bimonthly basis to effect a gradual Class II correction. The upper component involves torquing spurs in 0.7 mm spring hard stainless steel to the upper central incisors, limiting unwanted retroclination of the incisors, and therefore promoting maximal forward development of the mandible. A midline spring may be incorporated in the upper appliance to facilitate transverse increase; this was activated in the present case from the outset. The upper removable component also involves posterior capping with a 1 mm layer of acrylic, acting to disengage the occlusion and facilitating sagittal correction. By limiting vertical opening, vertical maxillary growth may theoretically be restrained allowing more horizontal expression of mandibular growth, reducing any downward–backward rotational effects of appliance therapy. Adjunctive use of orthopaedic headgear may have an additive effect in terms of restraining maxillary vertical growth, although there is little evidence to support this approach.

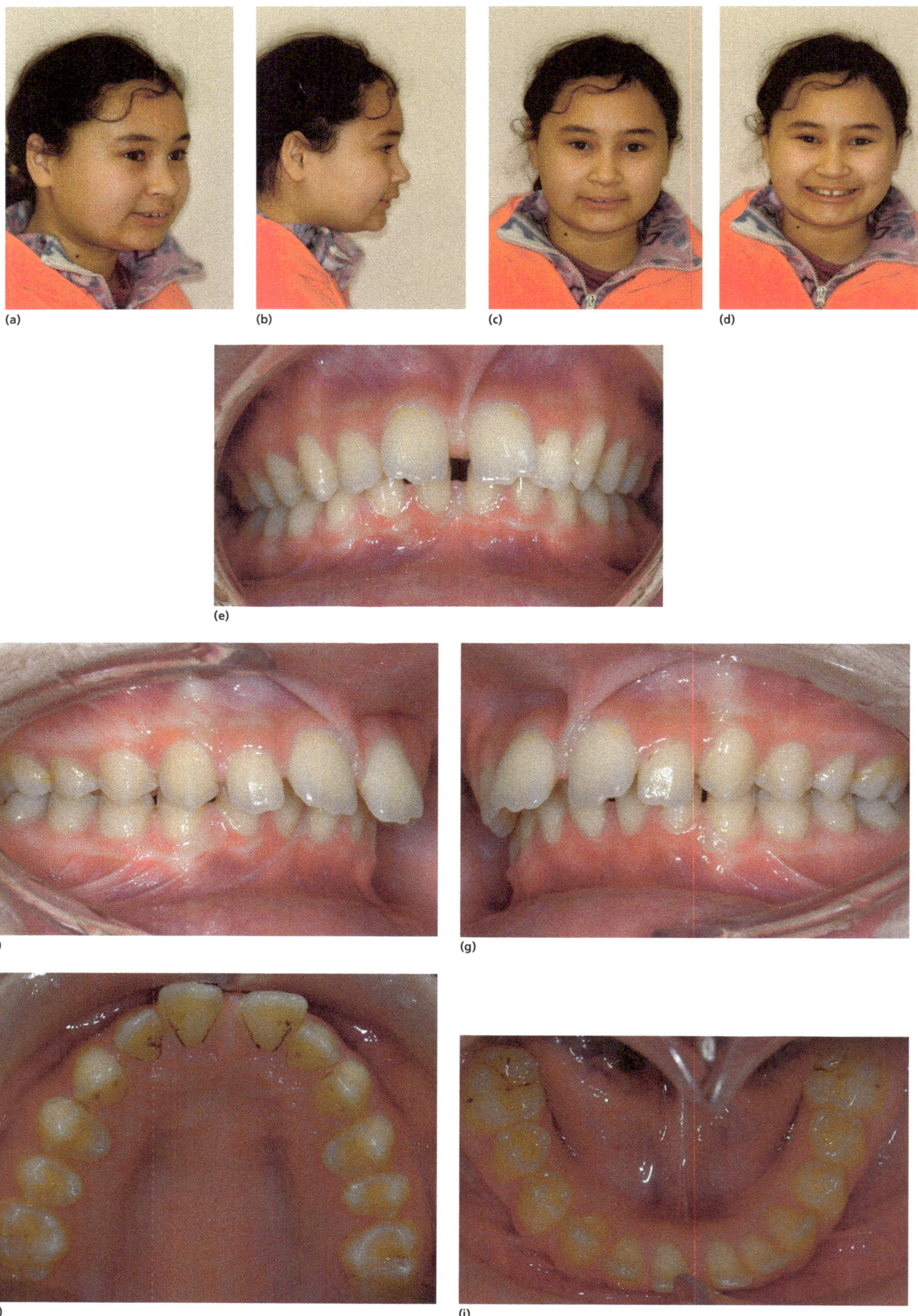

Figure 4.7 This 11-year-old female presented with a Class II division 1 incisor relationship on a moderate skeletal II pattern. She had an increased overjet of 11 mm with reduced vertical dimensions and an associated increased overbite. There was also generalized spacing and bimaxillary proclination, with the lower incisors at 113 degrees to the mandibular plane (a–i). A modified Twin Block was chosen to promote Class II correction with a concomitant increase in the vertical dimension. A lower sectional fixed appliance was placed in conjunction with the functional appliance to upright the lower incisors, promoting maximal skeletal correction of the Class II malocclusion by removing pre-existing dento-alveolar compensation (j). Comprehensive fixed appliance–based treatment was then undertaken over a period of 12 months to detail the final occlusion (k–s).

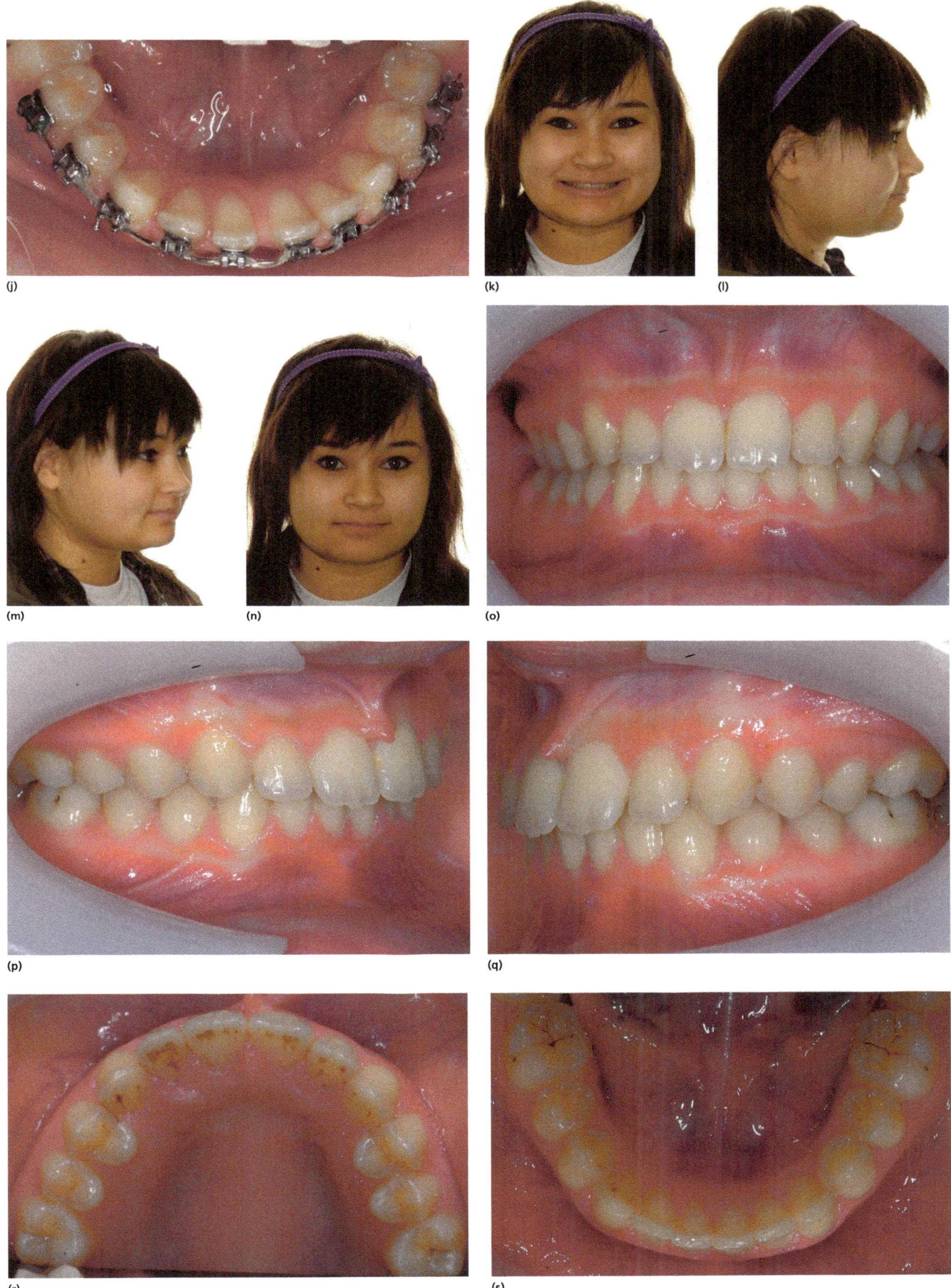

(j) (k) (l) (m) (n) (o) (p) (q) (r) (s)

Figure 4.7 (*Continued*)

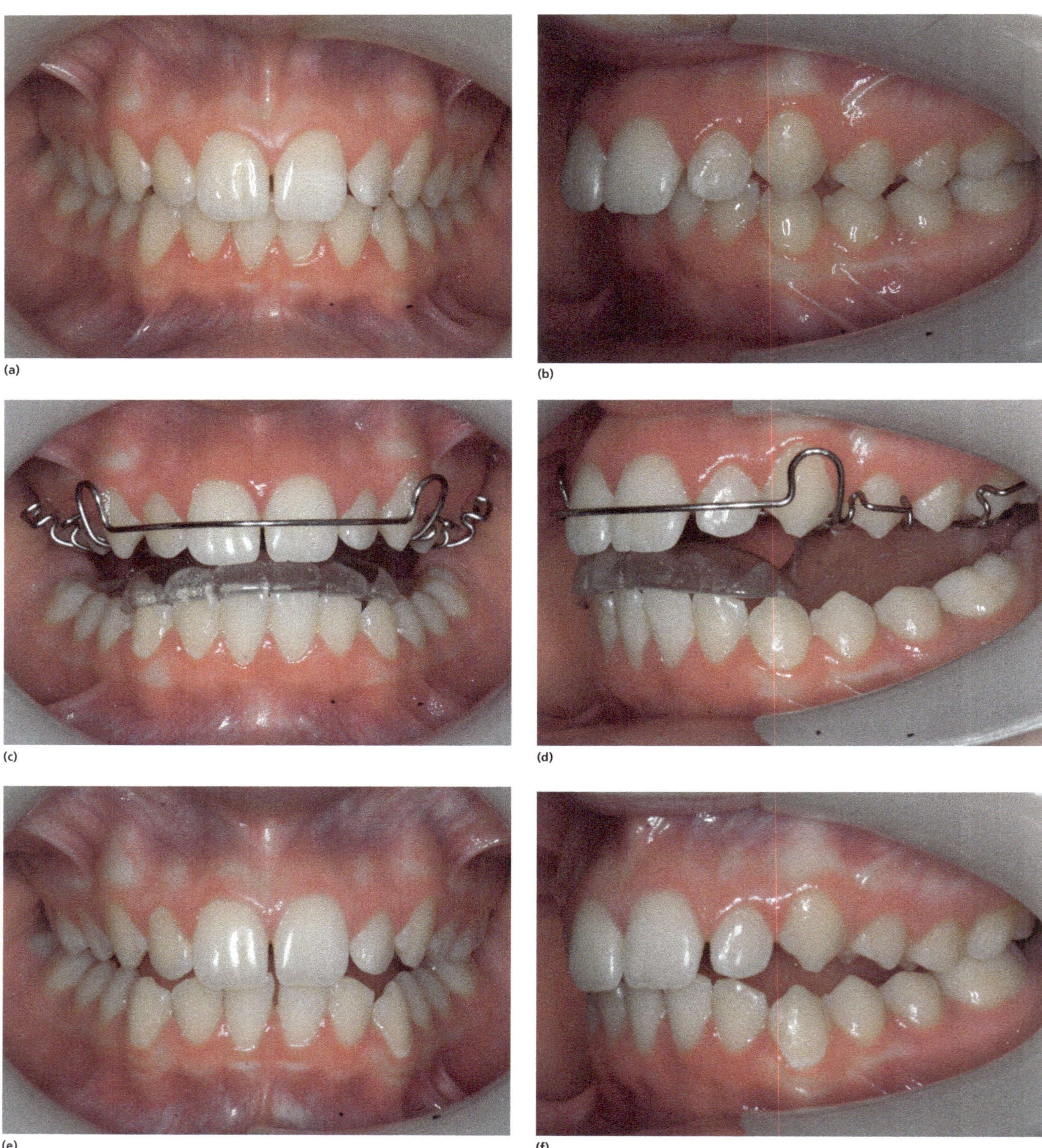

Figure 4.8 The median opening activator (a–d) has lower incisor capping, allowing posterior disclusion to facilitate overbite reduction (e, f). Posterior settling of the occlusal occurred over a 12-month period following withdrawal of the appliance (g, h). Cribs and occlusal rests are fabricated from 0.8 mm spring hard steel and a cingulum wire from 1 mm steel from canine to canine (i–n). The labial bow was described in 0.9 mm spring hard stainless steel. There are acrylic columns (l) in the canine–premolar region linked to a saddle upper plate, which is free of the upper anterior region.

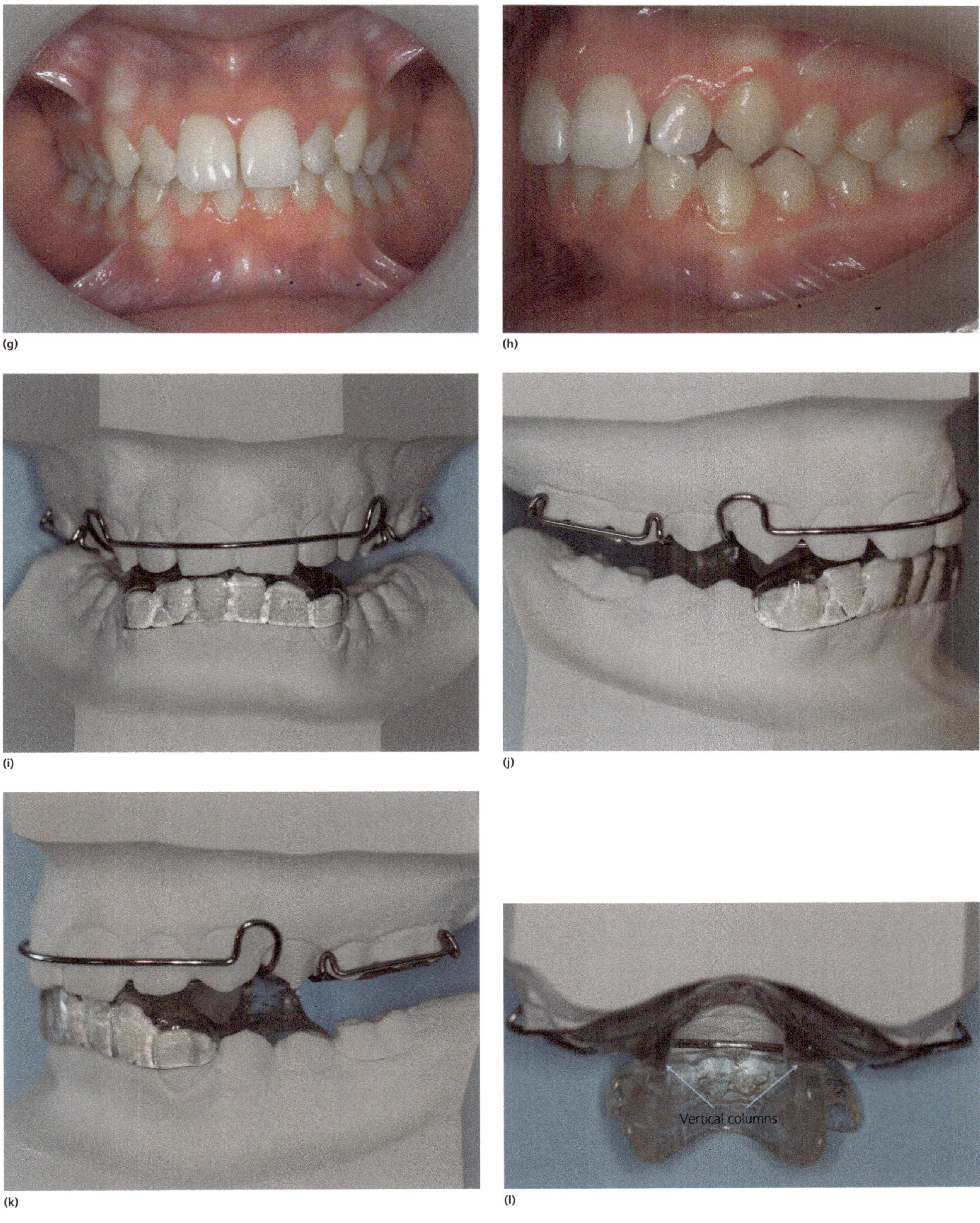

Figure 4.8 (*Continued*)

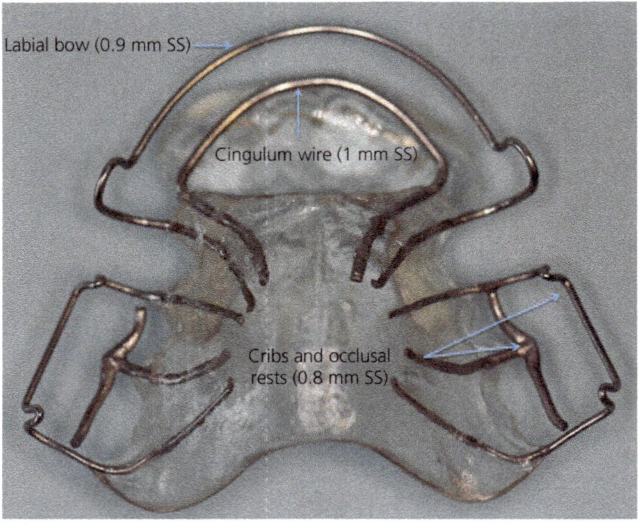

(m)

(n)

Figure 4.8 (*Continued*)

permitting eruption of these teeth and culminating in a reduction in the overbite. The Twin Block can also introduce a similar degree of overbite reduction; the mechanism by which it does so is different. In particular, treatment is associated with an increase in lower anterior face height, mesial eruption of the lower molars and restraint of incisal eruption. The presence of the occlusal blocks posteriorly results in impeded eruption of the lower posterior teeth in particular. Following withdrawal of the appliance the lateral open bites close routinely, facilitating consolidation of the decreased overbite and improved buccal interdigitation. The designer of the appliance advocates incremental trimming of the upper block throughout treatment to limit the development of lateral open bites,[72] leading to improved occlusal interdigitation following withdrawal of the appliance.

Summary

Functional appliances are now almost universally popular, being indicated in growing patients with skeletal II discrepancy associated with large overjets. In particular, functional appliances are thought to be most effective in the presence of average or reduced vertical dimensions. However, a number of appliances have been designed or may be tailored to manage patients with grossly increased or reduced vertical discrepancies effectively.

References

1. Keim RG, Gottlieb EL, Nelson AH, Vogels DS. 2008 JCO study of orthodontic diagnosis and treatment procedures: Part 1 Results and trends. J Clin Orthod. 2008; 32: 625–41.
2. Lee R, MacFarlane T, O'Brien K. Consistency of orthodontic treatment planning decisions. Clin Orthod Res. 1999; 2: 79–84.
3. Ribarevski R, Vig P, Vig KD, Weyant R, O'Brien K. Consistency of orthodontic extraction decisions. Eur J Orthod. 1996; 18: 77–80.
4. Baccetti T, Franchi L, Stahl F. Comparison of 2 comprehensive Class II treatment protocols including the bonded Herbst and headgear appliances: A double-blind study of consecutively treated patients at puberty. Am J Orthod Dentofacial Orthop. 2009; 135: 698.e1–10.
5. Sullivan PG. Prediction of the pubertal growth spurt by measurement of standing height. Eur J Orthod. 1983; 5: 189–97.
6. Tanner JM, Whitehouse RH, Takaishi M. Standards from birth to maturity for height, weight, height velocity, and weight velocity: British children, 1965. Arch Dis Child. 1966; 41: 454–71.
7. http://www.rcpch.ac.uk.
8. Houston WJB. The current status of growth prediction: A review. Br J Orthod. 1979; 6: 11–17.
9. Hunter WS, Baumrind S, Popovich F, Jorgensen G. Forecasting the timing of peak mandibular growth in males by using skeletal age. Am J Orthod Dentofacial Orthop. 2007; 131: 327–33.
10. Franchi L, Baccetti T, McNamara JA Jr. Mandibular growth as related to cervical vertebral maturation and body height. Am J Orthod Dentofacial Orthop. 2000; 118: 335–40.
11. Baccetti T, Franchi L, McNamara JA Jr. An improved version of the cervical vertebral maturation (CVM) method for the assessment of mandibular growth. Angle Orthod. 2002; 72: 316–23.
12. Nestman TS, Marshall SD, Qian F, Holton N, Franciscus RG, Southard TE. Cervical vertebrae maturation method morphologic criteria: Poor reproducibility. Am J Orthod Dentofacial Orthop. 2011; 140: 182–8.
13. Pasciuti E, Franchi L, Baccetti T, Milani S, Farronato G. Comparison of three methods to assess individual skeletal maturity. J Orofac Orthop. 2013; 74: 397–408.
14. Proffit WR. The timing of early treatment: An overview. Am J Orthod Dentofacial Orthop. 2006; 129: S47–9.
15. O'Brien K, Wright J, Conboy F, Appelbe P, Davies L et al. Early treatment for Class II Division 1 malocclusion with the Twin-block

appliance: A multi-center, randomized, controlled trial. Am J Orthod Dentofacial Orthop. 2009; 135: 573–9.
16. Cura N, Saraç M. The effect of treatment with the Bass appliance on skeletal Class II malocclusions: A cephalometric investigation. Eur J Orthod. 1997; 19: 691–702.
17. Malmgren O, Omblus J, Hägg U, Pancherz H. Treatment with an orthopedic appliance system in relation to treatment intensity and growth periods: A study of initial effects. Am J Orthod Dentofacial Orthop. 1987; 91: 143–51.
18. Omblus J, Malmgren O. Dental changes in the mandible during initial Bass appliance therapy. Eur J Orthod. 1998; 20: 17–23.
19. Hägg U, Pancherz H. Dentofacial orthopaedics in relation to chronological age, growth period and skeletal development: An analysis of 72 male patients with Class II division 1 malocclusion treated with the Herbst appliance. Eur J Orthod. 1988; 10: 169–76.
20. Baccetti T, Franchi L, Toth LR, McNamara JA Jr. Treatment timing for Twin-block therapy. Am J Orthod Dentofacial Orthop. 2000; 118: 159–70.
21. Konik M, Pancherz H, Hansen K. The mechanism of Class II correction in late Herbst treatment. Am J Orthod Dentofacial Orthop. 1997; 112: 87–91.
22. Ruf S. Pancherz H. Orthognathic surgery and dentofacial orthopedics in adult Class II Division 1 treatment: Mandibular sagittal split osteotomy versus Herbst appliance. Am J Orthod Dentofacial Orthop. 2004; 126:140–52.
23. Broadbent BH Sr, Broadbent BH Jr, Golden WG. Bolton standards of dentofacial development growth. St Louis, MO: CV Mosby; 1975.
24. Riolo ML, Moyers RE, McNamara JA, Hunter WS. An atlas of craniofacial growth. Ann Arbor, MI: Center for Human Growth and Development, University of Michigan; 1974.
25. Popovich F, Thompson GW. Craniofacial templates for orthodontic case analysis. Am J Orthod. 1977; 71: 406–20.
26. Ricketts RM, Bench RW, Hilgers JJ, Schulhof R. An overview of computerized cephalometrics. Am J Orthod. 1972; 61: 1–28.
27. Johnston LE. A simplified approach to prediction. Am J Orthod. 1975; 49: 1–14.
28. Björk A. Prediction of mandibular growth rotation. Am J Orthod. 1969; 55: 585–99.
29. Ari-Vivo A, Wisth PJ. An evaluation of the methods of structural growth prediction. Eur J Orthod. 1983; 5: 199–207.
30. Leslie LR, Southard TE, Southard KA, Casko JS, Jakobsen JR et al. Prediction of mandibular growth rotation: Assessment of the Skieller, Björk, and Linde-Hansen method. Am J Orthod Dentofacial Orthop. 1998; 114: 659–67.
31. von Bremen J, Pancherz H. Efficiency of early and late Class II Division 1 treatment. Am J Orthod Dentofacial Orthop. 2002; 121: 31–7.
32. Fleming PS, Qureshi U, Pandis N, DiBiase A, Lee RT. An investigation of cephalometric and morphological predictors of successful twin block therapy. Aust Orthod J. 2012; 28: 190–96.
33. Reynolds M, Reynolds M, Adeeb S, El-Bialy T. 3-d volumetric evaluation of human mandibular growth. Open Biomed Eng J. 2011; 5: 83–9.
34. Patel HP, Moseley HC, Noar JH. Cephalometric determinants of successful functional appliance therapy. Angle Orthod. 2002; 72: 410–17.
35. Caldwell S, Cook P. Predicting the outcome of twin block functional appliance treatment: A prospective study. Eur J Orthod. 1999; 21: 533–9.
36. Tulloch JF, Phillips C, Koch G, Proffit WR. The effect of early intervention on skeletal pattern in Class II malocclusion: A randomized clinical trial. Am J Orthod Dentofacial Orthop. 1997; 111: 391–400.
37. Illing HM, Morris DO, Lee RT. A prospective evaluation of Bass, Bionator and Twin Block appliances: Part 1 – The hard tissues. Eur J Orthod. 1998; 20: 501–16.
38. Yaqoob O, DiBiase AT, Fleming PS, Cobourne MT. Use of the Clark Twin Block functional appliance with and without an upper labial bow: A randomized controlled trial. Angle Orthod. 2011; 82: 363–9.
39. Patel HP, Moseley HC, Noar JH. Cephalometric determinants of successful functional appliance therapy. Angle Orthod. 2002; 72: 410–17.
40. Fleming PS, Qureshi U, Pandis N, DiBiase A, Lee RT. An investigation of cephalometric and morphological predictors of successful twin block therapy. Aust Orthod J. 2012; 28: 190–96.
41. Caldwell S, Cook P. Predicting the outcome of twin block functional appliance treatment: A prospective study. Eur J Orthod. 1999; 21: 533–9.
42. Franchi L, Baccetti T. Prediction of individual mandibular changes induced by functional jaw orthopedics followed by fixed appliances in Class II patients. Angle Orthod. 2006; 76: 950–54.
43. Baccetti T, Franchi L, Stahl F. Comparison of 2 comprehensive Class II treatment protocols including the bonded Herbst and headgear appliances: A double-blind study of consecutively treated patients at puberty. Am J Orthod Dentofacial Orthop. 2009; 135: 698.e1–10.
44. Harrison JE, O'Brien KD, Worthington HV. Orthodontic treatment for prominent upper front teeth in children. Cochrane Database Syst Rev. 2007; 18: CD003452.
45. Meazzini MC, Mazzoleni F, Bozzetti A, Brusati R. Does functional appliance treatment truly improve stability of mandibular vertical distraction osteogenesis in hemifacial microsomia? J Craniomaxillofac Surg. 2008; 36: 384–9.
46. Dyer FM, McKeown HF, Sandler PJ. The modified twin block appliance in the treatment of Class II division 2 malocclusions. J Orthod. 2001; 28: 271–80.
47. Van Spronsen PH, Weijs WA, Valk J, Prahl-Andersen B, Van Ginkel FC. A comparison of jaw muscle cross-sections of long-face and normal adults. J Dent Res. 1992; 71: 1279–85.
48. Ingervall B, Helkimo E. Masticatory muscle force and facial morphology in man. Arch Oral Biol. 1978; 23: 203–6.
49. Kreiborg S, Jenson B, Moller E, Bjork A. Craniofacial growth in a case of congenital muscular dystrophy. Am J Orthod. 1978; 74: 207–15.
50. Hall BK, Herring SW. Analysis and growth of the musculoskeletal system in the embryonic chick. J Morphol. 1990; 206: 45–56.
51. Herring SW, Lakars TC. Craniofacial development in the absence of muscle contraction. J Craniofac Genetics Devel Biol. 1981; 1: 341–84.
52. Byrd K, Stein ST, Sokoloff AJ, Shankar K. Craniofacial alterations following electrolytic lesions of the trigeminal motor nucleus in actively growing patients. Am J Anat. 1990; 189: 93–110.
53. Hunt N, Shah R, Sinanan A, Lewis M. Northcroft memorial lecture 2005: Muscling in on malocclusions: Current concepts on the role of muscles in the aetiology and treatment of malocclusion. J Orthod. 2006; 33: 187–97.
54. Adams GR, Hather BM, Baldwin KM, Dudley GA. Skeletal muscle myosin heavy chain composition and resistance training. J Appl Phys. 1993; 74: 911–15.

55. Korfage JA, Koolstra JH, Langenbach GE, van Eijden TM. Fiber-type composition of the human jaw muscles: (Part 1) Origin and functional significance of fiber-type diversity. J Dent Res. 2005; 84: 774–83.
56. Van Dyck C, Dekeyser A, Vantricht E, Manders E, Goeleven A et al. The effect of orofacial myofunctional treatment in children with anterior open bite and tongue dysfunction: A pilot study. Eur J Orthod. 2015; July 1 (epub).
57. Al-Khateeb SN, Abu Alhaija ES, Majzoub S. Occlusal bite force change after orthodontic treatment with Andresen functional appliance. Eur J Orthod. 2015; 37: 142–6.
58. Antonarakis GS, Kjellberg H, Kiliaridis S. Predictive value of molar bite force on Class II functional appliance treatment outcomes. Eur J Orthod. 2012; 34: 244–9.
59. Antonarakis GS, Kjellberg H, Kiliaridis S. Bite force and its association with stability following Class II/1 functional appliance treatment. Eur J Orthod. 2013; 35: 434–41.
60. Kadkhoda S, Nedjat S, Shirazi M. Comparison of oral-health-related quality of life during treatment with headgear and functional appliances. Int J Paediatr Dent. 2011; 21: 369–73.
61. O'Brien K, Wright J, Conboy F, Sanjie Y, Mandall N et al. Effectiveness of treatment for Class II malocclusion with the Herbst or twin-block appliances: A randomized, controlled trial. Am J Orthod Dentofacial Orthop. 2003; 124: 128–37.
62. Read MJ, Deacon S, O'Brien K. A prospective cohort study of a clip-on fixed functional appliance. Am J Orthod Dentofacial Orthop. 2004; 125: 444–9.
63. Sahm G, Bartsch A, Witt E. Micro-electronic monitoring of functional appliance wear. Eur J Orthod. 1990; 12: 297–301.
64. Cornelius-Schott T, Schlipf C, Glasl B, Schwarzer C, Weber J, Ludwig B. Quantification of patient compliance with Hawley retainers and removable functional appliances during the retention phase. Am J Orthod Dentofacial Orthop. 2013; 144: 433–40.
65. Tsomos G, Ludwig B, Grossen J, Pazera P, Gkantidis N. Objective assessment of patient compliance with removable orthodontic appliances: A cross-sectional cohort study. Angle Orthod. 2014; 84: 56–61.
66. Cirgic E, Kjellberg H, Hansen K, Lepp M. Adolescents' experience of using removable functional appliances. Orthod Craniofac Res. 2015; 18: 165–74.
67. Marşan G. Effects of activator and high-pull headgear combination therapy: Skeletal, dentoalveolar, and soft tissue profile changes. Eur J Orthod. 2007; 29: 140–48.
68. McDonagh S, Moss JP, Goodwin P, Lee RT. A prospective optical surface scanning and cephalometric assessment of the effect of functional appliances on the soft tissues. Eur J Orthod. 2001; 23: 115–26.
69. Ibitayo AO, Pangrazio-Kulbersh V, Berger J, Bayirli B. Dentoskeletal effects of functional appliances vs bimaxillary surgery in hyperdivergent Class II patients. Angle Orthod. 2011; 81: 304–11.
70. Parkin NA, McKeown HF, Sandler PJ. Comparison of 2 modifications of the twin-block appliance in matched Class II samples. Am J Orthod Dentofacial Orthop. 2001; 119: 572–7.
71. Gkantidis N, Halazonetis DJ, Alexandropoulos E, Haralabakis NB. Treatment strategies for patients with hyperdivergent Class II Division 1 malocclusion: Is vertical dimension affected? Am J Orthod Dentofacial Orthop. 2011; 140: 346–55.
72. Clark W. Design and management of Twin Blocks: Reflections after 30 years of clinical use. J Orthod. 2010; 37: 209–16.

CHAPTER 5

Clinical use of the Twin Block appliance

The Twin Block appliance was first developed by William Clark in 1977.[1] Since then the appliance has undergone considerable adaptation and streamlining, much of which has been prompted by the originator.[2] The initial appliance was described in conjunction with a Concorde facebow affording further sagittal and vertical control, but also permitting placement of an inter-maxillary elastic from the lower appliance to the facebow. The rationale for this was to encourage the mandible into a forward posture during sleep, maintaining forward position over a 24-hour period.[1] Originally, the intersecting blocks met at a 45-degree angle; a 70-degree angle is now recommended. A labial bow from maxillary first molar to first molar was also recommended initially; this is no longer considered necessary and is regarded as unaesthetic, potentially hampering patient compliance.[2]

Over the past 30 years the Twin Block has become the most popular removable functional appliance in the United Kingdom.[3] Its proposed advantages include the following:

- Efficiency: Overjet reduction is typically rapid.
- Simplicity and low cost: The appliance is relatively simple to fabricate with low associated laboratory costs.
- Versatility: It allows concomitant expansion, and there is the ability to add headgear and to vary the design depending on vertical skeletal and occlusal requirements.
- Good patient tolerance.

The most significant limitations, however, include its removable nature, placing an onus on excellent compliance to achieve Class II correction and leading to a limited capacity to integrate removable versions with fixed appliances. Fixed variants do exist,[4] however, and have been the subject of prospective research, but these have yet to meet with widespread use.[5,6]

Case selection

General features

The Twin Block appliance is particularly suited to patients in the late mixed or early permanent dentition, as there are sufficient erupted teeth to anchor and retain the appliance. Partially shed or partially erupted teeth will tend to prevent accurate fitting of the appliance after the impressions, and a loosely fitting appliance may deter the patient from full-time wear. Typically, therefore, complete eruption of the first premolars allied to the first permanent molars is desirable to allow optimal retention of the appliance. If the second primary molars are retained, these may be bypassed and allowed to exfoliate during the functional phase. The leeway space may subsequently be utilized during the later fixed appliance phase to address any residual space requirements. Patients should ideally be sufficiently mature to understand the objective of the appliance and the requirement to establish a forward habitual posture. There is, however, variable evidence in relation to the impact of age on the acceptability of appliances and the outcome of functional appliance therapy.[7] Nevertheless, compliance with Twin Blocks is favourable overall, with non-compliance rates of less than 10% reported.[8]

Skeletal features

As the appliance is primarily aimed at correction of mandibular retrognathia, the forward posture of the mandible should be aesthetically desirable. Moreover, it should ideally result in an apparently improved vertical dimension, and correction of any antero-posterior variation in the molar relationship. If the forward posture produces excessive lip incompetence, it is likely that the anterior vertical facial dimension is increased and a Twin Block is unlikely to be appropriate.

Soft tissue features

One of the objectives of the appliance is to encourage the development of an anterior oral seal, as described by Fränkel with the functional regulator.[9] Patients presenting with a deep labio-mental fold will have an unfurling of the lower lip with downward and forward posturing of the mandible, which has been shown to improve the aesthetics as perceived by patients and orthodontists.[10] Incompetent lips, particularly when associated with a lower lip trap behind the maxillary incisors, are commonly associated with mandibular retrognathia. This tends to improve during appliance therapy and lip competence following treatment is thought to contribute to the prolonged stability of the occlusal change. However, lip incompetence in the absence of a lip trap may also be indicative of an increased vertical skeletal dimension, hampering the response to Twin Block therapy.

Orthodontic Functional Appliances: Theory and Practice, First Edition. Padhraig Fleming and Robert Lee.

Dental features

The Twin Block appliance is not easily retained when a full fixed appliance is in place. Some preliminary alignment of the upper and lower labial segments can be undertaken prior to or in combination with the Twin Block phase with either removable or sectional fixed appliances (Figure 5.1). Severely malaligned upper incisors or retroclined incisors can present an obstruction to the required forward bite registration, and this is best resolved before fitting the appliances. Alternatively, an upper sectional fixed appliance or springs palatal to the maxillary central incisors may be added to procline the maxillary central incisors in Class II division 2 cases.[11]

Impressions

Good-quality alginate impressions are sufficient for the fabrication of the Twin Block. While other functional appliances require recording of areas of soft tissue where the functional appliance will extend or indeed stretch, this is not necessary with the Twin Block, as it is a tooth-borne appliance.

Bite registration

When the appliance is in place, it is essential that the lower block engages anterior to the upper block to maintain the forward posture of the mandible, otherwise the mandible may be maintained in a downward rather than forward position. The latter will fail to maintain the required forward posture necessary for Class II correction but may also impair the comfort of the appliance, leading to lip incompetence with the appliance *in situ* and ultimately risking poor patient compliance. This engagement is ensured by registering the bite open beyond the freeway space, and the general finding is that the posterior teeth are 5mm or more out of occlusion[12, 13] (see Figure 5.2).

Furthermore, a large anterior opening may preclude effective eating and may impair speech with the appliance in place. On the other hand, blocks lacking sufficient height may impair forward posture of the mandible, particularly at night, limiting the effectiveness of the forward posture. A method of producing a reproducible degree of bite opening is the use of a preformed plastic gauge, which is inserted between the incisors. In those patients with a deep overbite a significant posterior bite opening will ensue and the degree of forward posture that the patient can comfortably maintain can be assessed. An alternative technique involves a thickened block of wax moulded to the dental arches. This approach requires a measurement of the thickness of the wax in the premolar region, which should generally be 5–7 mm.

Considerable debate and disagreement have surrounded the merits of incremental mandibular advancement versus one-step advancement. Intuitively, it would be expected that larger initial advancement may result in greater soft tissue stretch, leading to more pronounced dental changes than with more gradual advancement. It appears, however, on the basis of prospective research that little difference in the relative proportion of skeletal to dento-alveolar effects is likely with either approach.[13–15] Therefore, single-step advancement may be preferable in view of the simplicity of this approach. The Twin Block lends itself to efficient, single-step Class II correction, with Clark advocating maximal activation of 10 mm in one phase.[2] Larger overjets may necessitate re-activation either at chair-side or in the laboratory to advance the mandible further.[16]

Appliance design

Clark's original design had the acrylic blocks cut at 45 degrees to the occlusal plane; this has since been modified to 70 degrees to provide better engagement of the blocks and more positive forward positioning. The upper appliance had a labial bow, but this has now largely been abandoned, as active retraction of the upper incisors is not necessary. Maxillary incisor uprighting usually occurs due to the altered resting position of the lower lip induced by appliance therapy.

Additionally, the appliance has been streamlined considerably since the original design and is therefore less visible and potentially more comfortable. Forces are not applied directly to the upper incisors. Retention is achieved by cribs to the maxillary first molars and additional cribs on maxillary first premolars if they are erupted. If individual cribs are fractured during wear, the supplementary cribs are often adequate to retain the appliance. Clark, however, advocates use of delta clasps rather than Adam's clasps, as the former may provide excellent retention with a lower risk of fracture due to a reduced requirement for adjustment.[2]

The lower appliance has Adam's cribs on the first premolars, typically made from 0.7 mm stainless steel. In earlier stages of dental development, the first primary molars may be clasped or indeed may be bypassed, with supplementary retention added anteriorly to maintain adequate retention (Figures 5.3 and 5.4). Clark does not recommend cribs on the mandibular first permanent molars, but does advise that the first molars be incorporated in the appliance. Additional retention afforded by ball clasps on the lower incisors or Adam's cribs on the first molars are widely used.[13] Acrylic capping of the lower incisors has been found to improve the lower retention, but also to increase the risk of demineralization of the lower incisors by retaining plaque and acid.[17] Methods to limit lower incisor proclination have been suggested, including the use of a lower labial bow. However, in the absence of lower arch spacing this has a limited capacity to upright the mandibular incisors during functional appliance therapy. An alternative involves bolstering posterior anchorage in the lower appliance (by incorporating first molars in the design) to limit the forces on the lower incisors, as mandibular incisors have limited anchorage value and capacity to resist

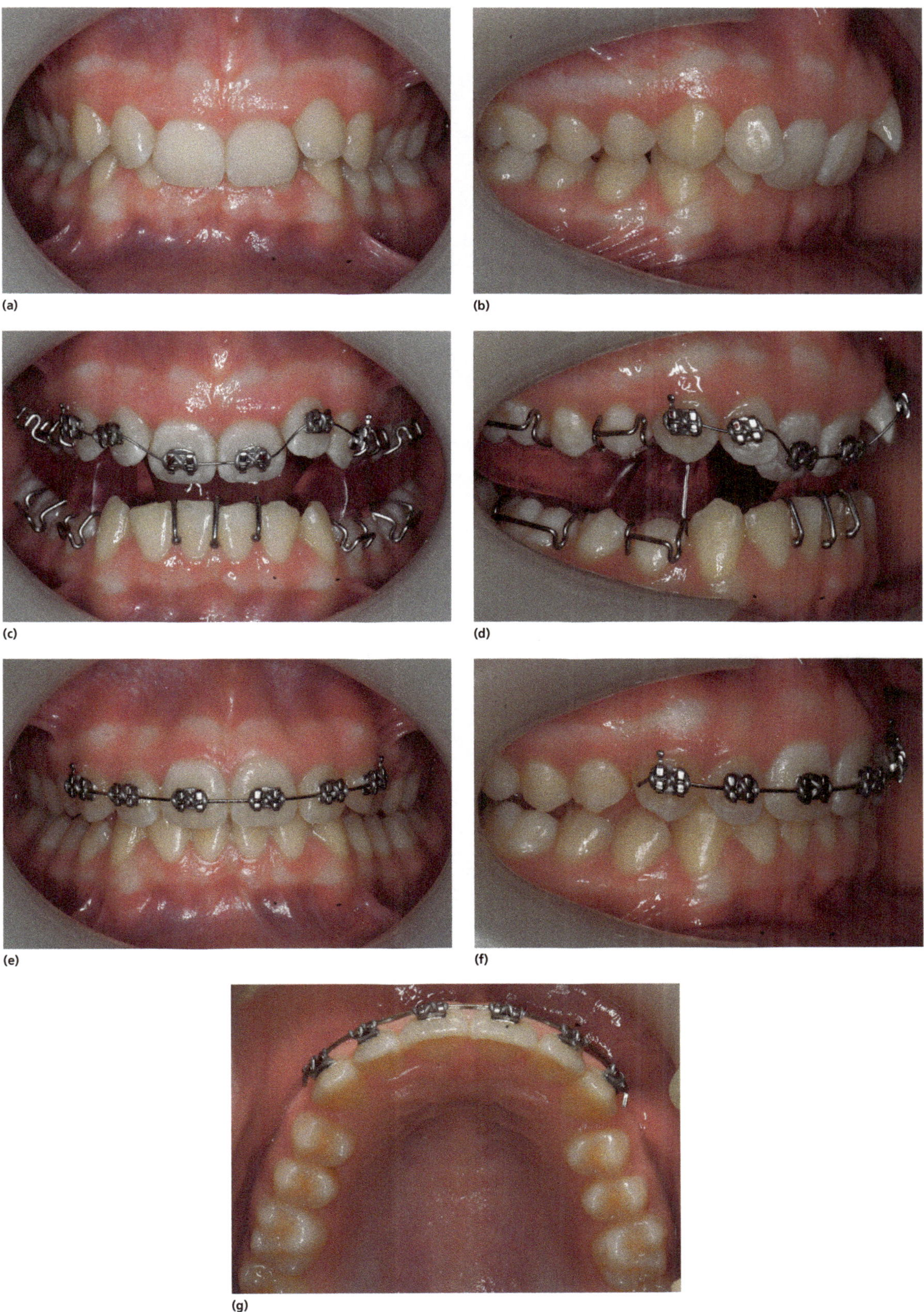

Figure 5.1 A Class II division 2 malocclusion with retroclined maxillary central incisors and Class II buccal segment relationships (a, b). A modified Twin Block was placed in conjunction with a sectional fixed appliance to advance the maxillary incisors during the fixed appliance phase (c, d). Consequently, Class II correction could be undertaken in concert with upper anterior alignment (e–g). A similar case is shown in h–l. A sectional fixed appliance was placed with progression into rectangular stainless steel wires to allow torque expression (m–o). Decompensation of the maxillary incisors was accomplished in conjunction with molar correction, with overcorrection of the molar and canine relationships and creation of lateral open bites after 8 months of therapy (p–s). Rotation of the maxillary canines may be reduced with incorporation of the maxillary premolars in the sectional fixed appliance during the functional phase, but alternatively can be easily addressed during the comprehensive fixed phase. The final occlusal result is shown in (t–x).

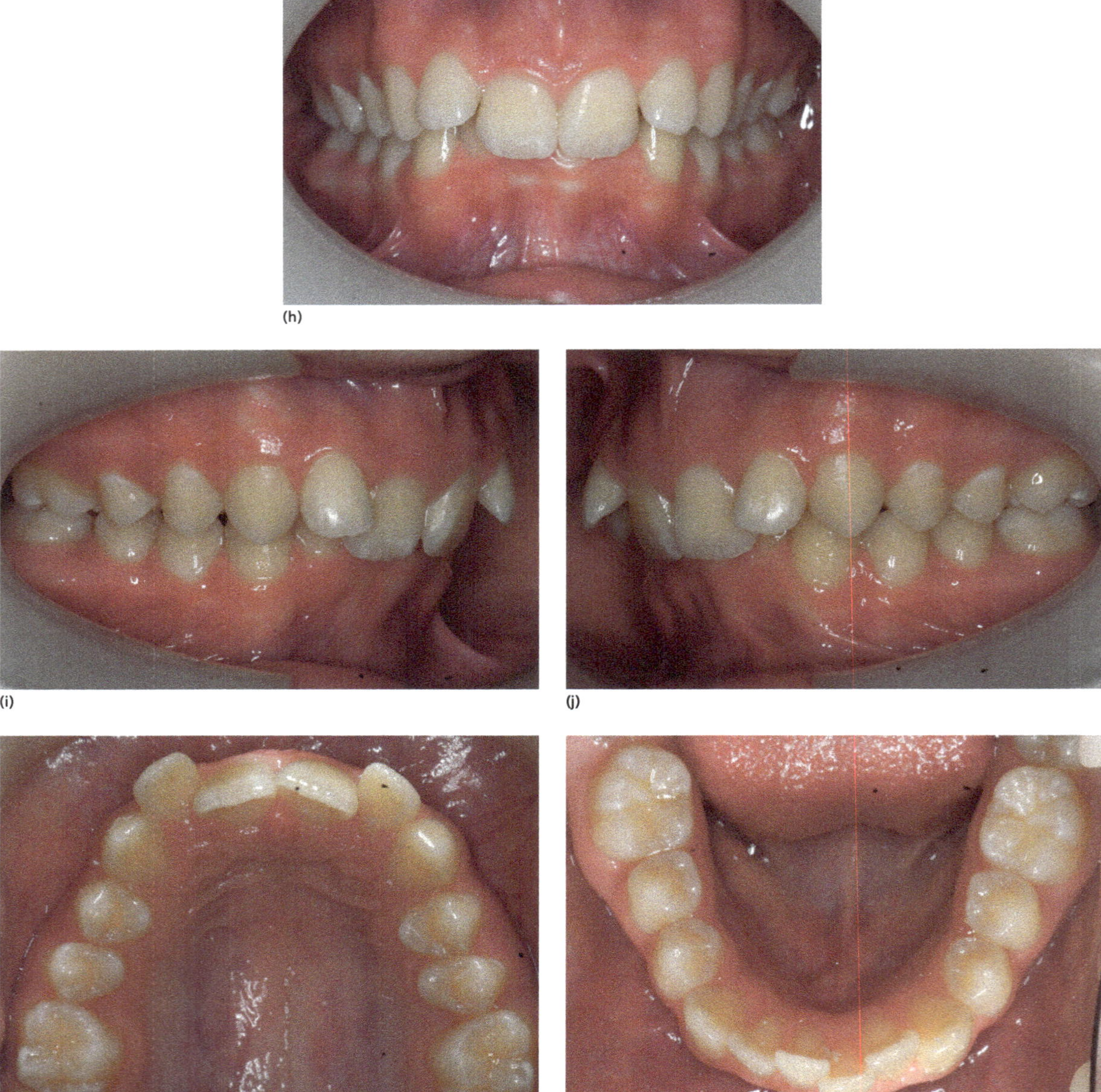

Figure 5.1 (*Continued*)

proclination. Nevertheless, some mandibular incisor proclination is typical with Twin Block therapy.[12–15]

While Twin Blocks are now typically considered most appropriate for patients with average or reduced vertical dimensions, modifications to promote vertical restraint have been developed. Such modifications include the following:

- Occlusal stops to second molars: These are directed at limiting eruption of the second molars, as this may result in further overbite reduction and increase in lower facial height.
- Flying headgear tubes: These may be incorporated in the upper appliance in the premolar region to permit adjunctive use of orthopaedic or high-pull headgear to restrict maxillary or vertical growth. However, there remains limited evidence of any associated benefit.[18]
- Torquing spurs: These may be added to the maxillary incisors to maintain an aesthetic inclination secondary to Class II correction with the functional appliance. From an aesthetic viewpoint, due to the orientation of the occlusal plane, the

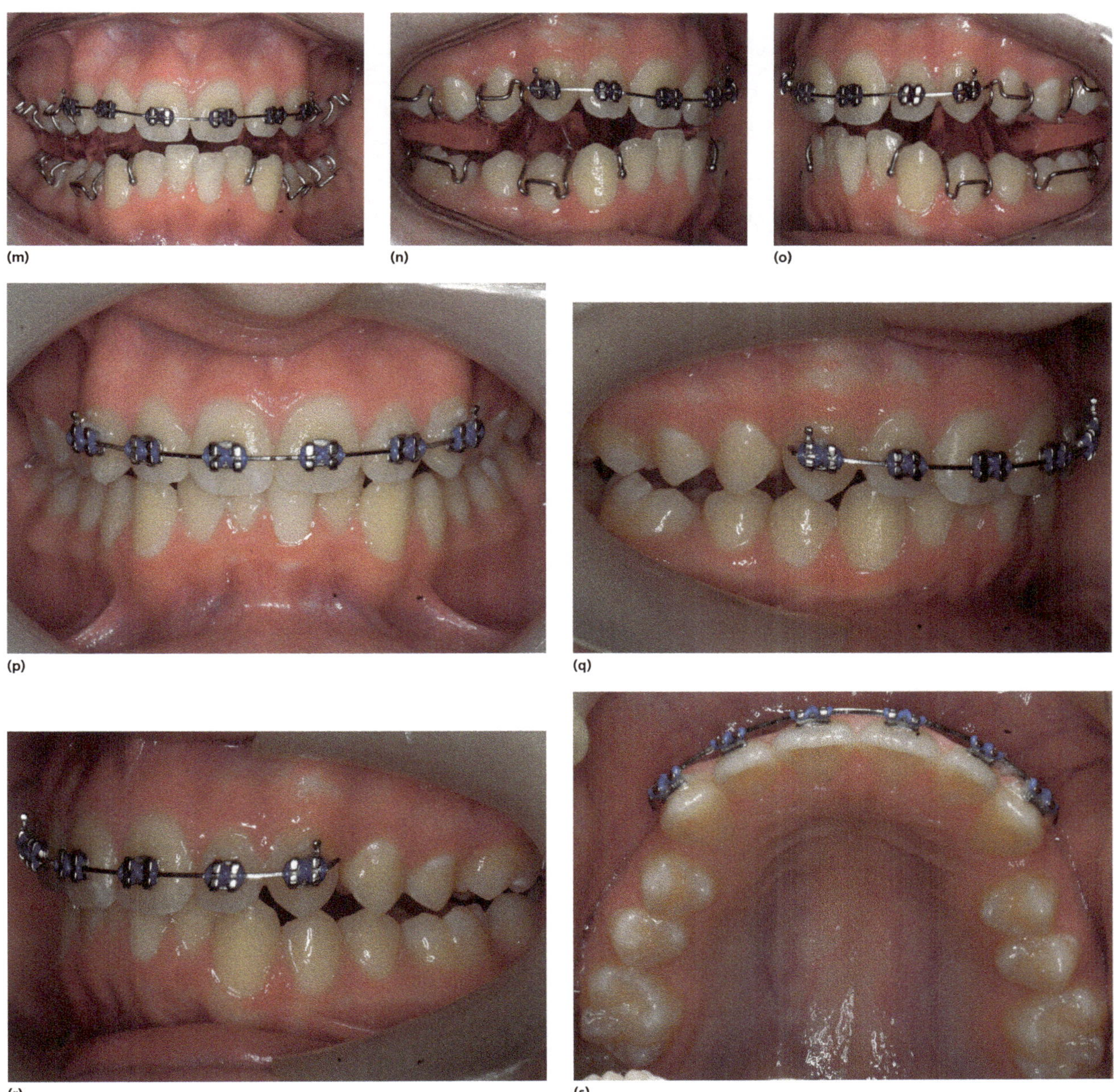

(m) (n) (o) (p) (q) (r) (s)

Figure 5.1 (*Continued*)

maxillary incisors may look upright in high-angle cases.[18] The torquing spurs are an attempt to counteract this and have been described in concert with other high-angle functional appliances also relying on headgear use, including the Teuscher and van Beek appliances.

The upper appliance also usually includes a midline expansion screw, permitting a degree of maxillary arch expansion. This allows expansion at the rate of 0.2–0.5 mm per week depending on the number of turns prescribed. The requirement for upper expansion should be gauged either on pre-treatment models or clinically following forward mandibular posture to a corrected incisal relationship, as an apparent transverse discrepancy may be related to the antero-posterior discrepancy. The inclusion of a midline screw does make the upper appliance more prone to fracture; breakages incorporating the midline tend to be catastrophic, necessitating laboratory input.

Fitting the appliance

The upper and lower components are fitted separately and the retention of each is checked. The patient should be able comfortably to position the mandible downward and forward with the

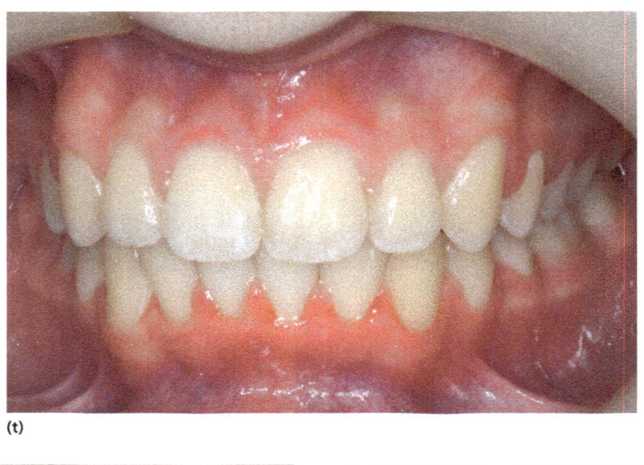

(t)

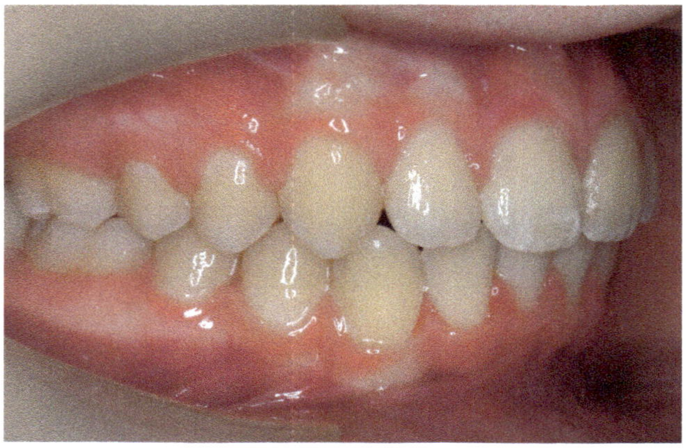

(u)

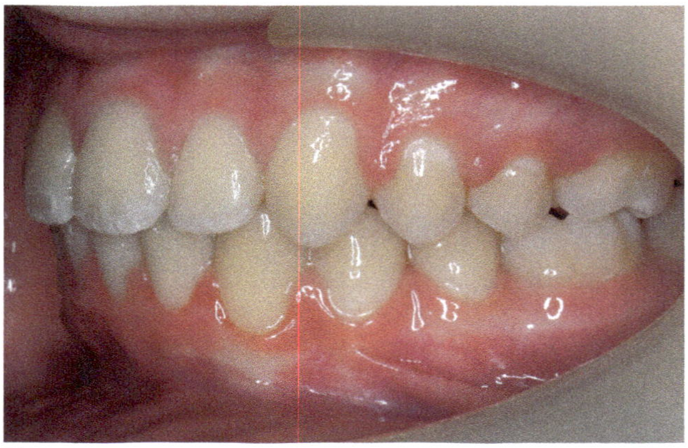

(v)

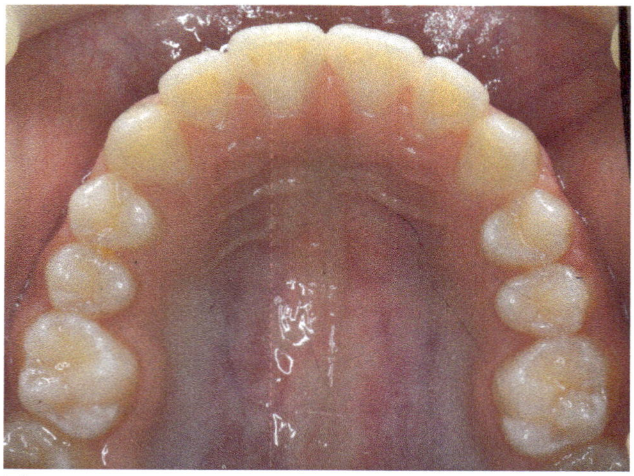

(w)

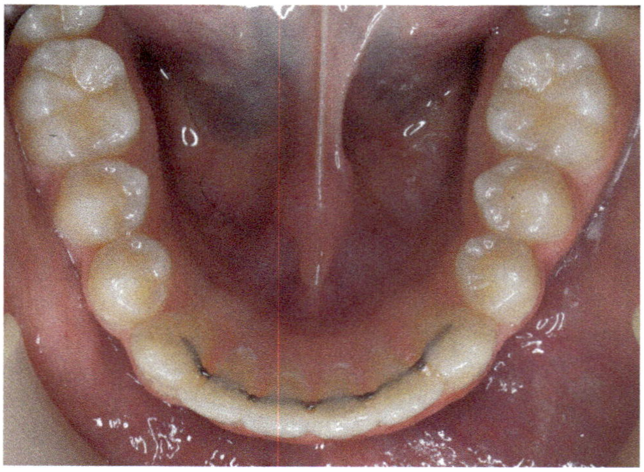

(x)

Figure 5.1 (*Continued*)

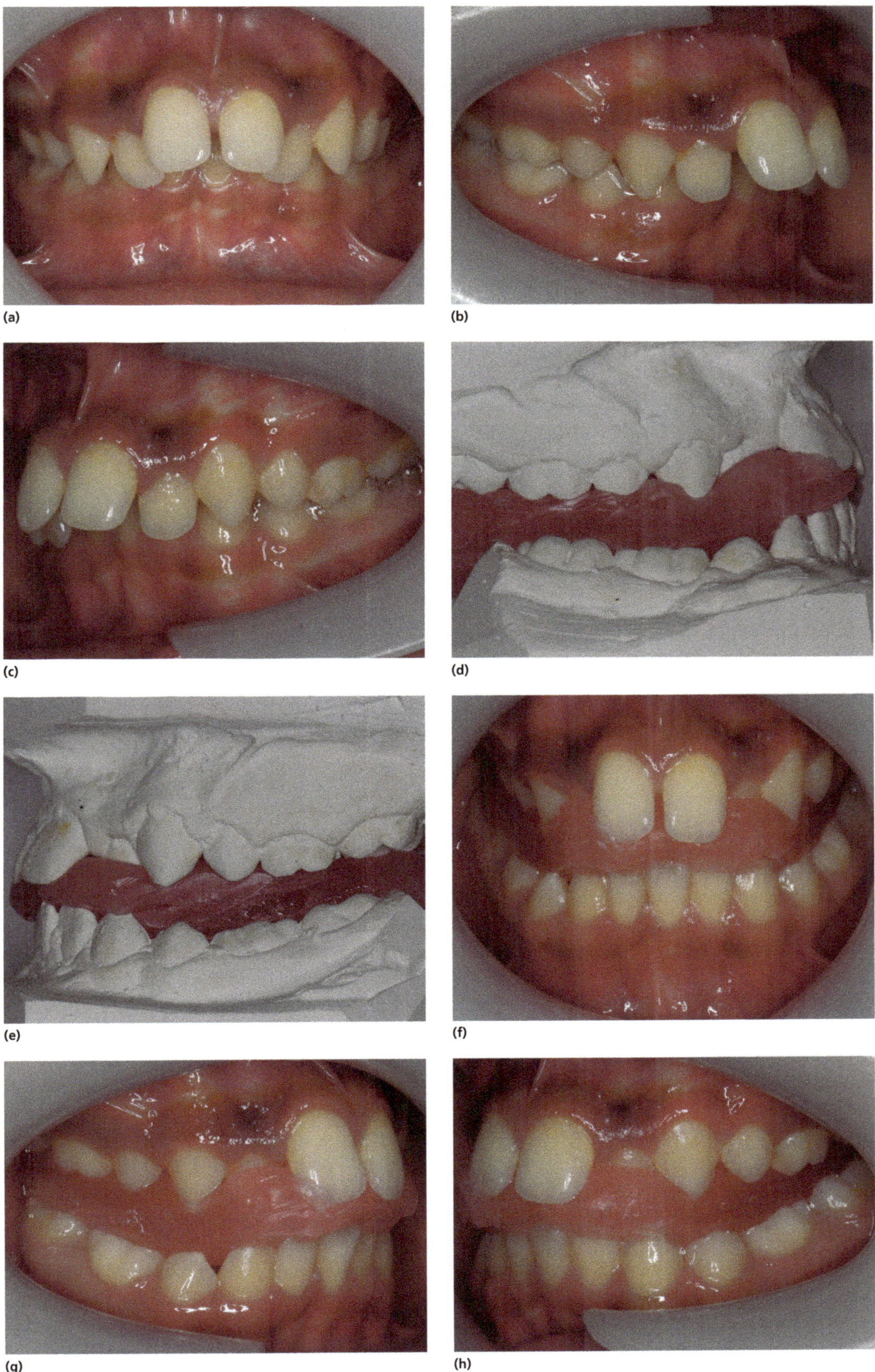

Figure 5.2 Wax bite registration on a patient with an increased overjet and overbite with an increased curve of Spee (a–c). Opening of 2–3 mm has been achieved anteriorly, with the wax approximately 6–7 mm thick in the premolar region to allow adequate block height without excessive anterior opening (d–h).

The use of a blue acrylic Exacto Bite Stick™ is also shown (i–k). The acrylic is 2 mm thick anteriorly and has grooved upper and lower surfaces. The maxillary incisors are allowed to seat into one of three upper grooves to control the amount of mandibular advancement. The mandibular incisors fit into the single groove on the lower surface. The anterior thickness of 2 mm should control the vertical opening anteriorly, resulting in a well-tolerated and comfortable appliance. In this instance full seating was not achieved anteriorly, resulting in a corresponding increase in the height in the premolar region (k). A further record is shown (l) with full seating anteriorly, corresponding to a minimal (2 mm) opening. The wax thickness is greatest in the premolar region before reducing in the molar region, reflecting the orientation and depth of the occlusal curve.

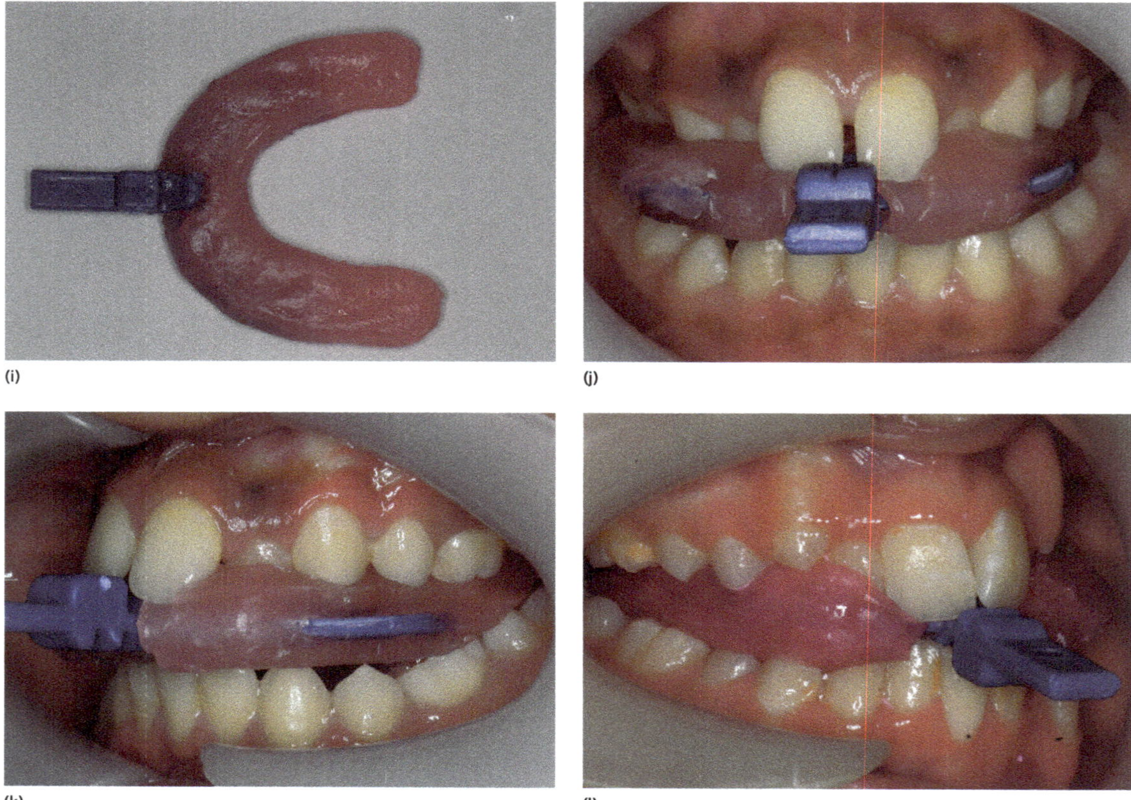

Figure 5.2 (*Continued*)

lower block in front of the upper. If this cannot be achieved, it is likely that the blocks are too deep or the protrusion excessive. It may be possible to reduce the blocks at the chair-side, but ideally the bite should be re-registered with either less bite opening or reduced forward protrusion. Full-time wear of the appliance from the outset is desirable, but often the appliance is removed for eating initially and then worn full time after the first follow-up appointment. A tapered increase in the wear of the appliance is advocated by some clinicians; there remains limited evidence on the relative merits of either approach, however.

Follow-up appointments

When the patient has worn the appliance for a few weeks, speech should be normal, the patient should be habitually posturing forwards and a small degree of lateral open bite should be present. The lateral open bite develops as a result of unimpeded incisal eruption and vertical growth, while eruption in the buccal segments is restrained due to the presence of the occlusal blocks.

Once it is clear that the appliance is being worn on a full-time basis, it is appropriate that the upper arch is expanded by turning the midline screw. Expansion is known to be unstable; early expansion therefore allows for a period of consolidation of the transverse changes during the latter period of functional appliance therapy.

The acrylic behind the upper incisors may be trimmed during the expansion phase to allow limited spontaneous alignment of the incisors or uprighting of the incisors from lower lip pressure on the labial surface of the maxillary incisor crowns. Depending on the severity of the initial problem, overjet reduction of the order of 2 mm may be anticipated at 6-week intervals over the initial 6 months of functional appliance therapy.

Within 6 months, complete overjet correction would be expected[13] and a marked lateral open bite will have developed. Failure of overjet reduction with associated lateral open bite is indicative of the patient not engaging the blocks to achieve adequate forward posture, and an increase in block thickness or additional advancement of the blocks is likely to be required.

After overjet correction, trimming the upper block posteriorly to allow the lower first molars to erupt is advocated, although lateral open bites do tend to close spontaneously following partial or complete withdrawal of the appliance (Figure 5.5). Indeed, resolution of lateral open bites tends to be unimpeded by the presence of fixed appliances (Figures 5.6 and 5.7). However, Clark recommends sequential trimming of the upper block to prevent the establishment of open bites in the first instance in an

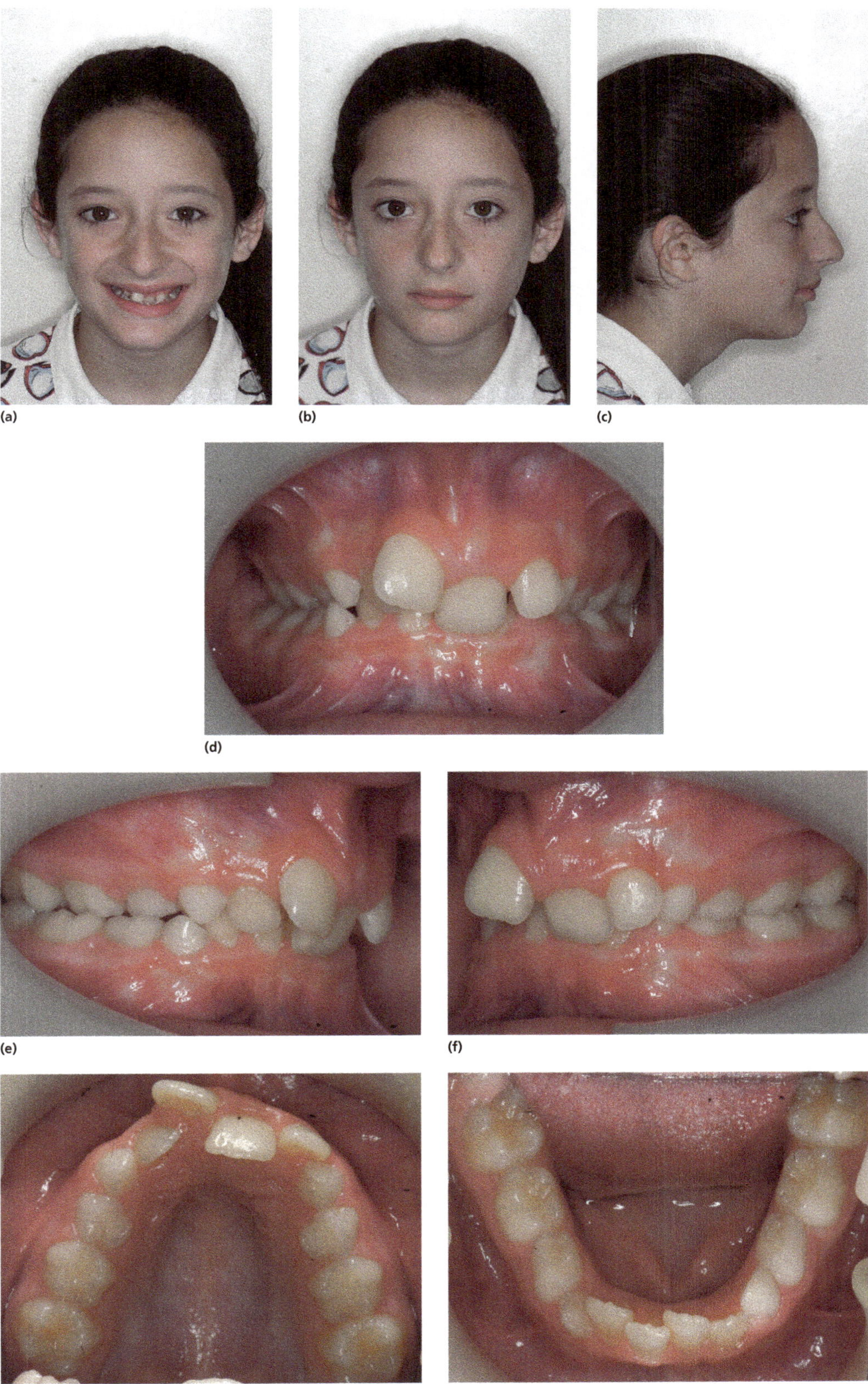

Figure 5.3 A 10-year-old female presented in the mixed dentition with an increased overjet of 10 mm to a proclined maxillary right central incisor with upper anterior crowding (a–h). A sectional fixed appliance was placed to align and locally decompensate the maxillary incisors, with concomitant use of a Twin Block to correct the Class II relationships as an interceptive treatment phase. Maxillary first permanent molars and first primary molars were used as retention. Adams' cribs were placed on the lower first molars with a lower anterior labial bow (i–l). After 9 months of appliance therapy, the initial phase was completed with placement of an upper bonded retainer prior to establishment of the permanent dentition and definitive treatment in the permanent dentition (m–t).

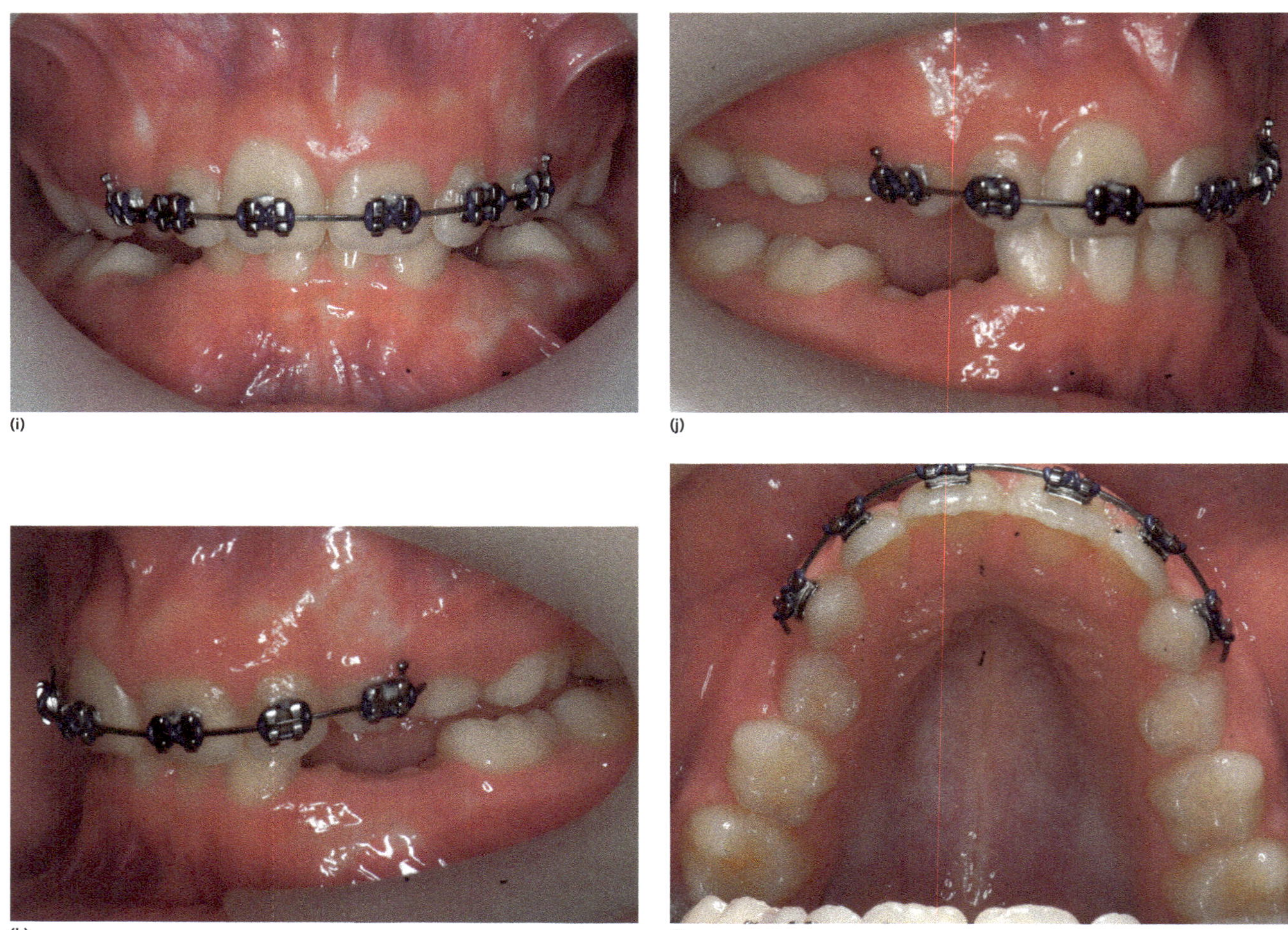

(i) (j) (k) (l)

Figure 5.3 (*Continued*)

effort to limit relapse post-treatment and to provide an adequate occlusal platform to preserve support for the temporo-mandibular joints. If the lower first molar erupts differentially ahead of the lower second premolar, there is a risk of reducing the available space for the second premolar, predisposing to localized crowding and displacement of the second premolar.

Clinical trials involving the authors have compared the results with full-time wear of the appliances for 9 months and 15 months, followed by withdrawal of the appliances for a period of 3 months to allow closure of the lateral open bites by eruption of upper and lower premolars and molars.[19, 20] In both circumstances the lateral open bite consistently closed spontaneously and it was felt that any habitual postural elements from the appliances would no longer be present. It is generally found after 1 year of full-time appliance wear that the overjet relapse is not more than 1 mm, the lateral open bite corrects and the antero-posterior correction of the molars is maintained during a 3-month observation period. Alternatively, phased withdrawal or direct progression to fixed appliance therapy can be undertaken.

Breakages

Appliance breakages are most frequently at the cribs on the lower appliance, with 56 breakages being reported in a cohort of 35 patients over the course of treatment.[13] These breakages did not generally result in withdrawal of the appliance, but rather removal of the fractured crib and maintenance of the appliance with the other retention cribs. Consequently, breakages with the Twin Block are generally not a significant problem and can be overcome at the chair-side with or without laboratory input. This is particularly beneficial during the active correction phase of therapy when full-time wear of the existing appliance or replacement without delay is required; relapse in the overjet will be apparent if the appliance is withdrawn for a prolonged period. Moreover, replacement

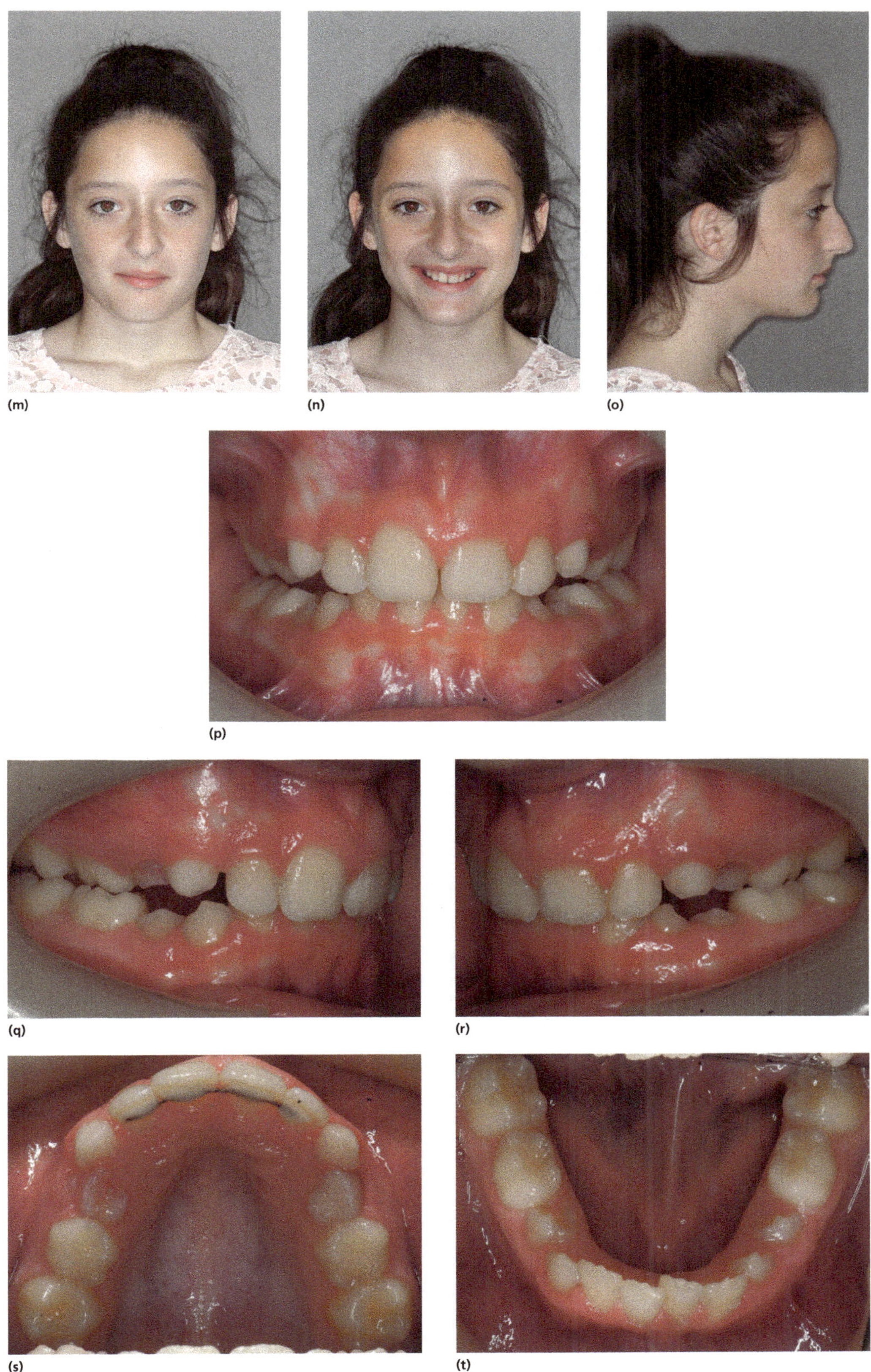

Figure 5.3 (*Continued*)

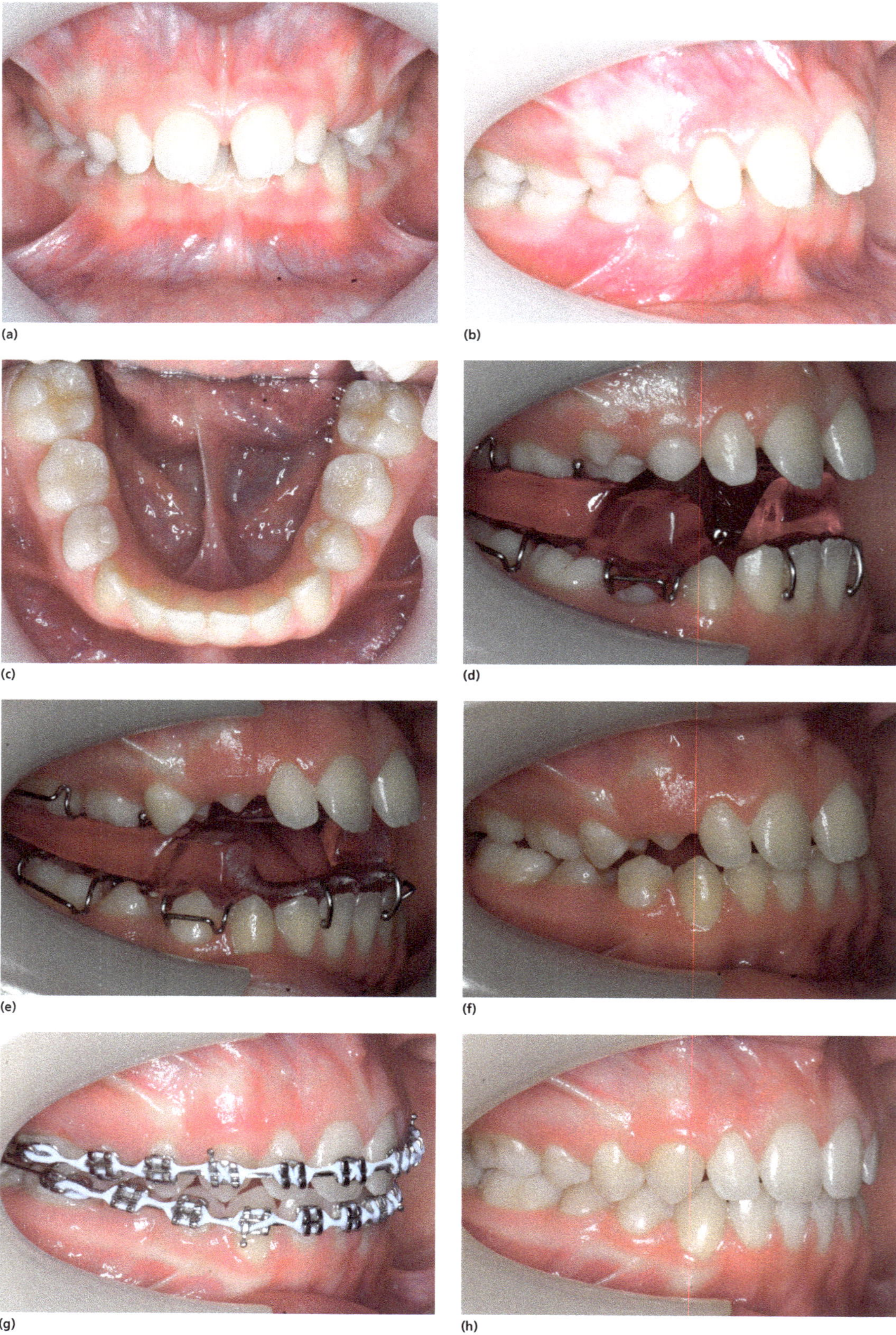

Figure 5.4 In this 13-year-old female with delayed dental development in the late mixed dentition, a ball-ended clasp was placed in the upper primary molar region as the first premolar had not erupted. As the lower right first premolar was close to erupting, an Adam's clasp was incorporated in the design and used at a later stage once the tooth had erupted sufficiently to offer retention (a–h).

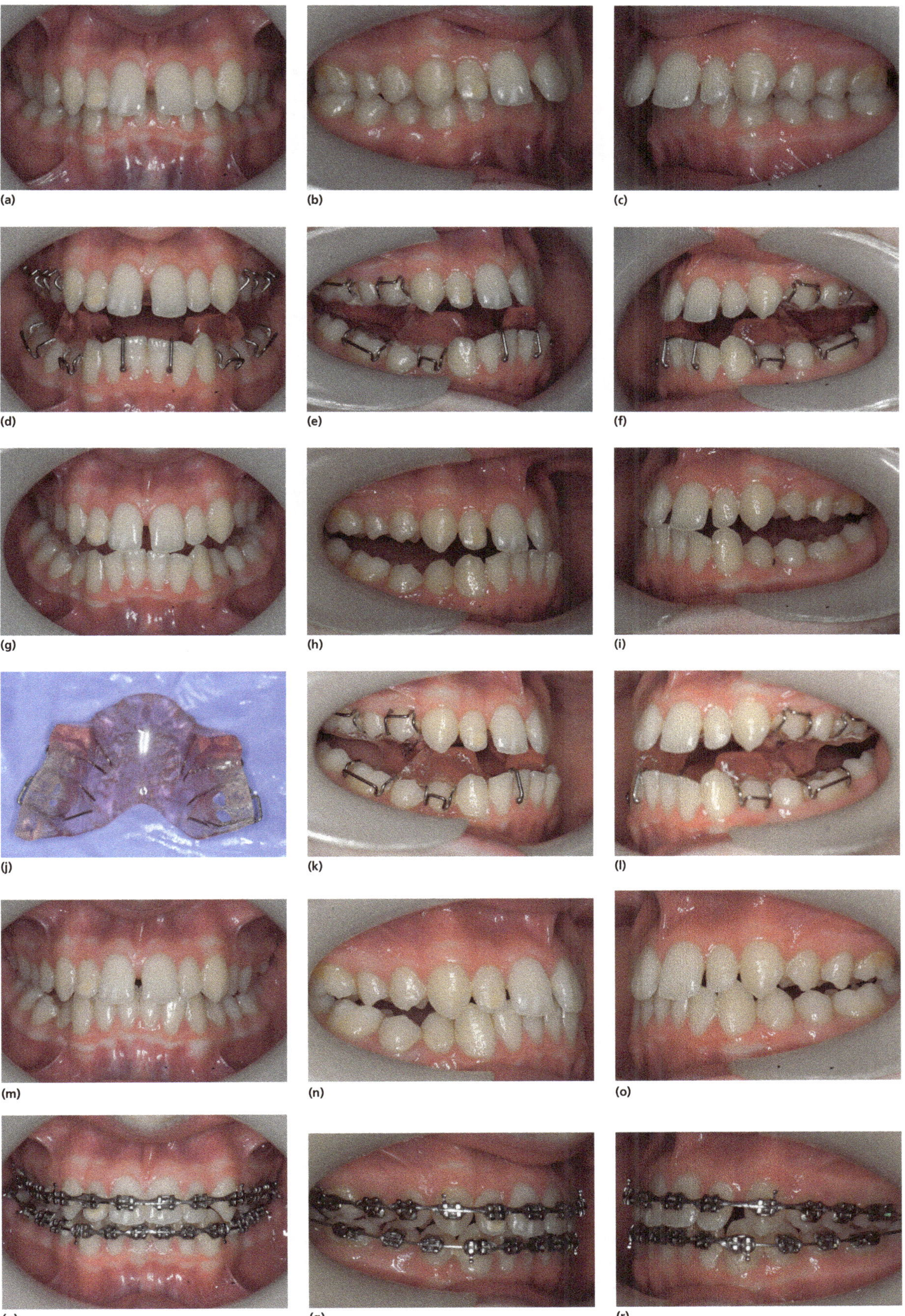

Figure 5.5 A 12-year-old male presented with a Class II division 1 incisor relationship in the early permanent dentition, with a large overjet of 12 mm and Class II molar relationships bilaterally (a–c). A modified Twin Block was fitted with one-step advancement to fully eliminate the overjet (d–i), resulting in overcorrection of the malocclusion to Class III molar relationships bilaterally. Significant lateral open bites arose due to the presence of the acrylic blocks allied to clasping of the first permanent molars. The upper appliance was trimmed to allow for regression of the lateral open bites prior to proceeding with fixed appliance therapy. This occurred over a 6-week period of part-time wear (j–o). Further resolution occurred without recourse to inter-arch elastics during the fixed appliance phase (p–u). The final occlusal result is shown in (v–x).

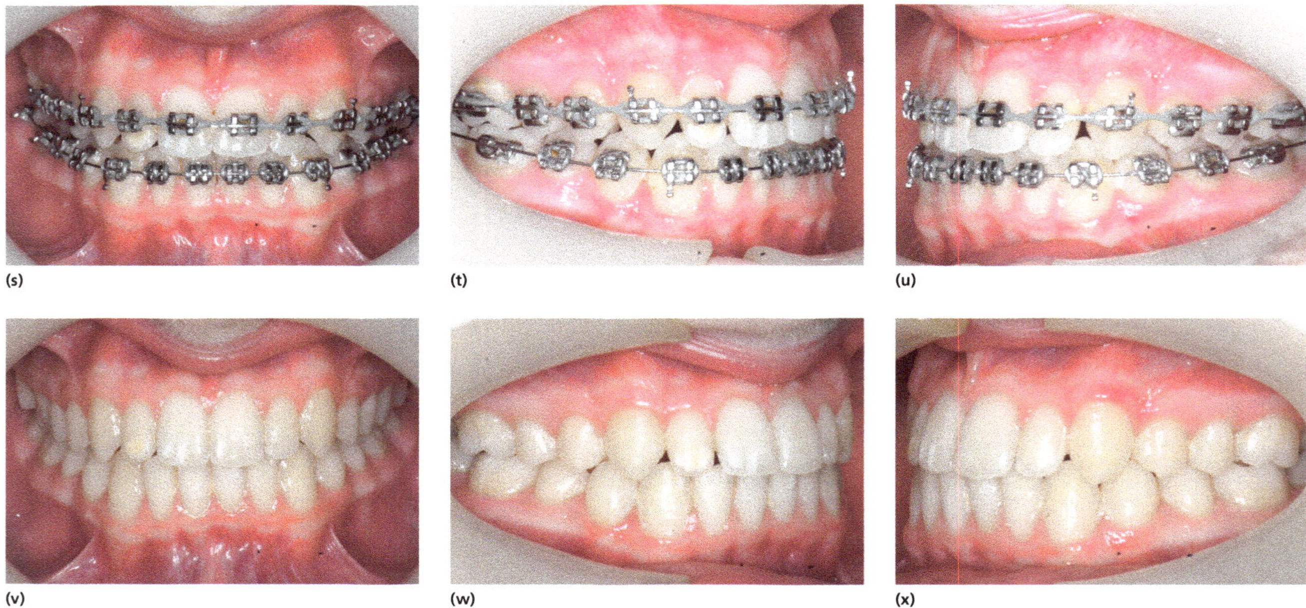

Figure 5.5 (*Continued*)

of the appliance will necessitate a period of re-acquaintance with the appliance, further taxing compliance.

Overjet and reversed overjet

It has been noted that the temporo-mandibular joint allows a relatively uniform degree of forward movement of the mandible and this is generally of the order of 9–11 mm.[21] At the outset of treatment this should be checked and will manifest as an overjet reduction of 9–11 mm with maximal forward mandibular posture. During the course of treatment a habitual forward posture may develop, which may be misinterpreted as supplementary mandibular growth. Provided that the difference between the resting overjet and the overjet on maximal posture, which will be a reversed overjet as treatment proceeds, does not reduce and is maintained at the initial amount, it can be assumed that the estimate of overjet correction is not postural and is genuine. It is then important that this change is maintained until stable condylar and glenoid fossa modification has been consolidated (Figure 5.8).

Length of retention

In both fixed and removable functional therapy, rapid overjet correction needs to be maintained for a reasonable period[22, 23] to avoid relapse. Accepted clinical practice involves use of a functional appliance for a period of approximately 12 months. The duration of appliance wear allied to the relative length of the active and retention phases of therapy has varied in clinical trials of functional appliance therapy. For example, O' Brien et al. involved wear of the appliance for up to 15 months, with clinicians using various protocols for retention once overjet correction was achieved.[24] A period of full-time wear of up to 15 months has been reported in a further trial comparing the Twin Block with a hybrid functional appliance. In the latter study a mean overjet relapse of 1 mm from an initial overjet of 10 mm was observed during the retention phase.[19]

Space planning for fixed therapy

Each individual patient will have a unique growth pattern and response to therapy and the nature and extent of this are best identified by a lateral cephalogram at the end of the functional phase of therapy. The changes in inclination of the lower incisors in particular should be identified, and unwanted proclination should be factored into the assessment of available space for the fixed appliance phase. If excessive proclination of lower incisors is accompanied by a significant degree of crowding, extractions might be indicated for stability, aesthetics and long-term gingival health around the lower incisors. The Twin Block, however, has been shown to result in a similar degree of lower incisor proclination to other removable functional appliances.

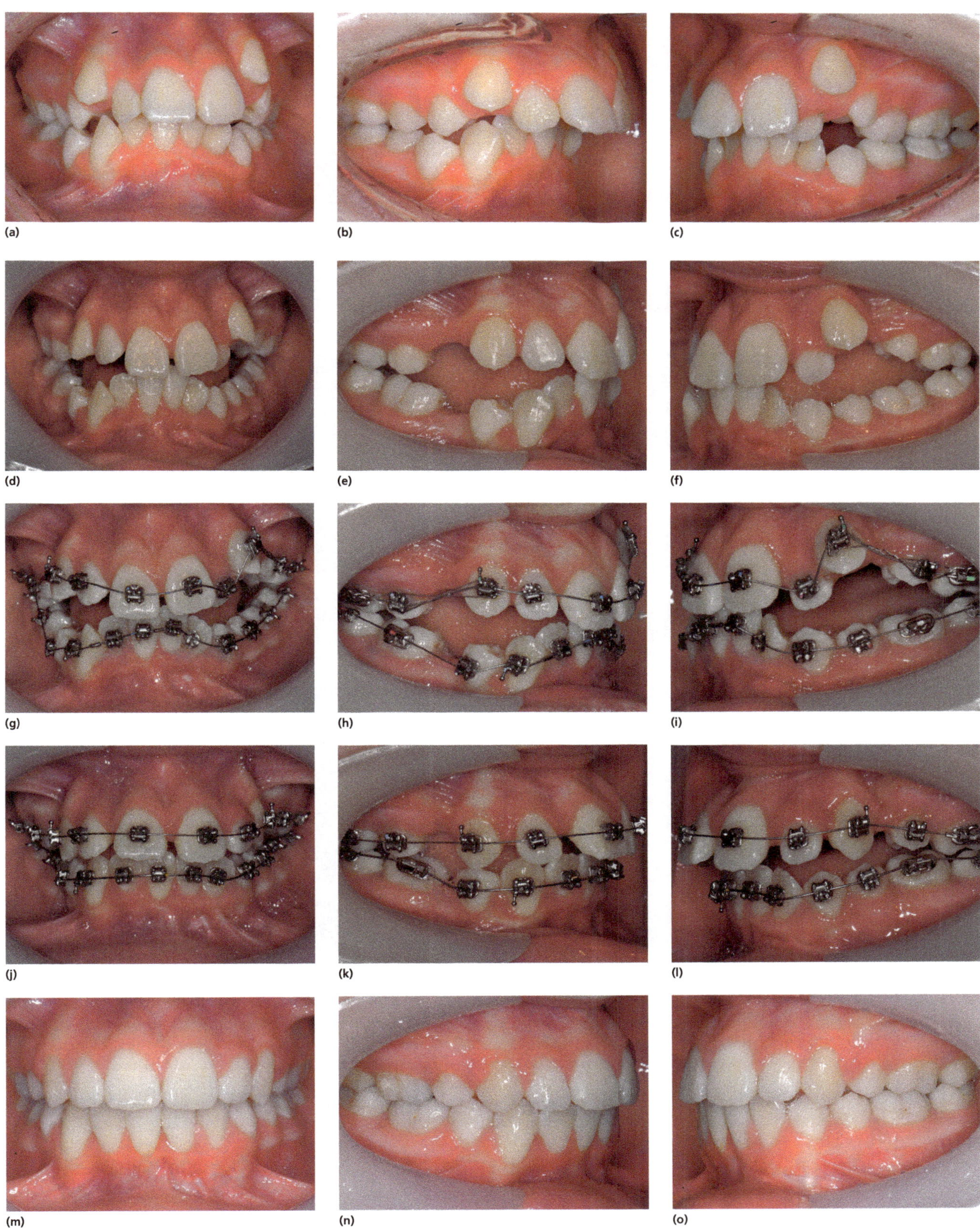

Figure 5.6 This female adolescent had a period of Twin Block wear to correct a significant Class II malocclusion with increased overjet of 12 mm. Trimming of the blocks was not undertaken during the functional phase, with pronounced resultant lateral open bites ensuing (a–f). Fixed appliances were placed without a pause to permit spontaneous resolution due to the likely need for a protracted fixed phase because of the degree of crowding and centre-line discrepancy (g–i). Spontaneous resolution of the lateral open bites occurred over a period of 10–12 weeks (j–l). Fixed appliance treatment was completed to enhance the posterior interdigitation, improving the prospect of prolonged stability (m–o).

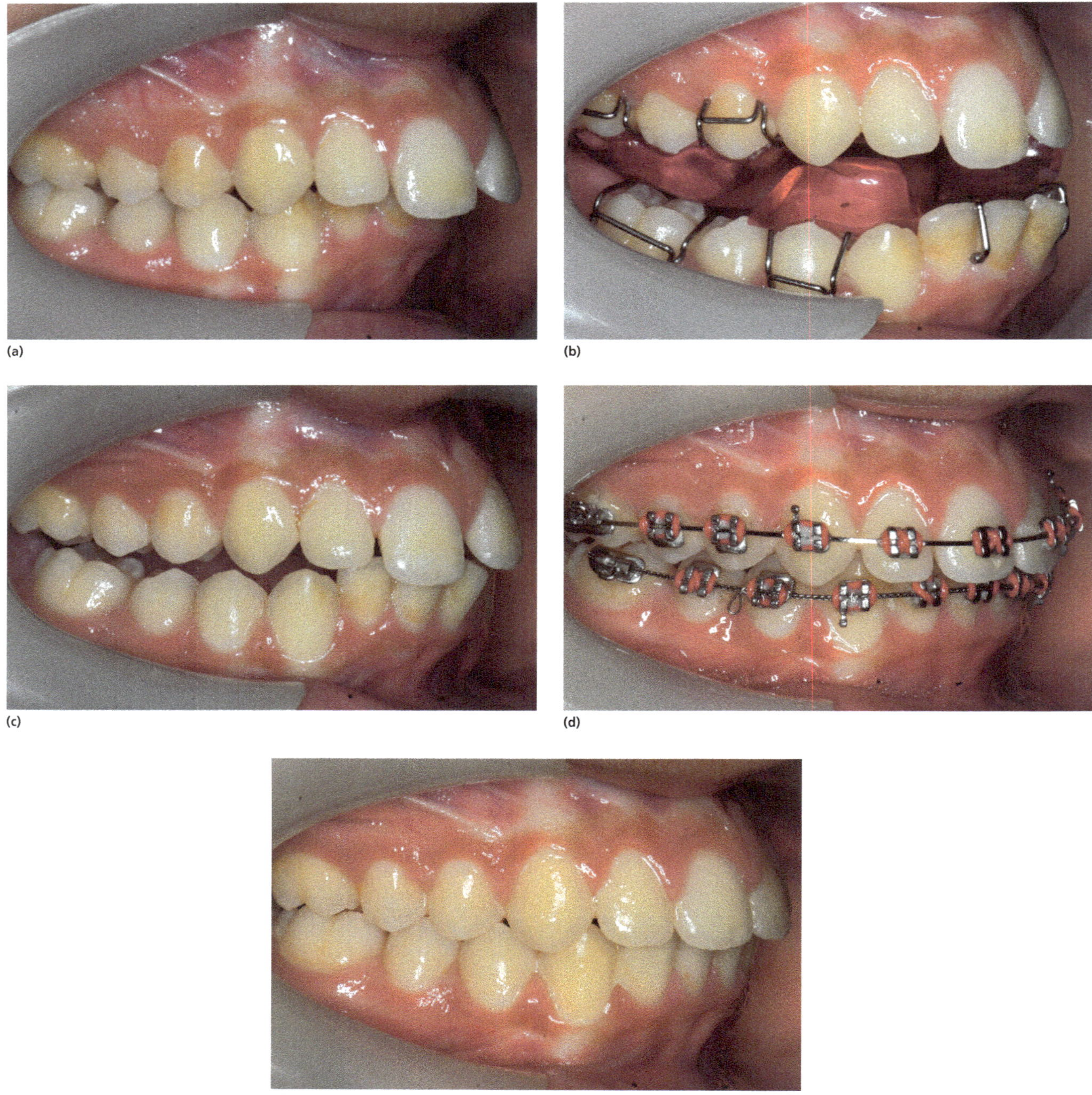

Figure 5.7 A further Class II division 1 case with an overjet of 9 mm (a). The malocclusion was fully corrected with a modified Twin Block (b). The blocks were relatively shallow, with limited lateral open bites accruing despite lack of acrylic trimming (c, d). Lateral open bites were closed during the fixed phase (d, e) due to their relatively limited extent and the presence of reasonable intercuspation; hence, condylar stability occurred relatively early in the fixed phase.

A similar situation with shallow (5 mm) blocks is given in f–i. The blocks also met at approximately 45 degrees rather than the recommended, more positive 70-degree intersection that Clark now recommends. Notwithstanding this, forward posture was maintained and the resultant lateral open bites were minimal despite diligent wear of the appliance.

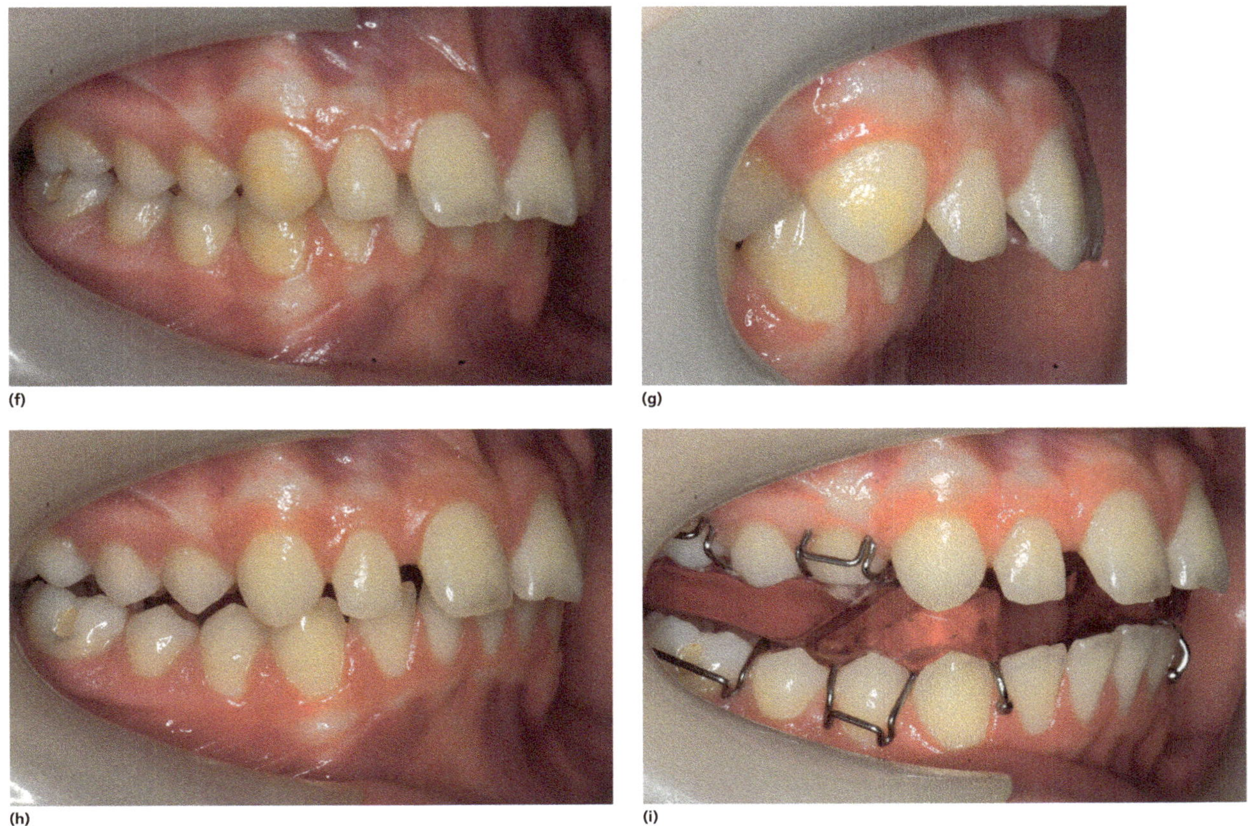

(f) (g) (h) (i)

Figure 5.7 (*Continued*)

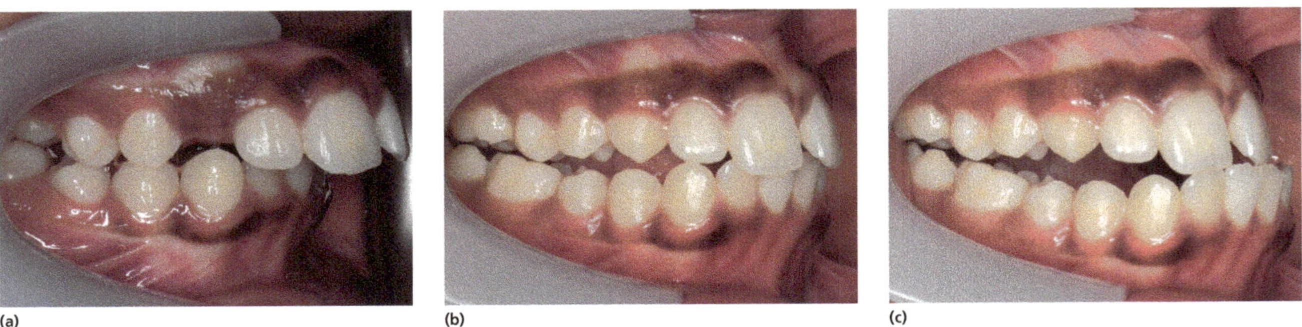

(a) (b) (c)

Figure 5.8 A significant Class II malocclusion with an overjet of 10 mm (a) was corrected fully with a Twin Block over a period of 9 months, resulting in lateral open bites and over-correction of the molar relationships (b). On maximum protrusion there was a reverse overjet of 3 mm (c), confirming that the Class II correction was genuine and not attributable to habitual posture.

A similar case with a slightly larger overjet (d–f) was treated with a Twin Block (g–i), resulting in full Class II correction (j–l). Maximal protrusion highlights the degree of genuine change, with a frank reverse overjet of 6 mm in the most protruded position. Maximal protrusion highlights the degree of genuine change, with a frank reverse overjet of 6 mm in the most protruded position (m, n).

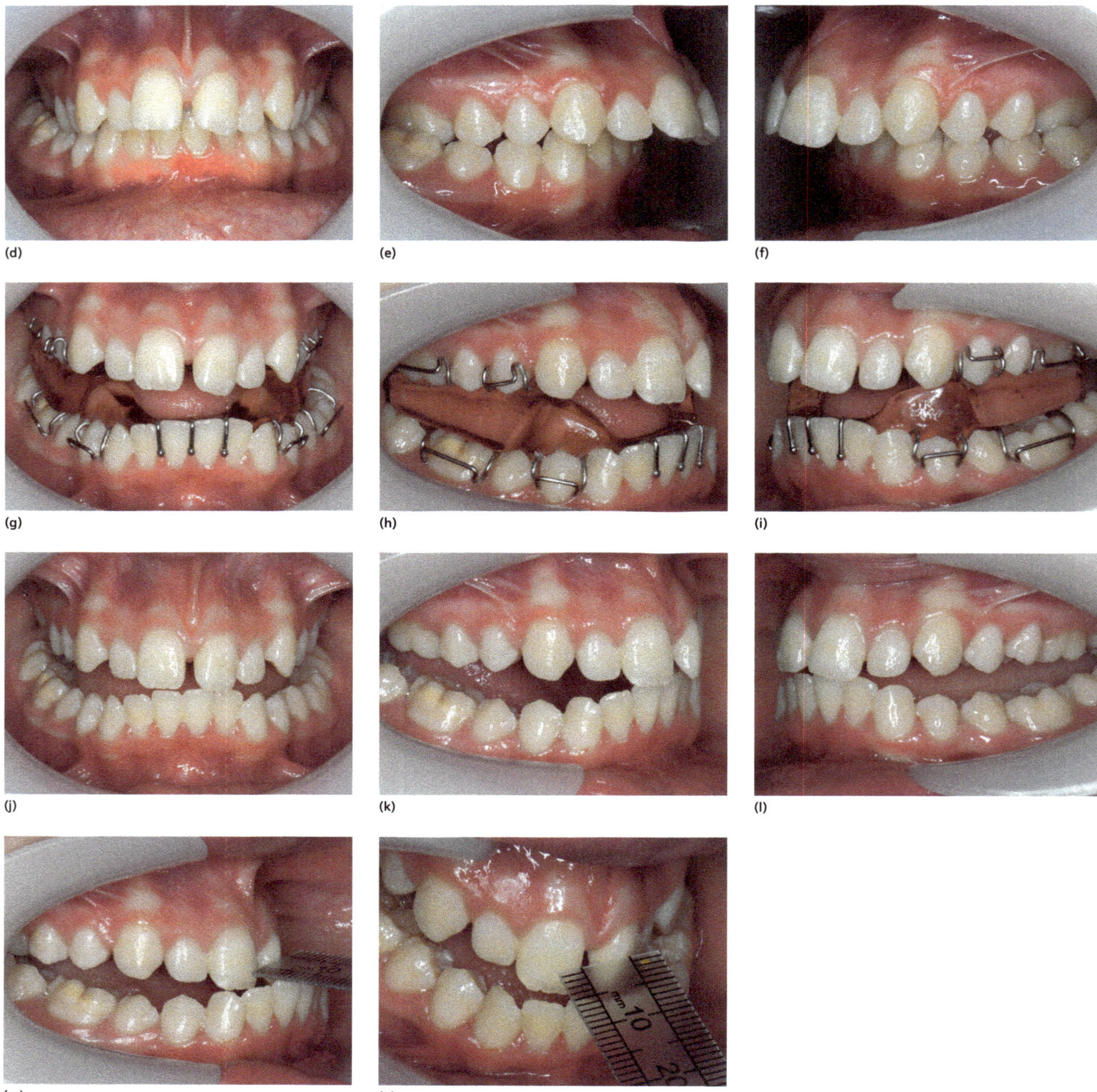

Figure 5.8 *(Continued)*

Post-treatment retention

On completion of fixed appliance therapy, the inherent skeletal discrepancy may tend to re-establish itself. Generally an ideal occlusion with good intercuspation will remain stable; however, a number of patients may have reduced mandibular growth in the post-treatment period. A Twin Block on a nocturnal basis may be considered to preserve antero-posterior correction, although a reduced vertical dimension may be considered to limit the risk of bite opening or impairment of posterior interdigitation where there is some evidence of relapse or incomplete antero-posterior correction. The objective, therefore, should be to establish and maintain good intercuspation of posterior teeth. Alternatives to the Twin Block including an activator or Bionator may also be considered for this purpose.

Summary

The Twin Block is an effective removable appliance for correcting antero-posterior discrepancies in the late mixed or early permanent dentition. It is versatile, robust and well tolerated on a full-time basis, resulting in efficient Class II correction. Overjet correction within 6 months can be expected with a Twin Block; however, an adequate period of retention is required to maintain this, as the posterior teeth are normally out of occlusion until the appliance is withdrawn. It is generally preferable to complete the growth modification before finishing fixed appliance therapy, and a degree of relapse should be anticipated during the fixed appliance phase.

References

1. Clark WJ. The twin block traction technique. Eur J Orthod. 1982; 4: 129–38.
2. Clark W. Design and management of Twin Blocks: Reflections after 30 years of clinical use. J Orthod. 2010; 37: 209–16.
3. Chadwick SM, Banks P, Wright JL. The use of myofunctional appliances in the UK: A survey of British orthodontists. Dent Update. 1998; 25: 302–8.
4. Clark WJ. New horizons in orthodontics & dentofacial orthopedics: Fixed Twin Blocks & TransForce lingual appliances. Int J Orthod Milwaukee. 2011; 22: 35–40.
5. Giuntini V, Vangelisti A, Masucci C, Defraia E, McNamara JA Jr, Franchi L. Treatment effects produced by the Twin-block appliance vs the Forsus Fatigue Resistant Device in growing Class II patients. Angle Orthod. 2015; 85: 784–9.
6. Read MJ, Deacon S, O'Brien K. A prospective cohort study of a clip-on fixed functional appliance. Am J Orthod Dentofacial Orthop. 2004; 125: 444–9.
7. Baccetti T, Franchi L, Toth LR, McNamara JA Jr. Treatment timing for Twin-block therapy. Am J Orthod Dentofacial Orthop. 2000; 118: 159–70.
8. Illing HM, Morris DO, Lee RT. A prospective evaluation of Bass, Bionator and Twin Block appliances. Part 1 – The hard tissues. Eur J Orthod. 1998; 20: 501–16.
9. Fränkel R. A functional approach to orofacial orthopaedics. Br J Orthod. 1980; 7: 41–51.
10. Sattarzadeh AP, Lee RT. Assessed facial normality after Twin Block therapy. Eur J Orthod. 2010; 32: 363–70.
11. Dyer FMV, McKeown HF, Sandler PJ. The modified Twin Block appliance in the treatment of class II division 2 malocclusions. J Orthod. 2001; 28: 271–80.
12. Lund DI, Sandler PJ. The effects of Twin Blocks: A prospective controlled study. Am J Orthod Dentofacial Orthop. 1998; 113: 104–10.
13. Gill DS, Lee RT. Prospective clinical trial comparing the effects of conventional Twin-block and mini-block appliances: Part 1. Hard tissue changes. Am J Orthod Dentofacial Orthop. 2005; 127: 465–72.
14. Banks P, Wright J, O'Brien K. Incremental versus maximum bite advancement during twin-block therapy: A randomized controlled clinical trial. Am J Orthod Dentofacial Orthop. 2004; 126: 583–8.
15. Sharma AA, Lee RT. Prospective clinical trial comparing the effects of conventional Twin-block and mini-block appliances: Part 2. Soft tissue changes. Am J Orthod Dentofacial Orthop. 2005; 127: 473–82.
16. Carmichael GJ, Banks PA, Chadwick SM. A modification to enable controlled advancement of the Twin Block appliance. Br J Orthodont. 1999; 26: 9–14.
17. Dixon M, Jones Y, Mackie IE, Derwent SK. Mandibular incisal edge demineralization and caries associated with Twin Block appliance design. J Orthod. 2005; 32: 3–10.
18. Parkin NA, McKeown HF, Sandler PJ. Comparison of 2 modifications of the twin-block appliance in matched Class II samples. Am J Orthod Dentofacial Orthop. 2001; 119: 572–7.
19. Lee RT, Barnes E, DiBiase A, Govender R, Qureshi U. An extended period of functional appliance therapy: A controlled clinical trial comparing the Twin Block and Dynamax appliances. Eur J Orthod. 2014; 36: 512–21.
20. Lee RT, Kyi CS, Mack GJ. A controlled clinical trial of the effects of the Twin Block and Dynamax appliances on the hard and soft tissues. Eur J Orthod. 2007; 29: 272–82.
21. Chateau M, Petit H, Roche M, Craig W. Functional orthopedics: The 'four pieces' and Class II treatment. Am J Orthod. 1983; 84: 191–203.
22. Pancherz H, Hansen K. Occlusal changes during and after Herbst treatment: A cephalometric investigation. Eur J Orthod. 198; 8: 215–28.
23. Chayanupatkul A, Rabie AB, Hägg U. Temporomandibular response to early and late removal of bite-jumping devices. Eur J Orthod. 2003; 25: 465–70.
24. O'Brien K, Wright J, Conboy F, Sanjie Y, Mandall N et al. Effectiveness of early orthodontic treatment with the Twin-block appliance: A multicenter, randomized, controlled trial. Part 1: Dental and skeletal effects. Am J Orthod Dentofacial Orthop. 2003; 124: 234–43.

CHAPTER 6

Rigid fixed functional appliances

Peter Miles

Class II treatment may be managed in either a one- or two-phased approach. Apart from the more invasive option of surgery, non-extraction options include the use of headgear, removable functional appliances (e.g. Twin Block, activator) or fixed functional appliances (e.g. Herbst; MARA – Allesee Orthodontic Appliances, Sturtevant, WI), often prior to comprehensive treatment with brackets in a two-phase approach. Alternatively, a single-phased approach is becoming increasingly popular in comprehensive treatment with brackets combined with headgear and/or elastics, which requires more cooperation from the patient, or to reduce the onus on compliance a fixed Class II corrector (e.g. Forsus FRD – 3M Unitek, Monrovia, CA; Jasper Jumper – American Orthodontics, Sheboygan, WI) may be used. Rigid fixed functional appliances including the Herbst and MARA will be discussed in this chapter, while flexible fixed variants (often termed Class II correctors) will be covered in Chapter 7.

A functional appliance is usually one that engages both dental arches and acts principally by holding the mandible away from its normal resting position.[1] This description would therefore best fit rigid appliances such as the Herbst and MARA. However, with non-rigid appliances such as the Forsus or even elastics, some forward posturing of the mandible may occur. A functional appliance may also be described as one aimed at modifying growth, but given that prospective clinical trials[2–4] have found that initial growth acceleration dissipates over time, perhaps the more appropriate description is fixed Class II correctors. However, the current convention is to term these fixed functional appliances (FFA).

Herbst

The Herbst appliance is by far the most researched of the fixed functional appliances, with the bite jumping phase of treatment usually completed within 6 to 8 months.[5] It was named after its developer, Emil Herbst, who according to Pancherz first described it in 1905.[6] The Herbst appliance (Figure 6.1) comes in various forms and may be cemented in place with crowns, bands or cast metal splints. Additionally, there is a bonded acrylic splint variant and a removable type.

The feature common to all designs is the rigid telescoping buccal tubes and rods, which keep the mandible in continuous protrusion both at rest and in function. A lingual arch is usually included in the lower arch and a trans-palatal arch (TPA) is often incorporated in the upper element, helping to maintain arch form while limiting potential unwanted movements such as the mesial tipping of the lower anchor teeth or buccal rolling of maxillary molars. As with other functional appliances, certain cases may require upper arch expansion, since a transverse discrepancy may be introduced when the mandible is advanced. It is usually best to carry out the expansion phase prior to addition of the telescopic arms. The possible requirement for expansion can be assessed by having the patient posture forward into an edge-to-edge bite and re-assessing the transverse relationships (Figure 6.1).

For maximal treatment effect, it has been proposed that the appliance should be constructed with an edge-to-edge incisal position.[7] However, other researchers have suggested that step-wise advancement may result in a greater change in the skeletal base relationship.[8,9] Step-wise advancement with the use of preformed spacers of known dimensions incrementally advances the mandible during treatment. In a retrospective comparison of step-wise and maximal advancement, a larger improvement in the sagittal jaw base relationship of 2.9 mm was recorded using step-wise advancement.[8] However, there were important differences between the groups, with, for example, step-wise advancement was used with a Herbst in combination with headgear for 12 months, compared with a standard Herbst appliance used for 10 months with maximal advancement. A large component of the recorded difference was due to a 1–1.5 mm distalizing/'headgear' effect on the maxilla, which may also relate to the additional 2 months of treatment allied to the use of headgear. Another study concluded that the amount of skeletal change was higher with step-wise advancement of the Herbst.[10] However, again this study was retrospective and involved comparison of step-wise advancement in adult Chinese subjects over 12 months, versus mandibular advancement to an incisal edge-to-edge position in German adult subjects over a shorter period (7–9 months). Outcomes may have been confounded by differences in centres, ethnic groups and treatment times. In contrast, a higher

Orthodontic Functional Appliances: Theory and Practice, First Edition. Padhraig Fleming and Robert Lee.

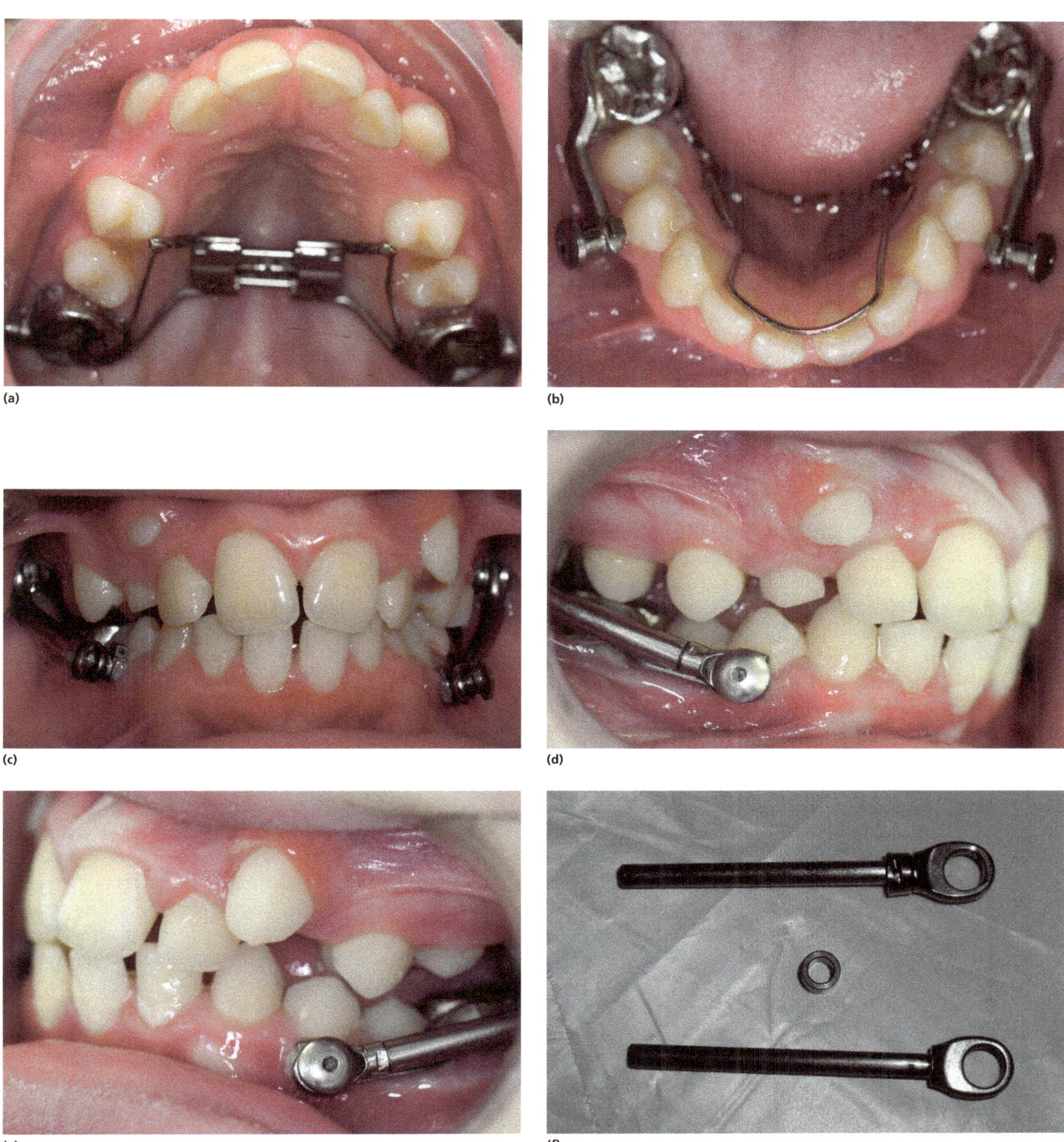

(a) (b) (c) (d) (e) (f)

Figure 6.1 This Herbst appliance incorporates crowns as anchorage on the molars (a, b) and is cantilevered in the lower arch. The upper component may include a trans-palatal arch to maintain arch form and reduce buccal flaring of the molars. In cases requiring transverse expansion to coordinate the arch width, an expansion device may be used (a). The expansion can be completed prior to adding the side arms (c–f), which consist of an upper tube and a lower rod. If the arms are added before the expansion, the angle of entry of the rod into the tube may cause binding and discomfort. The rods can be activated to advance the mandible further during treatment by the addition of pre-cut metal spacers (f), which slide onto the rod and can be crimped with a heavy set of pliers. The lower component includes a lingual arch (b) resting on the lower incisors to reduce mesial molar tipping.

level of evidence from the removable functional appliance literature involving the use of Twin Blocks in a randomized clinical trial (RCT) failed to show a difference in treatment effects with step-wise versus maximal advancement.[11] In view of the limited evidence concerning step-wise advancement with the Herbst appliance in terms of bite correction and an absence of data on patient comfort, currently either approach could be justified.

In terms of design options, Herbst appliances may be anchored to the teeth by either banding or bonding. Bonding may be augmented with adjunctive use of stainless steel crowns to enhance retention. Banded designs typically involve both maxillary and mandibular first permanent molars. Mandibular first premolars can also be included, with the pivot attached in this region. A continuous wire can be used to connect the lower first molars and premolars to increase the strength of the appliance. With crown Herbst appliances, the cantilever design has become popular, whereby a stiff, stainless steel bar projects mesially from the mandibular first molar to the first premolar where the pivot is sited. A lower lingual arch may be included to reinforce the lower appliance. Occlusal rests may also project distally from the lower first molar to control the eruption of the second molar. In the upper appliance the pivots may be soldered to the upper molar crowns. Again, bands may be added to the maxillary premolars for additional retention and durability.

Prefabricated appliances, such as the Hanks Herbst appliance™ (American Orthodontics, Sheboygan, WI) with bands fitted to the molar teeth, have been developed and marketed more recently. These incorporate telescoping attachment mechanisms in an effort to reduce the risk of disengagement and associated emergencies. Attempts have been made to increase the range of excursive movements to improve patient comfort and tolerance. The telescoping design has also been relocated mesially, ensuring easier access for placement, while reducing impingement of the appliance posteriorly and associated risks of ulceration and encroachment on the coronoid process. While traditional Herbst designs necessitated disengagement of the lower screw and piston for re-activation, recent alterations have also included use of slide-on shims to avoid this.

Mechanism of Class II correction

As with removable functional appliances, the original aim of Herbst therapy was to achieve increased mandibular growth. Initial studies of the Herbst appliance were favourable, reporting approximately 2 mm of increased mandibular length change over a 6-month period when compared with untreated controls, and a 5 mm reduction in the overjet.[6,7] One study[7] found molar correction averaging 6.7 mm attributed to a 2.2 mm increase in mandibular length, a 2.8 mm distal movement of the maxillary molars, and a 1 mm mesial movement of the mandibular molars. The 5.2 mm overjet correction was mainly due to the 2.2 mm increase in mandibular length and a 1.8 mm mesial movement of the mandibular incisors. The reported correction, therefore, seemed to be almost equally attributable to skeletal and dental change.

Class II subjects can present with a range of smaller to very large overjets. One study involved comparison of subjects requiring smaller advancement (<7 mm, average = 5.9 mm) with those requiring larger increments (>9.5 mm, average = 11.2 mm) using the Herbst followed by pre-adjusted Edgewise appliances.[12] The group requiring the larger advancement exhibited greater lower incisor intrusion, protrusion and proclination. This recovered somewhat during the pre-adjusted Edgewise appliance phase, but was still larger in the greater advancement group. The ANB angle reduced by 1.3 degrees in the small advancement group and 1.9 degrees in the large advancement group during Herbst treatment; after pre-adjusted Edgewise appliances, the overall change reduced to 1 and 1.3 degrees, respectively. The greater correction in overjet, therefore, appears to come largely from a greater dental change, to which lower incisor protrusion (1.3 mm more) and proclination (4.8 degrees more) is a major contributor. Unfortunately, any 'headgear' effect on the maxilla or molar distalization was not assessed.

The Herbst appliance appears to be effective at correcting Class II malocclusions at least in the short term, but there is debate as to whether this improvement is sustained in the longer term. One study involved evaluation of patients receiving the Herbst appliance in the mixed dentition for 8 months in conjunction with partial 2 × 4 Edgewise brackets, with follow-up 16 months after Herbst removal.[13] Initially, the overjet reduced by 8.3 mm and molar correction of 7.5 mm arose. However, during the following 16-month period, the overjet and molar relationship relapsed, so that when compared with a historical control group, the net change in overjet was 2.4 mm and molar change was 2.8 mm. When examining subjects treated with a Herbst approximately 6 years after treatment, it was found that the observed headgear effect related to Herbst therapy relapsed considerably during the first 6 months following withdrawal of the appliance.[14] When examining a group of children age 8 years 8 months treated with the headgear–Herbst combination for 5 months followed by a 3–5-year period of activator retention, then re-examined at a mean age of 17 years 4 months, the initial protrusive effect on the mandible decreased from 3.9 mm to a less significant 1.5 mm.[15] Most of the retained 5.5 mm reduction in overjet was attributed to an ongoing headgear effect on the maxilla. This continued restraint in the forward growth of the maxilla was also found by Wigal et al.[16] However, the forward movement of the mandibular base returned to the pre-treatment position after fixed appliance therapy.

In a systematic review[17] of fixed and removable Herbst appliances, the authors found only three papers that met their inclusion criteria and the methodological quality of the studies was rated as poor. The magnitude of the mandibular skeletal change was in the range of 2–3 mm and there was minimal maxillary skeletal headgear effect. Most of the correction of the Class II was dental in nature, chiefly distalization of the upper molars and retroclination of the upper incisors, in addition to proclination of the lower incisors and mesial movement of the lower molars. The authors also compared previous reviews of bonded-type versus crown-type Herbsts. They noted that the magnitude of any differences was small, likely to be associated with the inter-occlusal acrylic layer and unlikely to be of clinical significance. They therefore concluded that the selection of Herbst design is really a clinical decision, as skeletal and dental differences between designs do not have a clinically significant impact. Similarly, when examining the cast-splint type Herbst with a premolar banded Herbst and a premolar/molar banded Herbst, no difference was noted in terms of anchorage loss and similar relapse was noted with all three types.[18]

Lower incisor changes

In a sample of 24 Class II division 1 subjects (mean age = 13.2 years), the lower incisors were proclined 10.8 degrees during treatment, but during the following 6 months post Herbst the incisal inclination reduced by 7.9 degrees.[19] After this time little change occurred and only 2.6 degrees of incisor proclination remained 5 years after treatment. Overall, the available space in the lower anterior region reduced by 0.6 mm and the irregularity index increased by 0.9 mm, but these changes arose during the observation period from 6 months to 5 years after the Herbst treatment was complete. The authors therefore concluded that this incisor crowding was unrelated to treatment or incisor uprighting and was due to normal craniofacial growth and associated occlusal maturation.

Another study examining the Herbst followed by placement of pre-adjusted Edgewise brackets found that during the Herbst phase the lower incisors were significantly protruded and proclined, with greater incisor movement arising with larger degrees of advancement.[12] Once the Herbst was removed and all teeth were bracketed, some recovery of the incisor position occurred; however, no association was found between treatment growth phase (pre-pubertal, pubertal, post-pubertal) and positional changes of the incisors. The consistent finding is that the lower incisors are advanced and proclined during treatment with the Herbst appliance and that this tendency does appear to reverse partially over time.

A concern relating to proclination of lower incisors is the potential for gingival recession.[20] When evaluating 98 children (mean age = 12.8 years) treated with the Herbst, varying degrees of incisor proclination were found (mean = 8.9 degrees, range = 0.5–19.5 degrees), but only 3% developed recession or experienced exacerbation of pre-existing recession. No association was found between the amount of incisor proclination and the development of gingival recession.[21] The authors concluded that at least in children and adolescents, orthodontic proclination did not seem to cause gingival recession in the short term. This was supported in another study that found no difference when comparing pre-adjusted Edgewise appliance treatment of Class II adolescents where the incisal edges were advanced an average of 3.9 mm with those that did not have the lower incisors advanced.[22] In a retrospective evaluation of patients undergoing pre-adjusted Edgewise appliance non-extraction treatment, no orthodontic variable was linked to recession,[23] with thin gingival biotype, visual plaque and inflammation useful predictors of gingival recession. Another retrospective study[24] in adult patients found that greater proclination (>95 degrees) and especially free gingival margin thickness (biotype) was linked to the risk of recession.

In a systematic review of gingival recession,[25] no association was found between appliance-induced labial movement of mandibular incisors and gingival recession. Important factors that may predispose to gingival recession included reduced thickness of the free gingival margin (biotype), a narrow mandibular symphysis, inadequate plaque control and aggressive tooth brushing. However, another systematic review[26] found that in most studies more proclined teeth risked recession, but that differences between proclined and non-proclined incisors were small and the clinical consequence was questionable, with the level of evidence being low. Thinner labial cortical bone has been demonstrated in untreated hyperdivergent facial types[27] along with a slightly higher rate of dehiscence.[28] There is, therefore, a potentially elevated risk of recession when advancing lower incisors in hyperdivergent facial types. As with many areas of orthodontics, more quality RCTs are required, but care should be exercised to maintain excellent oral hygiene, particularly in those with a thin tissue biotype and/or a hyperdivergent facial type.

Vertical effects

The success of functional appliance treatment of Class II subjects has been claimed to be associated with the vertical jaw base relationship, with higher-angle cases expected to respond poorly to functional jaw orthopaedics.[29] A criticism of Class II clinical trials such as those conducted in the United Kingdom[3] and United States[4] is that subjects should have been separated into hypodivergent, neutral and hyperdivergent facial types.[30] It has also been stated that hyperdivergent or long facial types are contraindicated for functional appliances, as they are more likely to exhibit an unfavourable growth pattern during treatment due to posterior mandibular growth rotation.[31, 32] Based on this premise, it has been suggested that the Herbst appliance is more suited to deep bite cases with retroclined lower incisors,[33, 34] with some researchers suggesting it to be contraindicated in patients with a high mandibular plane angle and excess lower facial height.[35] This is not dissimilar to the indications for most removable functional appliances.

When comparing a conventional banded Herbst in subjects with normal vertical proportions with a headgear reinforced acrylic splint type Herbst in subjects with increased vertical dimension, both groups were found to achieve a Class I relationship in the 9-month treatment period.[36] Although the authors stated that the splint-type Herbst with headgear in hyperdivergent patients offered more control of the vertical dimension, minimal difference (1 degree) in Frankfurt–mandibular plane angle (FMPA) between the groups was observed. When examining the mandibular plane angle in 24 Class II division 1 subjects, Herbst therapy was found to increase it only slightly (0.4 degrees), and during the 6 months post Herbst it reverted to baseline.[19] Over the ensuing 5 years, the mandibular plane angle actually reduced further, resulting in a total decrease of 2.2 degrees. When assessing the vertical effects of the Herbst on the mandibular plane angle in 10–14-year-olds during treatment, shortly after (6 months) and over the long term (4.5–5 years), the appliance was found to have minimal effect during treatment, while after treatment a decrease occurred.[37] Interestingly, no statistically significant differences were found with varying vertical dimensions.

In another study by the same group examining hyper- and hypodivergent Class II subjects aged 11 to 14 years, skeletal and dental changes were independent of the vertical facial type.[32] Similarly, when using an acrylic splint Herbst, although the lower anterior face height increased by 2.4 mm, both the Y-axis and mandibular plane angle remained essentially unchanged.[38] Thus, the overall vertical skeletal pattern did not change, in keeping with other research.[20] It therefore seems that functional appliance therapy with the Herbst appliance is equally effective and vertically neutral regardless of the pre-treatment vertical jaw base relationship. Increase in the anterior facial height dimension can, however, occur without an increase in the FMPA, and this could have implications for soft tissues and lip competence, with a long-term effect on stability and facial aesthetics.

When retrospectively comparing subjects treated in the early mixed, late mixed and permanent dentitions, it was concluded that treatment of Class II division 1 malocclusions in the permanent dentition is more efficient in terms of treatment time and PAR (Peer Assessment Rating) score reduction.[41] In adolescent (average age = 13.5 years) versus adult patients (average age = 20.7 years) undergoing Herbst treatment followed by pre-adjusted Edgewise appliances, treatment was considered equally efficient in adolescent and in adult Class II division 1 subjects, with similar reductions in PAR scores over comparable treatment times.[42] Similarly, when comparing surgical correction of Class II division 1 in adults with a Herbst and pre-adjusted Edgewise appliances, it was found that the Herbst appliance could achieve a molar correction averaging 4.1 mm and an average overjet reduction of 6.8 mm.[43] As would be expected, the amount of skeletal change contributing to overjet and molar correction was larger in the surgery group (63% and 80%, respectively) than in the Herbst group (13% and 22%). The authors therefore concluded that Herbst treatment could be considered an alternative to orthognathic surgery in borderline adult skeletal Class II malocclusions, especially when a large facial change is not the main goal of treatment.

Another study comparing Herbst correction with surgery in adult Class II subjects found that the Herbst achieved an average 5.3 mm overjet correction and a 2.3 mm molar correction, and concluded that the Herbst could be used in borderline skeletal Class II adult subjects.[44] Clearly, Herbst appliances may be useful in the non-surgical correction of Class II malocclusion in adults, particularly where the skeletal discrepancy is mild and dento-alveolar change would be sufficient to address the malocclusion (Figure 6.5).

Timing of Herbst treatment

Typically treatment with the Herbst appliance is recommended either during the pre-pubertal peak or in early adolescence (Figures 6.2–6.4). However, the Herbst has been suggested as early as 8 years of age during the early mixed dentition.[39] Although it was initially recommended for pre-pubertal patients, a later study demonstrated that the Herbst could be used just as effectively for overjet and molar correction after the pubertal growth peak.[40] However, there was less skeletal contribution to molar change and overjet correction, with the majority of the change being dento-alveolar. The late treatment group had a larger correction in overjet than the early group (8.4 mm vs 5.1 mm); this larger reduction partly explains the greater retraction of the upper incisors (+2.1 mm) and lower incisor advancement (+1.7 mm) in the late treatment group. This is supported by Martin and Pancherz,[12] in a study in which a group with larger advancements (average = 11.2 mm) exhibited more incisor advancement and proclination than those subjects with less advancement (average = 5.9 mm).

Soft tissue effects

In a systematic review of fixed functional appliances, an improvement of the facial convexity was confirmed.[45] Fixed functionals were shown to restrict the forward movement of the upper lip. No change in the antero-posterior position of the lower lip and soft tissue Menton was found, and soft tissue changes were similar among non-growing young adult and growing adolescent samples. However, the review relied on a secondary level of evidence.[45]

In a more recent RCT[46] of Class II division 1 patients, 60 subjects were randomly allocated to either a Herbst appliance, Twin Block or an untreated control group. Both appliances reduced the soft tissue profile convexity, but greater advancement of soft tissue Pogonion and the lower lip were observed in the Twin Block group, with a greater proportion of overall change attributed to mandibular elongation and advancement in that group.[47] The main difference in dental change was 3 degrees greater proclination of the lower incisors in the Herbst group than in the Twin Block group. As discussed in previous long-term studies,

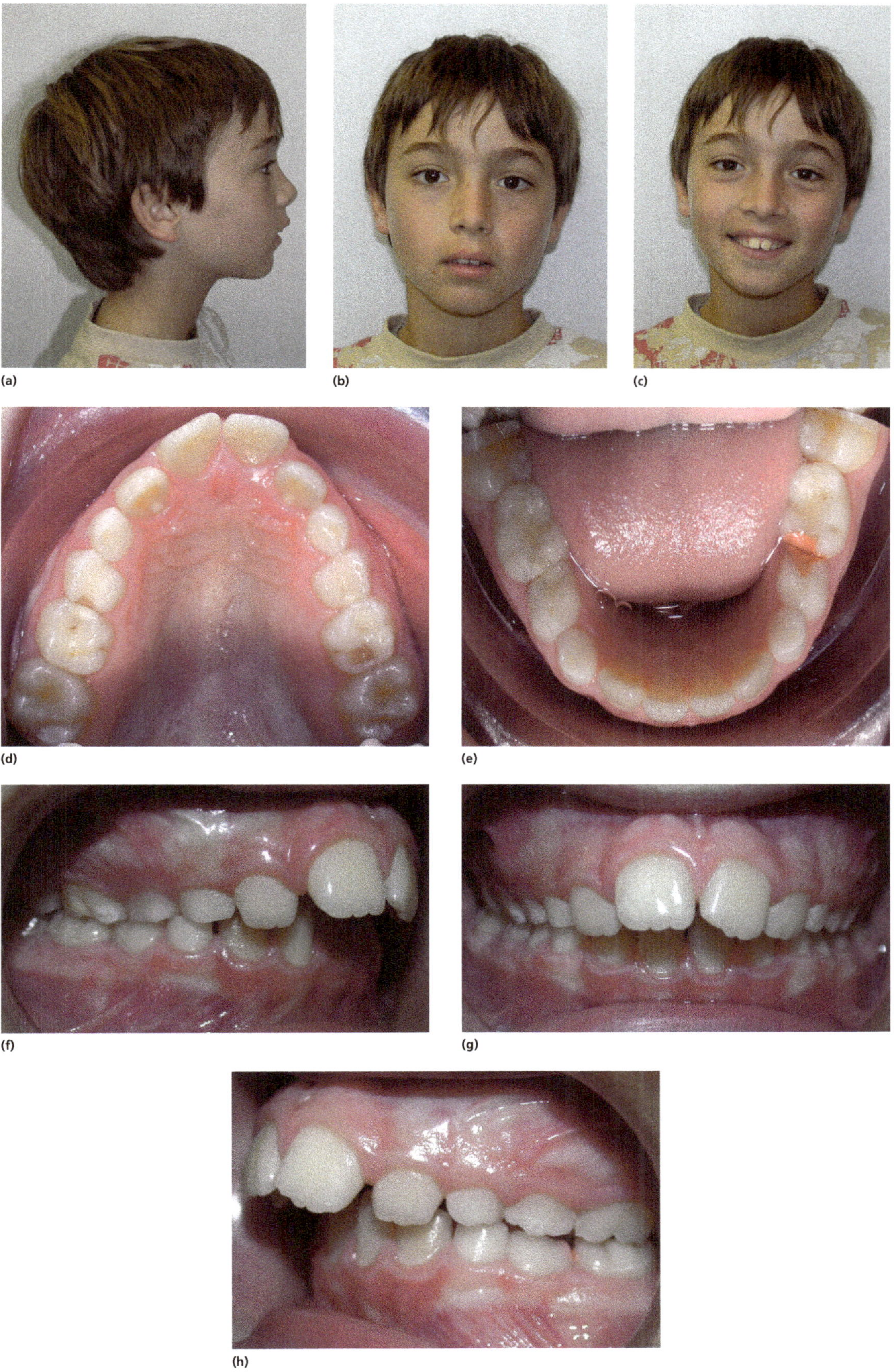

Figure 6.2 This 11-year-old male was treated with a Herbst appliance in conjunction with an upper expander (a–h). After 1 month of expansion and 8 months with the Herbst, a significant improvement in the overjet was achieved and the appliances removed. An upper Hawley retainer was made to retract the upper incisors slightly (i–p). The patient was then monitored until he was 14-years-old and on eruption of the remaining permanent dentition, the patient and his family chose to accept the final alignment and occlusion (q–x).

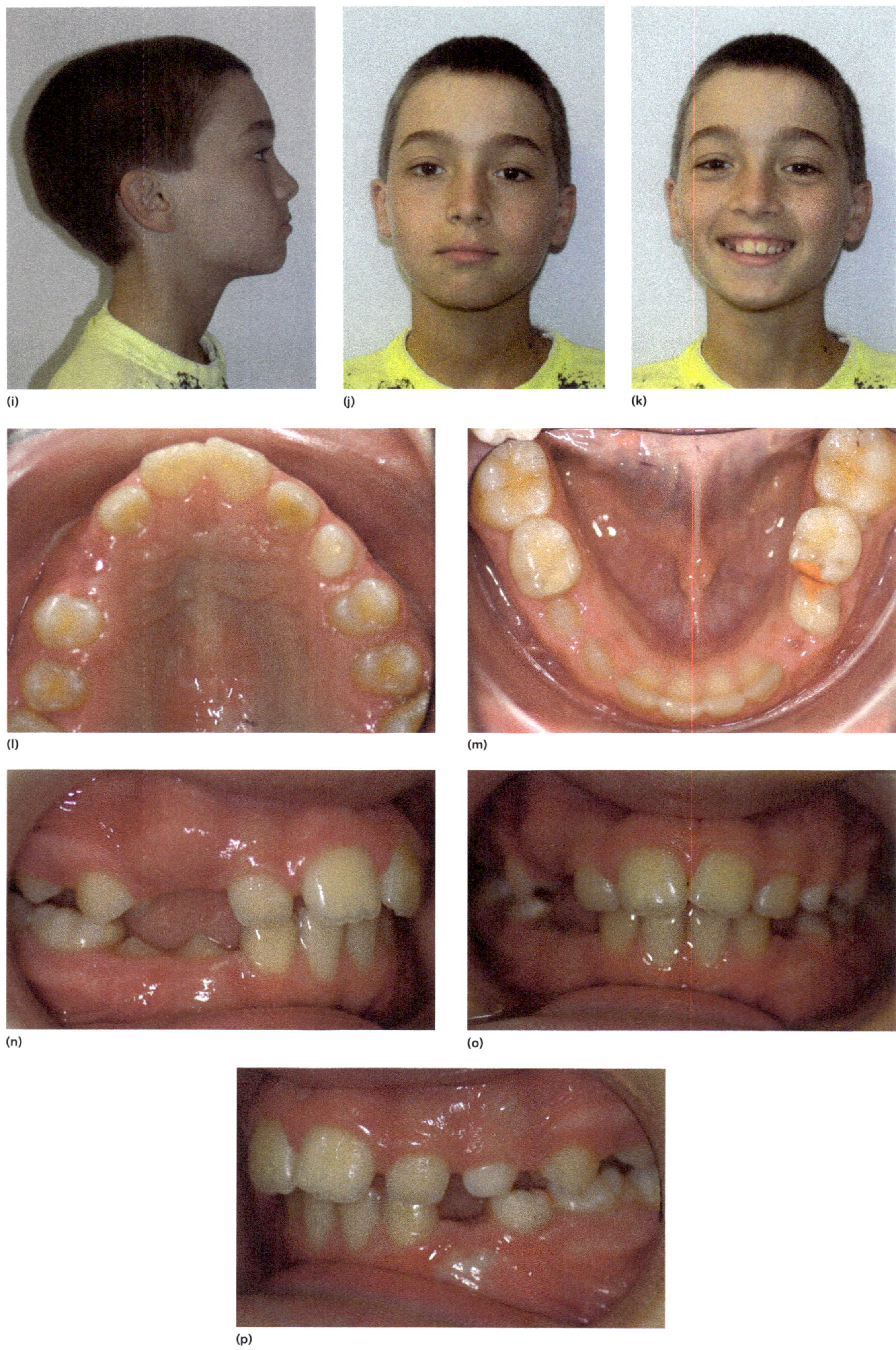

(i) (j) (k) (l) (m) (n) (o) (p)

Figure 6.2 (*Continued*)

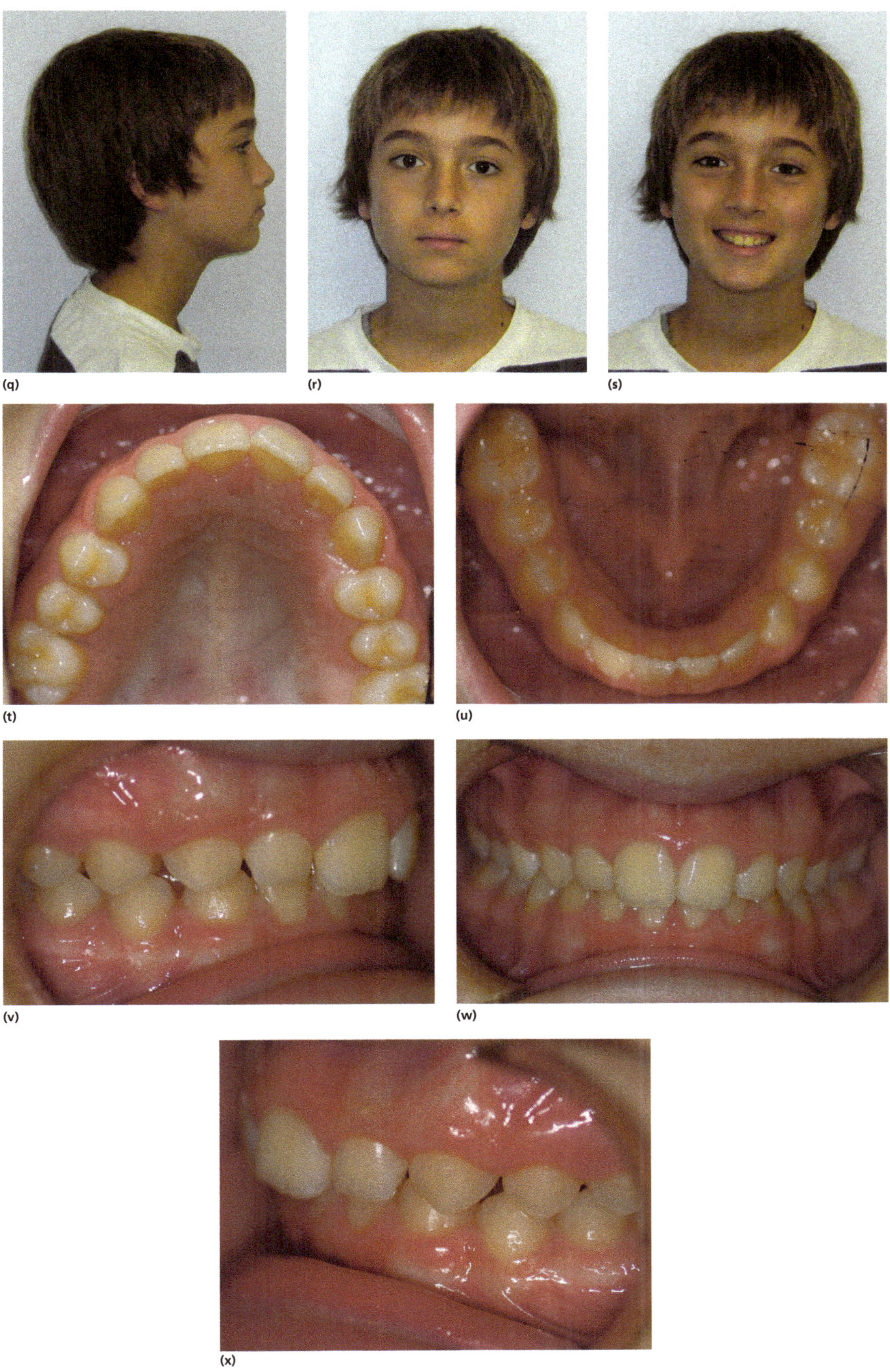

Figure 6.2 (*Continued*)

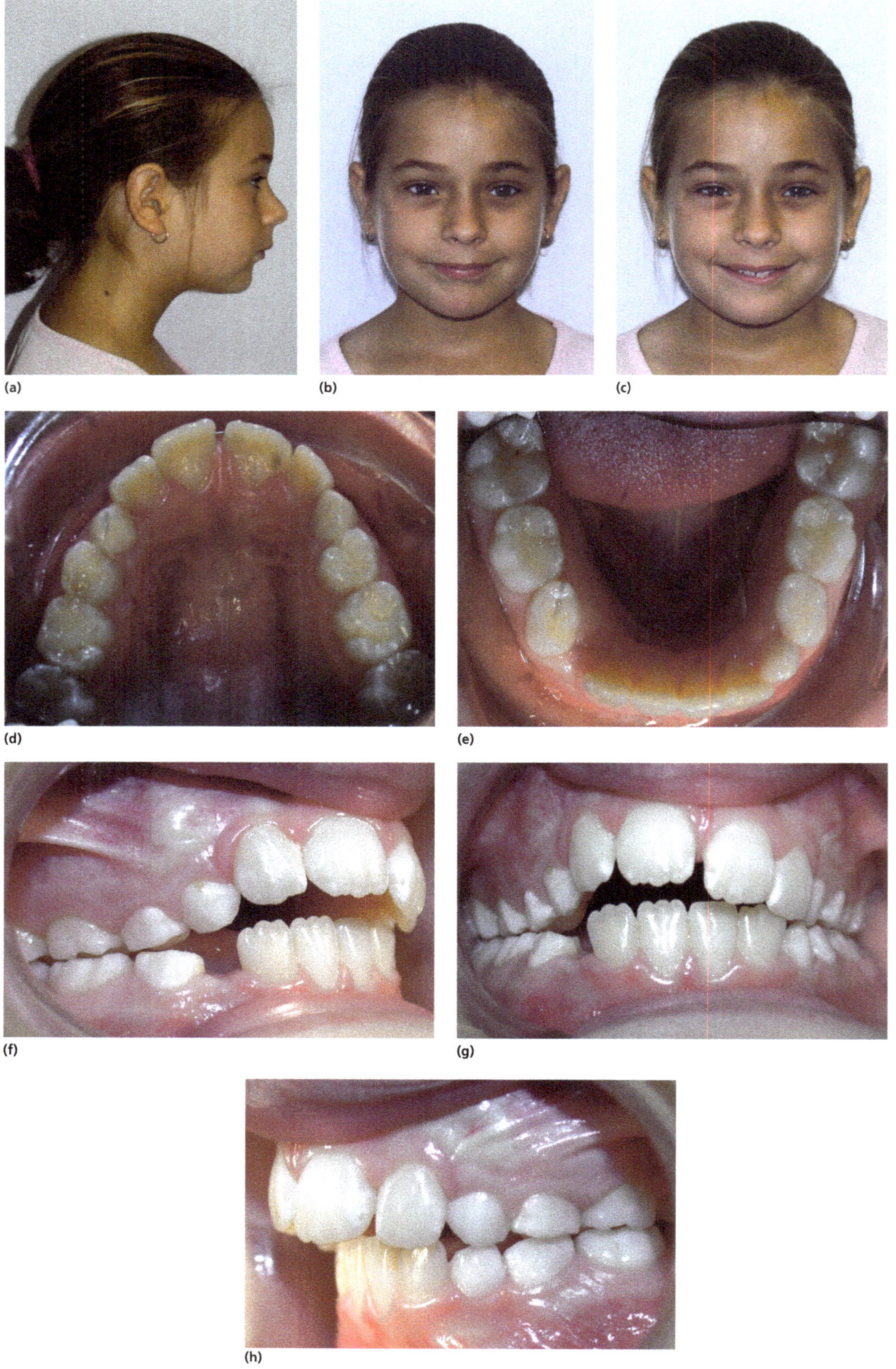

Figure 6.3 The patient presented at age 11 years with a persistent thumb habit and associated open bite and constricted maxillary arch in addition to a Class II malocclusion. To reduce reliance on compliance, a Herbst appliance was chosen in conjunction with a maxillary rapid palatal expander, which was activated over 5 weeks. After 2 months the side arms were added to the Herbst to advance the mandible into an edge-to-edge occlusion. The Herbst was activated by an additional 2 mm once during treatment spanning 8 months to achieve the desired molar correction and then removed (a–h). The habit had reduced by 2 months and stopped completely by 7 months into treatment. After the Herbst treatment the family and child chose to accept the alignment and occlusion. The patient was monitored for 6 months while the occlusion settled and retainers made (i–p). Five years later the patient returned. Class II correction had been stable; however, retainers had not been worn and some crowding had occurred (q–x). The patient elected to finalize the alignment with Invisalign sequential aligners over a period of 19 months. This was followed by provision of fixed and removable retainers (y–af).

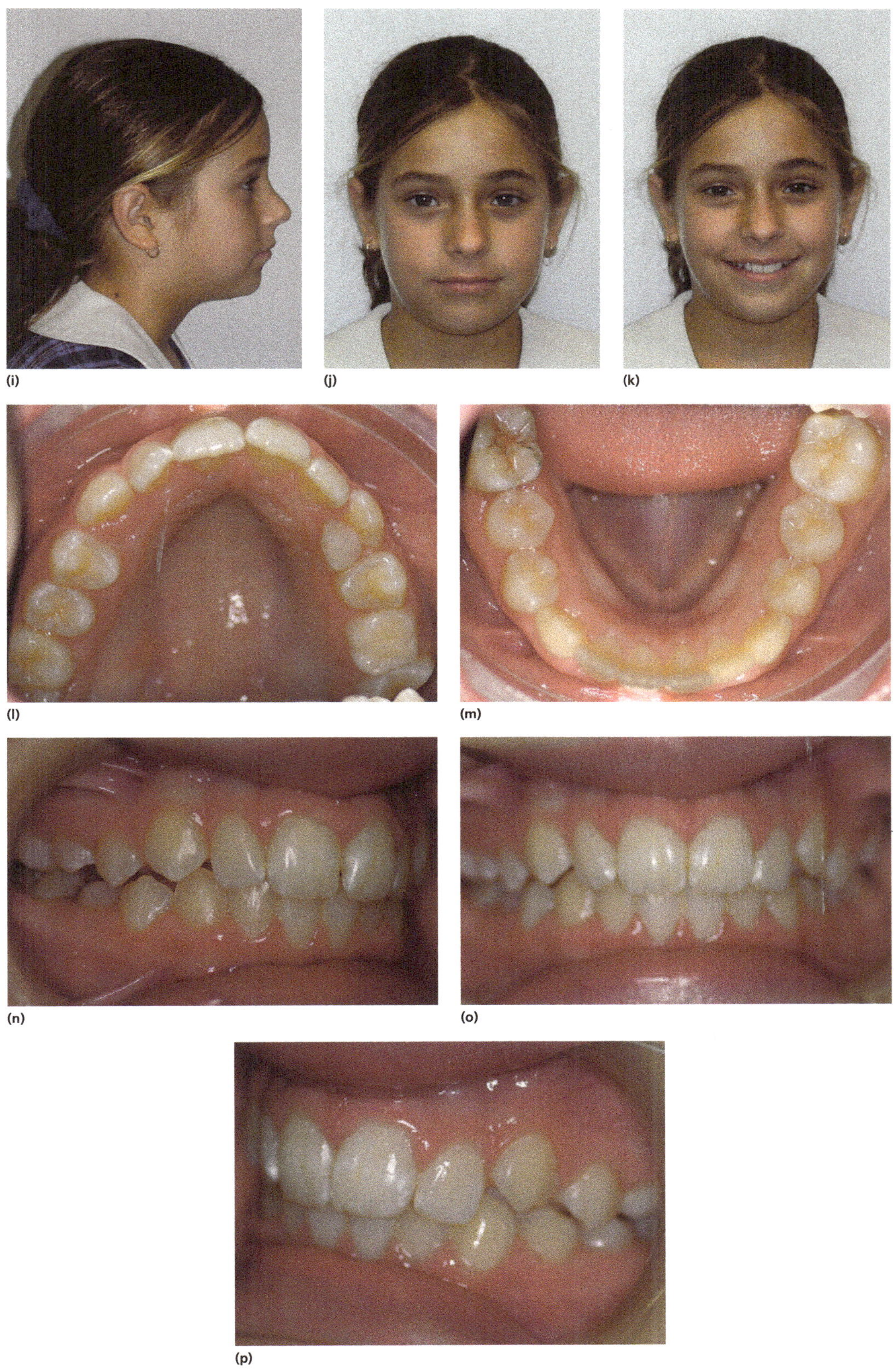

Figure 6.3 (*Continued*)

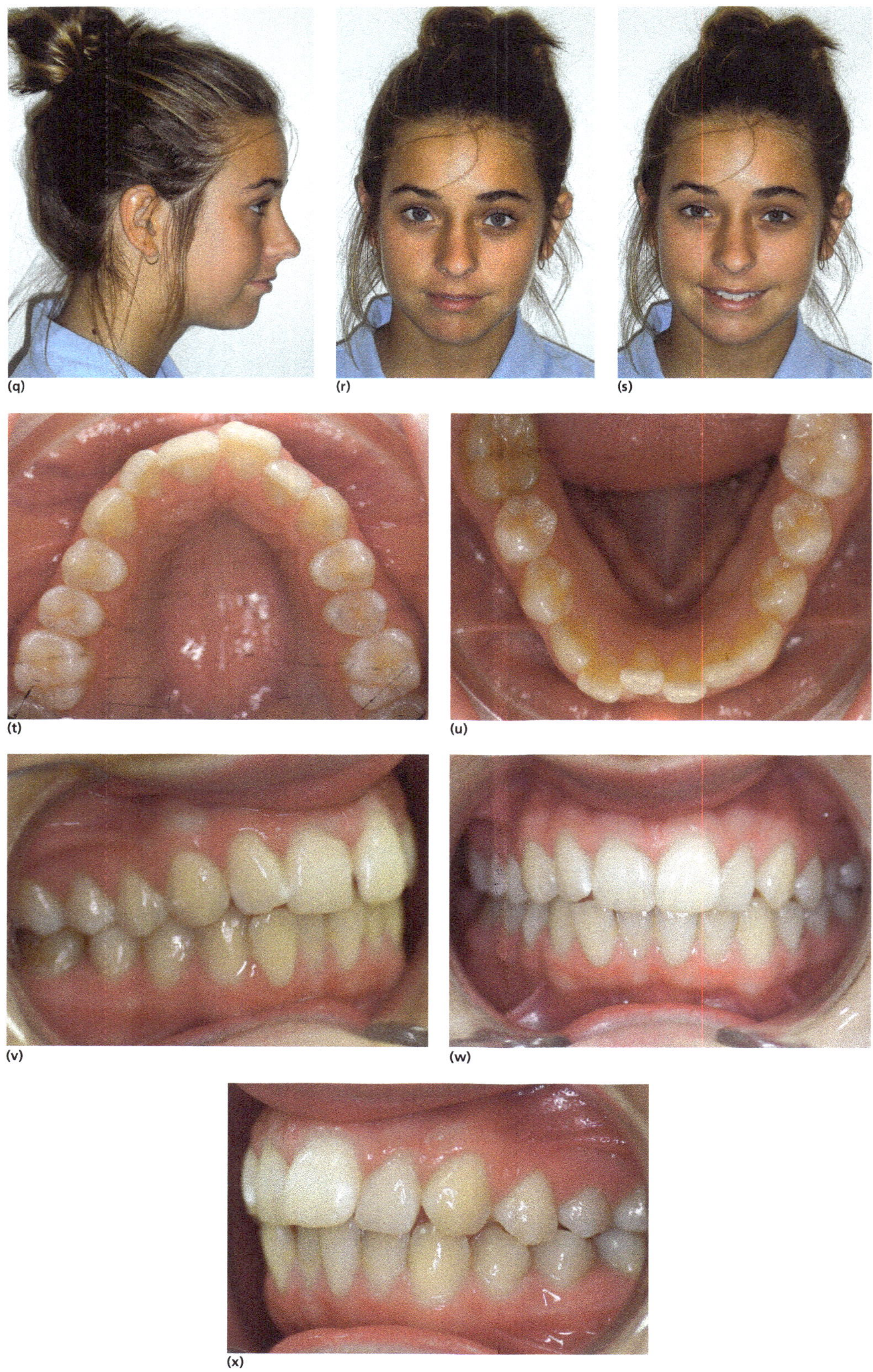

Figure 6.3 (*Continued*)

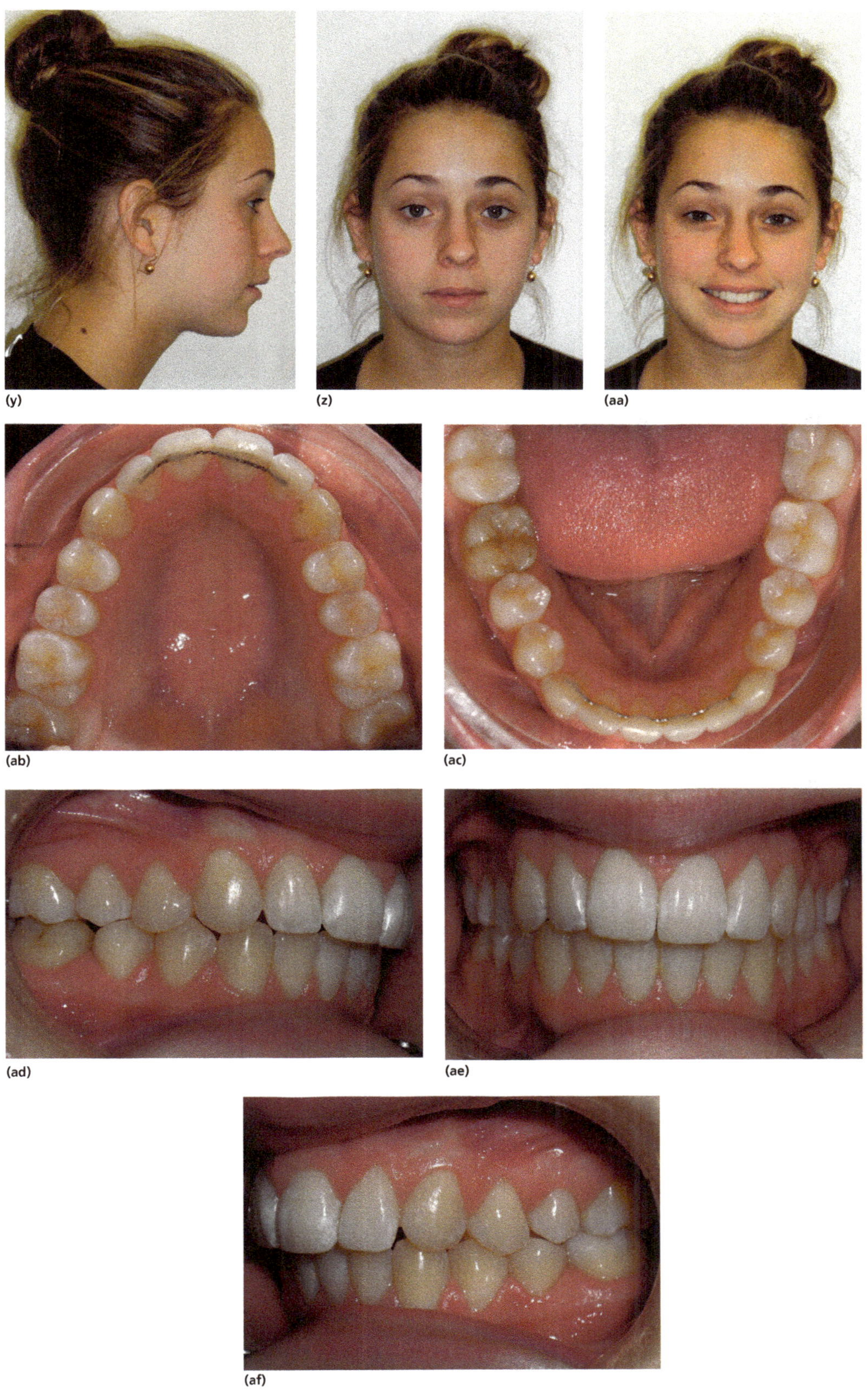

Figure 6.3 (*Continued*)

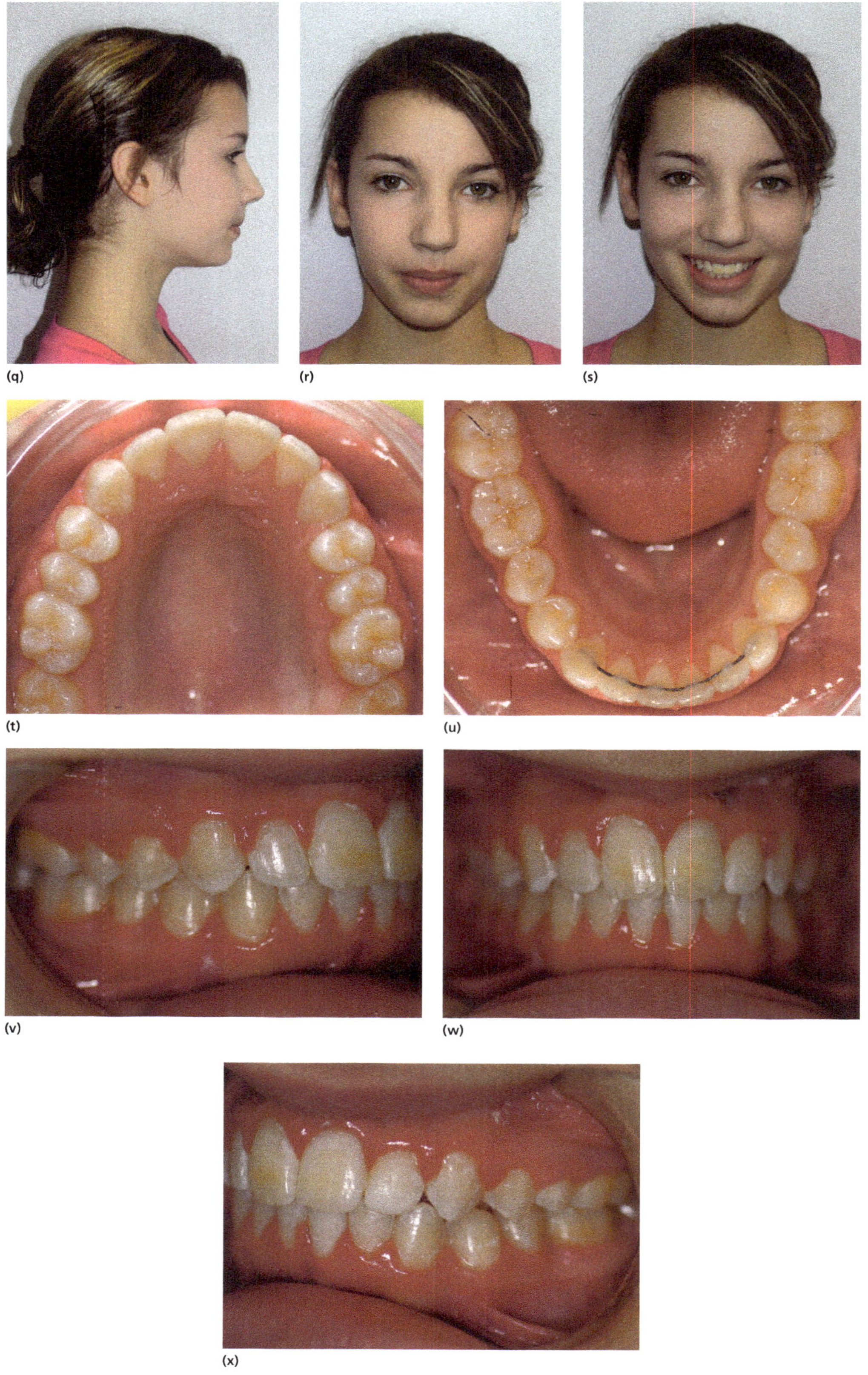

Figure 6.4 (*Continued*)

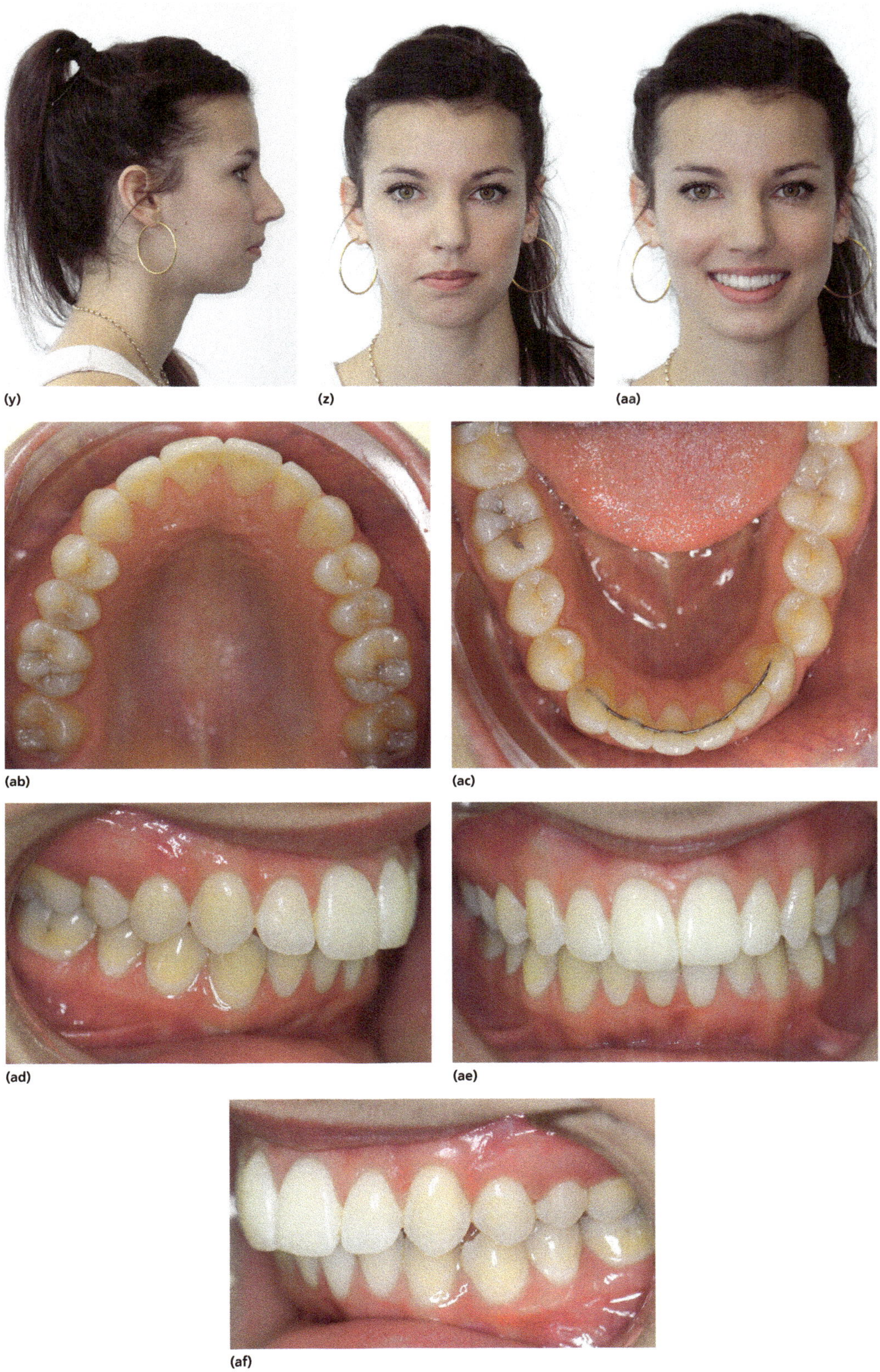

Figure 6.4 (*Continued*)

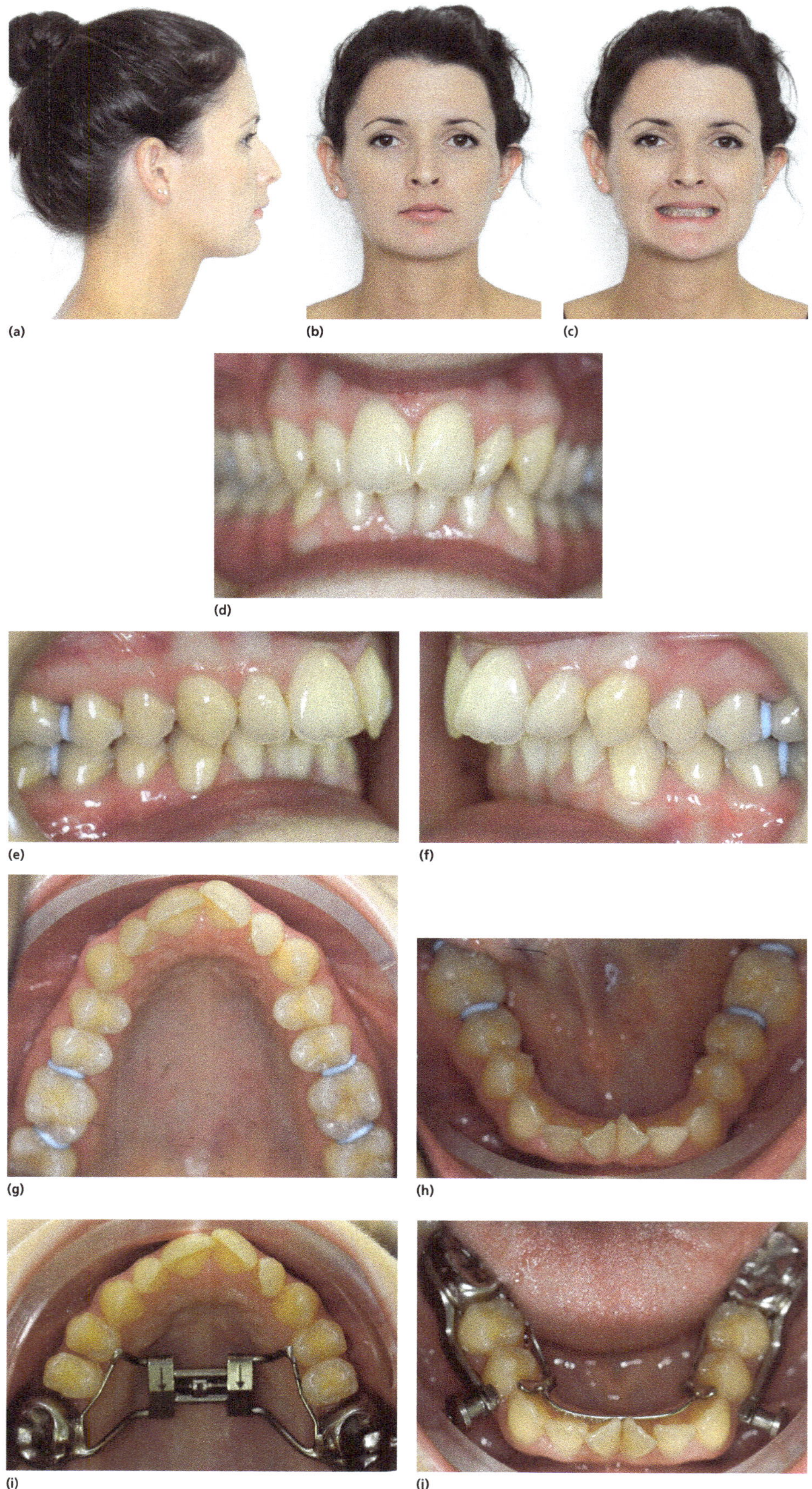

Figure 6.5 Herbst and Invisalign case. An adult female presented with a Class II division 2 malocclusion on a skeletal II pattern (a–h). A cast Herbst appliance was fitted with maxillary expansion (i, j). The appliance was in place for 9 months leading to over-correction of the Class II malocclusion with upper arch spacing (k–r). Thereafter, a clear aligner system (Invisalign™) was used to address some Class II occlusal relapse (s, t) and to detail the occlusion (u–ab).

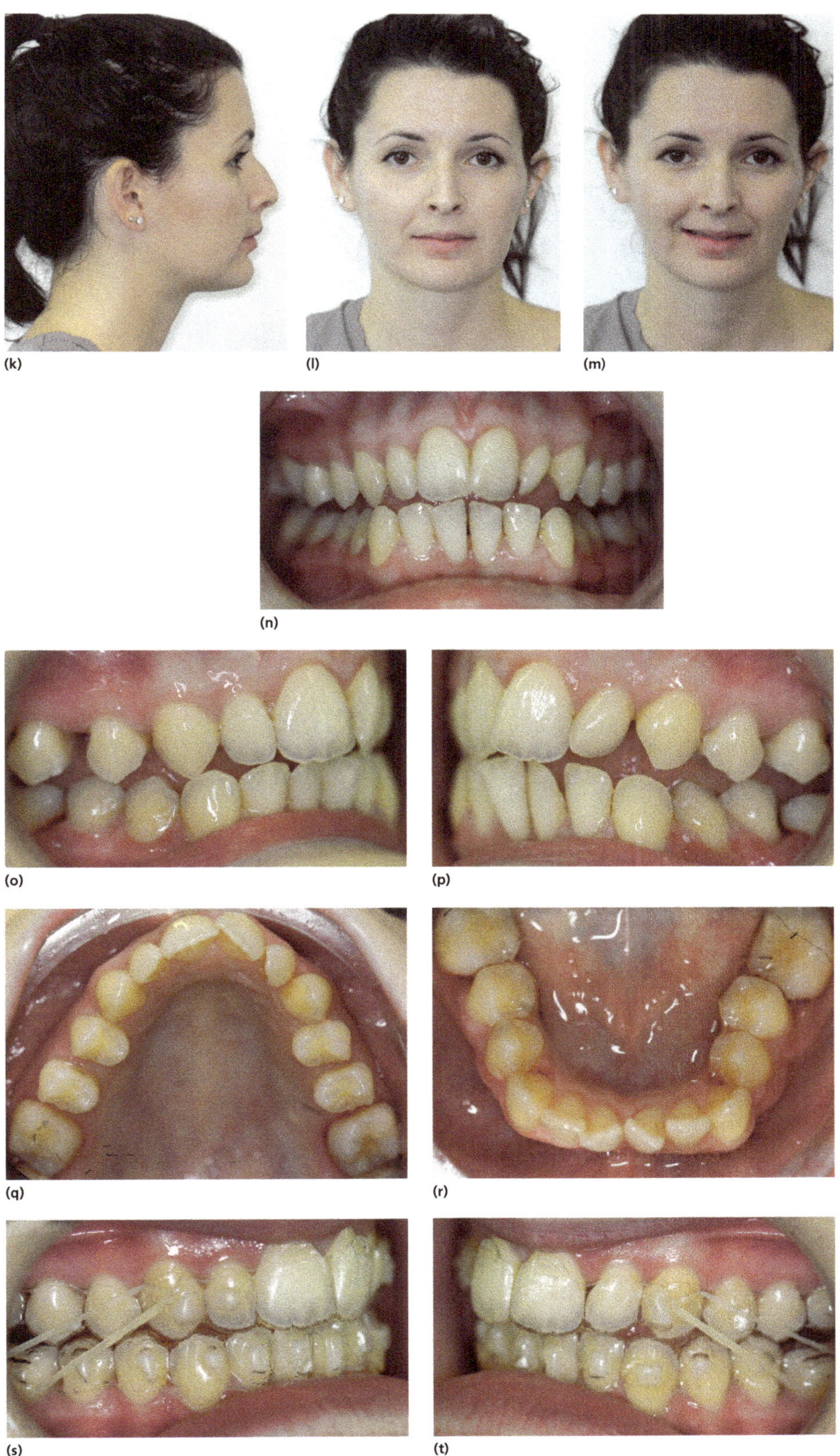

Figure 6.5 (*Continued*)

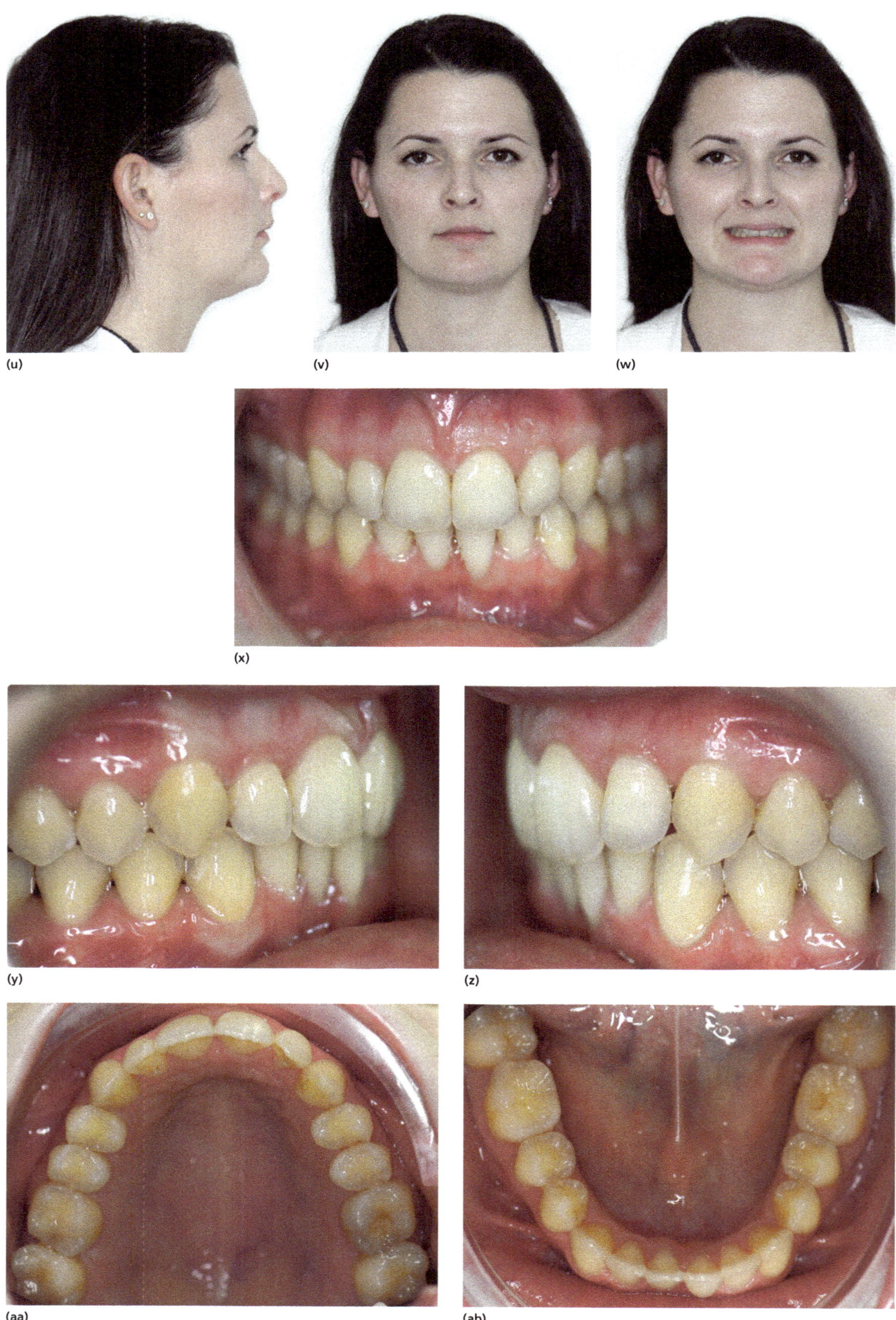

Figure 6.5 (*Continued*)

this proclination may dissipate over time as the incisors become upright. In a retrospective study of matched cases to evaluate the soft tissue profile silhouettes when treated with a Herbst or headgear, both followed by pre-adjusted Edgewise appliances, Herbst and headgear produced similar improvements in the soft tissue profile.[47] However, despite matching, there were some problems in that the pre-treatment profiles were rated less attractive in the headgear group than in the Herbst group.

Mandibular Anterior Repositioning Appliance (MARA)

Similar to the crowned cantilevered Herbst, the MARA involves crowns fitted to both upper and lower first molar teeth, with a lingual arch soldered to the lower crowns. An inclined plane is included to produce interference on closing, resulting in protrusion of the mandible. In view of this design, it can be used in concert with fixed Edgewise appliances.

In a study evaluating 30 selected pre-adolescent patients treated with the MARA over an average of 10.7 months, a 5.8 mm molar discrepancy was corrected by 47% skeletal and 53% dental change.[48] The skeletal change was purely in the mandible (no headgear effect), whereas most of the dental change resulted in maxillary molar distalization. Another retrospective study involved comparison of 4 groups of 20 consecutive patients treated with a Bionator, Herbst, Twin Block or MARA.[49] Although the initial chronological mean ages differed (10.6, 12.2, 10.9 and 11.1 years, respectively), the subjects were matched for growth stages using the cervical vertebral maturation technique. In contrast to the previous study, the MARA as well as the Herbst restricted maxillary growth (headgear effect). The average treatment times from the start of functional appliance therapy to the completion of comprehensive pre-adjusted Edgewise appliance therapy were 49 months for the Bionator, 41.6 months for the Herbst, 41.6 months for the Twin Block and 43.7 months for the MARA.[50] When examining 23 consecutively treated MARA subjects, again a headgear effect was noted along with mandibular elongation.[51]

A further study evaluating the effect of treatment timing examined pre-pubertal, peak pubertal and post-pubertal subjects undergoing MARA treatment in conjunction with fixed appliances.[52] The authors concluded that the ideal timing for treatment was during the pubertal growth peak as assessed by the cervical vertebral maturation (CVM), as mandibular length gains were larger (1.4–1.5 mm greater increase in Co-Gn than the other treatment groups) and dental compensations were lower. From a different perspective, in terms of the rate of molar correction, the peak pubertal group was least efficient at 1.26 mm/year versus 1.52 mm/year and 1.45 mm/year for the pre- and post-pubertal groups, respectively, although between-group differences were minor.

In an unpublished thesis comparing the MARA appliance with Forsus, both were effective in Class II correction.[53] However, the effects were different, as the Forsus had a greater restraint on the maxilla and resulted in more lower incisor proclination, while the MARA produced greater forward displacement of the mandible. The treatment period was 7 months greater with the MARA followed by pre-adjusted Edgewise appliances (33 months) compared with the Forsus which was used simultaneously with pre-adjusted Edgewise appliances (26 months). Similarly, a longer total treatment time (39.6 months) was found with the MARA when compared with the Herbst-like AdvancSync™ appliance (27.6 months).[54]

Both the MARA and the Herbst can be used simultaneously with pre-adjusted Edgewise appliances; however, when the appliance is removed some levelling of the molars and premolars may be required, necessitating a return to more flexible archwires, thereby potentially extending the overall treatment time. In terms of preferred fixed functional appliance, given that there appears to be minimal difference in the dento-skeletal effects related to the various appliances, the relative effectiveness in terms of time, cost and breakage rates in addition to patient comfort needs to be considered.

Comparison of fixed functional appliances

The research comparing fixed with removable functional appliances has been predominantly observational in nature. For example, in a retrospective study comparing the Herbst with the Twin Block in the correction of Class II malocclusion, only minor differences were detected in terms of treatment and post-treatment cephalometric effects.[55] An RCT comparing the Twin Block with the Herbst revealed no differences in skeletal and dental changes between the appliances.[2] However, Twin Block subjects were 2.4 times more likely not to complete the first phase of functional appliance therapy than the Herbst subjects. This study was undertaken in a more mature group of subjects (mean age = 12.5 years) and the results may not apply to younger subjects; patients aged 12.3 years or less have been shown to be three times more likely to complete Twin Block treatment than older patients.[11] Although the functional appliance phase of treatment was shorter with the Herbst by 1.5–2.2 months, there was no significant difference in the overall treatment time as the second phase in the Herbst group was longer, possibly due to greater bite settling having already occurred in the Twin Block group because of block trimming. However, the breakage rate of the cast Co-Cr Herbst was higher and the repair time was considerable (~3 more appointments). Alternative designs such as those using crowns on the lower premolars or cantilevered off the lower molars may have been associated with fewer breakages, but this has not yet been considered in a randomized controlled trial.

In a retrospective study comparing the activator appliance with the Herbst, the Herbst advanced the chin more in a shorter period of time (0.6 years vs 2.6 years). A review of functional appliances concluded that the Herbst was slightly more efficient in terms of the rate of mandibular length change (Co-Gn or Co-Pg; 0.28 mm per month) than the Twin Block (0.23 mm per month).[56] The Bionator (0.17 mm per month) and activator (0.12 mm per month) were less efficient again and the FR2 the least efficient (0.09 mm per month) in terms of the rate of change. There was a slight anterior mandibular rotation in the activator group, whereas the Herbst group demonstrated a slight posterior rotation. However, the age groups differed significantly, so the conclusions should be considered with some caution due to the quality of the primary studies assessed; stability of the change was also not assessed.

In a comparison of headgear and Herbst appliances both followed by pre-adjusted Edgewise appliances,[34] the occlusal success rate was 93% in both groups. However, the Herbst followed by pre-adjusted Edgewise appliance groups demonstrated greater advancement of the soft (1.8 mm) and hard (1.5 mm) tissue chin than the headgear and fixed pre-adjusted Edgewise group. The study was potentially biased by patients being able to choose their preferred treatment protocol. It would be interesting to see whether these changes would be maintained over the long term, as RCTs involving removable functional appliances suggest that the changes tend to dissipate.[3, 4] One such study comparing Herbst with Begg treatment[57] found that initially the Herbst provided a better skeletal change than the Begg with elastics (2 mm), but that the Begg group demonstrated a 2 mm greater reduction in overjet, mainly due to dental movements. The contribution of skeletal change to overjet reduction in the Herbst group was 51%, while it was only 4% in the Begg group. Although there was this initial difference in favour of the Herbst, it was not preserved 5–8 years later.[57] Similar findings of relatively stable occlusal change but hard tissue change towards baseline after Herbst treatment have been reported by others.[16, 38, 58]

Summary

As with removable functional appliances, although initial skeletal changes seem quite favourable with the Herbst appliance, they tend to diminish over time, leaving a mainly dentoalveolar change in the long term. Indeed, although the Herbst appliance has been used for larger overjet corrections of ~11 mm,[12] much of this improvement is attributable to dental change, to which lower incisor advancement is a major contributor. In view of equivocal research findings in terms of the relative merits of step-wise advancement over maximal advancement with the Herbst and other appliances and an absence of data on patient comfort, currently either approach could be justified. Further good-quality studies are required to assess the effect of lower incisor proclination and the risk of gingival recession, particularly in those patients with a thin gingival tissue biotype or a hyperdivergent facial type.

References

1. Isaacson KG, Reed RT, Stephens CD. The role of functional appliances. In: Isaacson KG, Reed RT, Stephens CD, eds, Functional orthodontic appliances. Oxford: Blackwell Scientific; 1990: 1.
2. O'Brien K, Wright J, Conboy F, Sanjie Y, Mandall N et al. Effectiveness of treatment for Class II malocclusion with the Herbst or twin-block appliances: A randomized, controlled trial. Am J Orthod Dentofacial Orthop. 2003; 124: 128–37.
3. O'Brien K, Wright J, Conboy F, Sanjie Y, Mandall N, et al. Effectiveness of early orthodontic treatment with the Twin-block appliance: A multicenter, randomized, controlled trial. Part 1: dental and skeletal effects. Am J Orthod Dentofacial Orthop. 2003: 124: 234–43.
4. Tulloch JF, Phillips C, Koch G, Proffit WR. The effect of early intervention on skeletal pattern in Class II malocclusion: A randomized clinical trial. Am J Orthod Dentofacial Orthop. 1997; 111: 391–400.
5. Pancherz H. The nature of Class II relapse after Herbst appliance treatment: A cephalometric long-term investigation. Am J Orthod Dentofac Orthop. 1991; 100: 220–33.
6. Pancherz H. Treatment of Class II malocclusions by jumping the bite with the Herbst appliance: A cephalometric investigation. Am J Orthod. 1979; 76: 423–42.
7. Pancherz H. The mechanism of Class II correction in Herbst appliance treatment: A cephalometric investigation. Am J Orthod. 1982; 82: 104–13.
8. Du X, Hägg U, Rabie ABM. Effects of headgear Herbst and mandibular step-by-step advancement versus conventional Herbst appliance and maximal jumping of the mandible. Eur J Orthod. 2002; 24: 167–74.
9. Hägg U, Du X, Rabie ABM. Initial and late treatment effects of headgear-Herbst appliance with mandibular step-by-step advancement. Am J Orthod Dentofac Orthop. 2002; 122: 477–85.
10. Purkayastha S, Rabie AB, Wong R. Treatment of skeletal Class II malocclusion in adults: Stepwise vs single-step advancement with the Herbst appliance. World J Orthod. 2008; 9: 233–43.
11. Banks P, Wright J, O'Brien K. Incremental versus maximum bite advancement during Twin-block therapy: A randomized controlled clinical trial. Am J Orthod Dentofac Orthop. 2004; 126: 583–8.
12. Martin J, Pancherz H. Mandibular incisor position changes in relation to amount of bite jumping during Herbst/multibracket appliance treatment: A radiographic-cephalometric study. Am J Orthod Dentofac Orthop. 2009; 136: 44–51.
13. VanLaecken R, Martin CA, Dischinger T, Razmus T, Ngan P. Treatment effects of the Edgewise Herbst appliance: A cephalometric and tomographic investigation. Am J Orthod Dentofac Orthop. 2006; 130: 582–93.
14. Pancherz H, Anehus-Pancherz M. The headgear effect of the Herbst appliance: A long-term cephalometric study. Am J Orthod Dentofac Orthop. 1993; 103: 510–20.
15. Wieslander L. Long-term effect of treatment with the headgear-Herbst appliance in the early mixed dentition. Stability or relapse? Am J Orthod Dentofac Orthop. 1993; 104: 319–29.
16. Wigal TG, Dischinger T, Martin C, Razmus T, Gunel E, Ngan P. Stability of Class II treatment with an Edgewise crowned Herbst appliance in the early mixed dentition: Skeletal and dental changes. Am J Orthod Dentofac Orthop. 2011; 140: 210–23.

17. Barnett GA, Higgins DW, Major PW, Flores-Mir C. Immediate skeletal and dentoalveolar effects of the crown- or banded type Herbst appliance on Class II division 1 malocclusion: A systematic review. Angle Orthod. 2008; 78: 361–9.
18. Weschler D, Pancherz H. Efficiency of three mandibular anchorage forms in Herbst treatment: A cephalometric investigation. Angle Orthod. 2004; 75: 23–7.
19. Hansen K, Koutsanas TG, Pancherz H. Long-term effects of Herbst treatment on the mandibular incisor segment: A cephalometric and biometric investigation. Am J Orthod. Dentofac Orthop. 1991; 112: 92–103.
20. Wehrbein H, Bauer W, Diedrich P. Mandibular incisors, alveolar bone, and symphysis after orthodontic treatment: A retrospective study. Am J Orthod Dentofac Orthop. 1996; 110: 239–46.
21. Ruf S, Hansen K, Pancherz H. Does orthodontic proclination of lower incisors in children and adolescents cause gingival recession? Am J Orthod Dentofac Orthop. 1998; 114: 100–6.
22. Årtun J, Grobéty D. Periodontal status of mandibular incisors after pronounced orthodontic advancement during adolescence: A follow-up evaluation. Am J Orthod Dentofac Orthop. 2001; 119: 2–10.
23. Melsen B, Allais D. Factors of importance for the development of dehiscences during labial movement of mandibular incisors: A retrospective study of adult orthodontic patients. Am J Orthod Dentofac Orthop. 2005; 127: 552–61.
24. Yared K, Zenobio EG, Pacheco W. Periodontal status of mandibular central incisors after orthodontic proclination in adults. Am J Orthod Dentofac Orthop. 2006; 130: 6.e1–e8.
25. Aziz T, Flores-Mir C. A systematic review of the association between appliance-induced labial movement of mandibular incisors and gingival recession. Aus Orthod J. 2011; 27: 33–9.
26. JossVassalli I, Grebenstein C, Topouzelis N, Sculean A, Katsaros C. Orthodontic therapy and gingival recession: A systematic review. Orth Craniofac Res. 2010; 13: 127–41.
27. Handelman C. The anterior alveolus: Its importance in limiting orthodontic treatment and its influence on the occurrence of iatrogenic sequelae. Angle Orthod. 1996; 66: 95–109.
28. Enhos S, Uysal T, Yagci A, Veli I, Ucar FI, Ozer T. Dehiscence and fenestration in patients with different vertical growth patterns assessed with cone-beam computed tomography. Angle Orthod. 2012; 82: 868–74.
29. Franchi L, Baccetti T. Prediction of individual mandibular changes induced by functional jaw orthopedics followed by fixed appliances in Class II patients. Angle Orthod. 2006; 76: 950–54.
30. Marsico E, Gatto E, Burrascano M, Matarese G, Cordasco G. Effectiveness of orthodontic treatment with functional appliances on mandibular growth in the short term. Am J Orthod Dentofac Orthop. 2011; 139: 24–36.
31. Tulley, W. The scope and limitations of treatment with the activator. Am J Orthod. 1972; 61: 562–77.
32. Ruf S, Pancherz, H. The mechanism of Class II correction during herbst therapy in relation to the vertical jaw base relationship: A cephalometric roentgenographic study. Angle Orthod. 1997; 67: 271–6.
33. Sfondrini MF, Cacciafesta V, Sfondrini G. Upper molar distalization: A critical analysis. Orth Craniofac Res. 2002; 5: 114–26.
34. Baccetti T, Franchi L, Stahl F. Comparison of 2 comprehensive Class II treatment protocols including the bonded Herbst and headgear appliances: A double-blind study of consecutively treated patients at puberty. Am J Orthod Dentofac Orthop. 2009; 135: 698–e1.
35. McSherry P, Bradley H. Class II correction-reducing patient compliance: A review of the available techniques. J Orthod. 2000; 27: 219–25.
36. Schiavon R, Grenga V, Macri V. Treatment of Class II high angle malocclusions with the Herbst appliance: A cephalometric investigation. Am J Orthod Dentofac Orthop. 1992; 102: 393–409.
37. Ruf S, Pancherz H. The effect of Herbst appliance treatment on the mandibular plane angle: A cephalometric roentgenographic study. Am J Orthod Dentofac Orthop. 1996; 110: 225–9.
38. Windmiller E. The acrylic-splint Herbst appliance: A cephalometric evaluation. Am J Orthod Dentofac Orthop. 1993; 104: 73–84.
39. Wieslander L. Intensive treatment of severe Class II malocclusions with a headgear-Herbst appliance in the early mixed dentition. Am J Orthod. 1984; 86: 1–13.
40. Konik M, Pancherz H, Hansen K. The mechanism of Class II correction in late Herbst treatment. Am J Orthod Dentofac Orthop. 1997; 112: 87–91.
41. von Bremen J, Pancherz H. Efficiency of early and late Class II Division 1 treatment. Am J Orthod Dentofac Orthop. 2002; 121: 31–7.
42. von Bremen J, Bock N, Ruf S. Is Herbst-multibracket appliance treatment more efficient in adolescents than in adults? A dental cast study. Angle Orthod. 2009; 79: 173–7.
43. Ruf S, Pancherz H. Orthognathic surgery and dentofacial orthopedics in adult Class II Division 1 treatment: Mandibular sagittal split osteotomy versus Herbst appliance. Am J Orthod Dentofac Orthop. 2004; 126: 140–52.
44. Chaiyongsirisern A, Rabie AB, Wong RWK. Stepwise advancement Herbst appliance versus mandibular sagittal split osteotomy: Treatment effects and long-term stability of adult Class II patients. Angle Orthod. 2009; 79: 1084–94.
45. Flores-Mir C, Major MP, Major PW. Soft tissue changes with fixed functional appliances in Class II division 1: A systematic review. Angle Orthod. 2006; 76: 712–20.
46. Baysal A, Uysal T. Soft tissue effects of Twin Block and Herbst appliances in patients with Class II division 1 mandibular retrognathy. Eur J Orthod. 2013; 35: 71–81.
47. Baysal A, Uysal T. Dentoskeletal effects of Twin Block and Herbst appliances in patients with Class II division 1 mandibular retrognathy. Eur J Orthod. 2014; 36: 164–72.
48. Sloss EA, Southard KA, Qian F, Stock SE, Mann KR et al. Comparison of soft-tissue profiles after treatment with headgear or Herbst appliance. Am J Orthod Dentofac Orthop. 2008; 133: 509–14.
49. Pangrazio-Kulbersh V, Berger JL, Chermak DS, Kaczynski R, Simon ES, Haerian A. Treatment effects of the mandibular anterior repositioning appliance on patients with Class II malocclusion. Am J Orthod Dentofac Orthop. 2003; 123: 286–95.
50. Siara-Olds N, Pangrazio-Kulbersh V, Berger J, Bayirli B. Long-term dentoskeletal changes with the Bionator, Herbst, Twin Block, and MARA functional appliances. Angle Orthod. 2010; 80: 18–29.
51. Ghislanzoni LTH, Toll DE, Defraia E, Baccetti T, Franchi L. Treatment and posttreatment outcomes induced by the Mandibular Advancement Repositioning Appliance: A controlled clinical study. Angle Orthod. 2011; 81: 684–91.

52. Ghislanzoni L, Baccetti T, Toll D, Defraia E, McNamara JA, Franchi L. Treatment timing of MARA and fixed appliance therapy of Class II malocclusion. Eur J Orthod. 2013; 35: 394–400.
53. Azizollahi S. Comparison of skeletal and dentoalveolar effects of the Forsus and MARA in treatment of Class II malocclusions. Doctoral dissertation, Saint Louis University, 2012.
54. Al-Jewair TS, Preston CB, Moll EM, Dischinger T. A comparison of the MARA and the AdvanSync functional appliances in the treatment of Class II malocclusion. Angle Orthod. 2012; 82: 907–14.
55. Schaefer AT, McNamara JA, Franchi L, Baccetti T. A cephalometric comparison of treatment with the Twin-block and stainless steel crown Herbst appliances followed by fixed appliance therapy. Am J Orthod Dentofac Orthop. 2004; 126: 7–15.
56. Cozza P, Baccetti T, Franchi L, De Toffol L, McNamara JA. Mandibular changes produced by functional appliances in Class II malocclusion: A systematic review. Am J Orthod Dentofac Orthop. 2006; 129: 599.e1–e12.
57. Nelson B, Hägg U, Hansen K, Bendeus M. A long-term follow-up study of Class II malocclusion correction after treatment with Class II elastics or fixed functional appliances. Am J Orthod Dentofac Orthop. 2007; 132: 499–503.
58. Bock N, Ruf S. Dentoskeletal changes in adult Class II division 1 Herbst treatment: How much is left after the retention period? Eur J Orthod. 2012; 34: 747–53.

CHAPTER 7

Flexible fixed functional appliances

Peter Miles

The most popular functional appliance in the United States is the Herbst appliance (crown type), used by 19.2% of orthodontists, followed by the Forsus at 17.4%.[1] However, preferences vary between countries, with a British survey[2] and an Australian survey[3] indicating that the Twin Block is the most commonly used functional appliance. In Australia the Twin Block is currently used by 70% of orthodontists, with spring type correctors (which include the Forsus, Jasper Jumper etc.) being the next most popular at 61%.

Fixed or non-compliance Class II correctors can be grouped into two categories:

- 'Rigid' fixed functional appliances (e.g. Herbst, MARA), meaning those that posture the mandible into one fixed position without any flexibility in the system, often but not exclusively used prior to comprehensive pre-adjusted Edgewise appliances in a two-phase approach. These have been discussed in Chapter 6.
- 'Flexible' fixed functional appliances (e.g. Forsus FRD, Jasper Jumper), encompassing those that have a component such as a spring allowing some give in the system when posturing the mandible forward, usually used concomitantly with fixed pre-adjusted Edgewise appliances in one comprehensive phase of treatment.

With prospective clinical trials of removable functional appliances finding no long-term benefit in terms of the final clinical result and longer treatment times with two-phase or a single comprehensive phase of treatment,[4,5] there is an argument for comprehensive pre-adjusted Edgewise appliances in parallel with the functional phase to improve efficiency in the majority of cases. Consequently, the alignment and the molar correction can be addressed simultaneously. Obviously there are exceptions where psychosocial or other reasons may prevail, indicating an early phase of treatment. However, when employing a single comprehensive phase of treatment, molar and overjet correction can be undertaken in a variety of ways, ranging from use of elastics and headgear to some form of flexible fixed functional appliance, or indeed a combination of these approaches.

Jasper Jumper

The eponymous Jasper Jumper was developed in 1987 by J.J. Jasper and was popularized thereafter.[6] It was the first flexible fixed functional appliance to apply a distal and intrusive force to the maxillary molars along with a mesial and intrusive force on the lower incisors. It consists of vinyl-coated springs attached to the maxillary molar headgear tubes and attached either directly to the lower archwire just distal to the canines, or to a sectional bypass wire from an auxiliary tube on the lower molar to just distal to the lower canine. As it applies a mesial force to the lower anteriors, it is essential that the lower wire is cinched or tied back to prevent excessive proclination of the lower incisors. There has also been a recommendation to use or add lingual root torque in the lower anteriors to enhance anchorage and reduce flaring, although the effect of this approach has not been assessed in a clinical trial.

In a study comparing the Jasper Jumper with the Herren activator and a headgear–activator combination, the Jasper Jumper consistently resulted in correction of the occlusion, while activator use resulted in a Class I occlusion in 43% of cases. However, as this was a non-randomized study, subjects were not matched for occlusion type or stage of dental development at the outset. The Jasper Jumper led to the greatest skeletal contribution to overjet correction (48%) but the least skeletal contribution to molar correction (38%).[7] As a proportion of the overall change, the amount of dental molar correction was lower with the Jasper Jumper but the magnitude was slightly (0.3 mm) greater in the Jasper Jumper group, as the appliance resulted in a bigger overall change. However, the difference was not found to be clinically significant. The Jasper Jumper subjects also demonstrated a marked intrusion of the lower incisors. As no brackets were placed on the lower canines and premolars, the 0.017 inch × 0.025 inch stainless steel archwires (0.018 inch slot brackets) effectively acted as utility arches or 2 × 4 appliances, potentially leading to a greater intrusive effect on the lower incisors than would have been the case with a fully bonded arch.

Orthodontic Functional Appliances: Theory and Practice, First Edition. Padhraig Fleming and Robert Lee.

Another study evaluated 31 consecutive cases (mean age = 12.9 years) from three orthodontic practices using 0.018 inch slot brackets apparently bonded to all teeth, although the Jasper Jumper was attached to the sectional bypass wire design.[8] The authors only assessed the effect of the Jasper Jumper; levelling and alignment had already taken place prior to the initial cephalogram and the second radiograph was taken on removal of the Jasper Jumper but before finishing/detailing. The Jasper Jumper phase took an average of 4.8 months. Although there was some maxillary restraint/headgear effect, the main effects of the appliance during this active phase were dental movements, with significant maxillary molar and incisor distal tipping and mesial bodily movement and tipping of the lower molars, with associated lower incisor tipping of 6.4 degrees. An intrusive effect was also noted on the upper molars and lower incisors.

A further study has evaluated the effects of the Jasper Jumper during the entire course of treatment involving full pre-adjusted Edgewise appliances in addition.[9] The same distalization effects were noted on the upper incisors and molars as well as some headgear effect. In the lower arch, mesialization of the lower molars and an 8.6-degree proclination of the lower incisors were noted, with no growth effect. After the subsequent fixed phase, molar tipping and maxillary incisor retroclination were corrected, although the lower incisors remained proclined by 6.5 degrees. A later study evaluating the Jasper Jumper in comparison to a headgear group used simultaneously with a fully bonded 0.022 inch pre-adjusted Edgewise appliance found that maxillary growth was restricted in the headgear group, while the Jasper Jumper resulted in labial tipping and protrusion of the lower incisors, with a modest 1–1.5 mm mandibular advancement.[10] Both appliances produced satisfactory Class II correction. A more recent study[11] evaluated the effects of the Jasper Jumper during treatment as well as the overall effect of treatment in 24 subjects (average age = 12.6 years). Again, the Jasper Jumper demonstrated mesial movement of the lower molars and 5-degree flaring with intrusion of the lower incisors. The correction was then held during the remainder of treatment with Class II elastics, during which time increases in overbite and overjet were recorded as the lower incisors uprighted and extruded.

Forsus

The original Forsus was developed by Bill Vogt in 2001 and was attached to the maxillary molar tubes and lower archwire, similar to the Jasper Jumper but consisting of a Nitinol flat spring or ribbon. When comparing the Jasper Jumper with the Forsus flat spring, they were found to yield similar results over just over 5 months.[12] Both appliances resulted in some accelerated mandibular growth with an inhibition of maxillary growth, but the major changes in attaining a Class I molar relationship were attributed to significant incisor and molar movements. When used in 0.018 inch Edgewise brackets with 0.017 inch × 0.025 inch stainless steel wires, both appliances expanded the dental arches despite adding buccal root torque to the posterior of the maxillary archwire. The authors concluded that if this expansion effect is not desired, a trans-palatal arch or other measure should be considered.

The later design of the Forsus FRD (fatigue resistant device) consists of an inter-maxillary push spring attached to the maxillary molar headgear tube and a push rod attached distal to the lower canine or first premolar, in conjunction with pre-adjusted Edgewise appliances (Figures 7.1 and 7.2).[13] Alternatively, the spring can be attached to a sectional bypass wire, as is the case with the Jasper Jumper. Typically, the appliances are fitted to working steel archwires following initial alignment. Elastomeric chain may be added to the upper appliance to prevent space opening in the maxillary arch, as these springs tend to be potent in terms of molar distalization. Consequently, upper arch distal movement can be effected *en masse*. The maxillary second molars should be incorporated in the fixed appliance to reduce buccal flaring of the maxillary first molars. Alternatively, a trans-palatal arch may also be used.

In a retrospective study comparing the use of the Forsus FRD with Class II elastics, 34 non-extraction Forsus patients were matched for gender, age and pre-treatment skeletal relationships with patients treated non-extraction with elastics.[14] Class II elastics and the Forsus FRD achieved similar reductions in overjet (2.8 mm and 3.2 mm, respectively), molar correction (2.4 mm and 3.2 mm) and skeletal change (2.3 mm and 2.6 mm) during correction of the Class II malocclusion (Table 7.1). There were no significant differences between the two methods, apart from a greater lower molar mesial movement and total molar correction in the Forsus FRD group. The predominant factor contributing to the treatment success in both groups was the greater forward displacement of the mandible. Another study described the effects of the Forsus FRD on 32 consecutive Class II subjects.[15] The Forsus FRD was attached directly to the mandibular archwire (0.019 inch x 0.025 inch stainless steel) and distal to the lower first premolars instead of the canines, and was in place an average of 5.2 months to achieve an edge-to-edge incisor relationship. Similar to the Jasper Jumper, a maxillary restraint or headgear effect was noted in the maxilla, while the effect on the mandible was mainly dento-alveolar, with mesial movement of the lower first molars and incisors with 6.1 degrees of proclination.

When evaluating the Forsus appliance in a group of peak pubertal and late pubertal subjects,[16] no significant difference was noted in the amount of overjet or molar correction, although the peak pubertal group exhibited significantly greater increase in ramal height (Co-Go = 0.9 mm) and mandibular length (Co-Gn = 1.3 mm). However, given the absence of a control group, it is not possible to conclude that this difference is not attributable to normal growth or a transient acceleration in growth. Cephalograms were taken immediately before and after the Forsus was placed and removed, so any subsequent deceleration in the peak pubertal group growth would also not have been recorded.

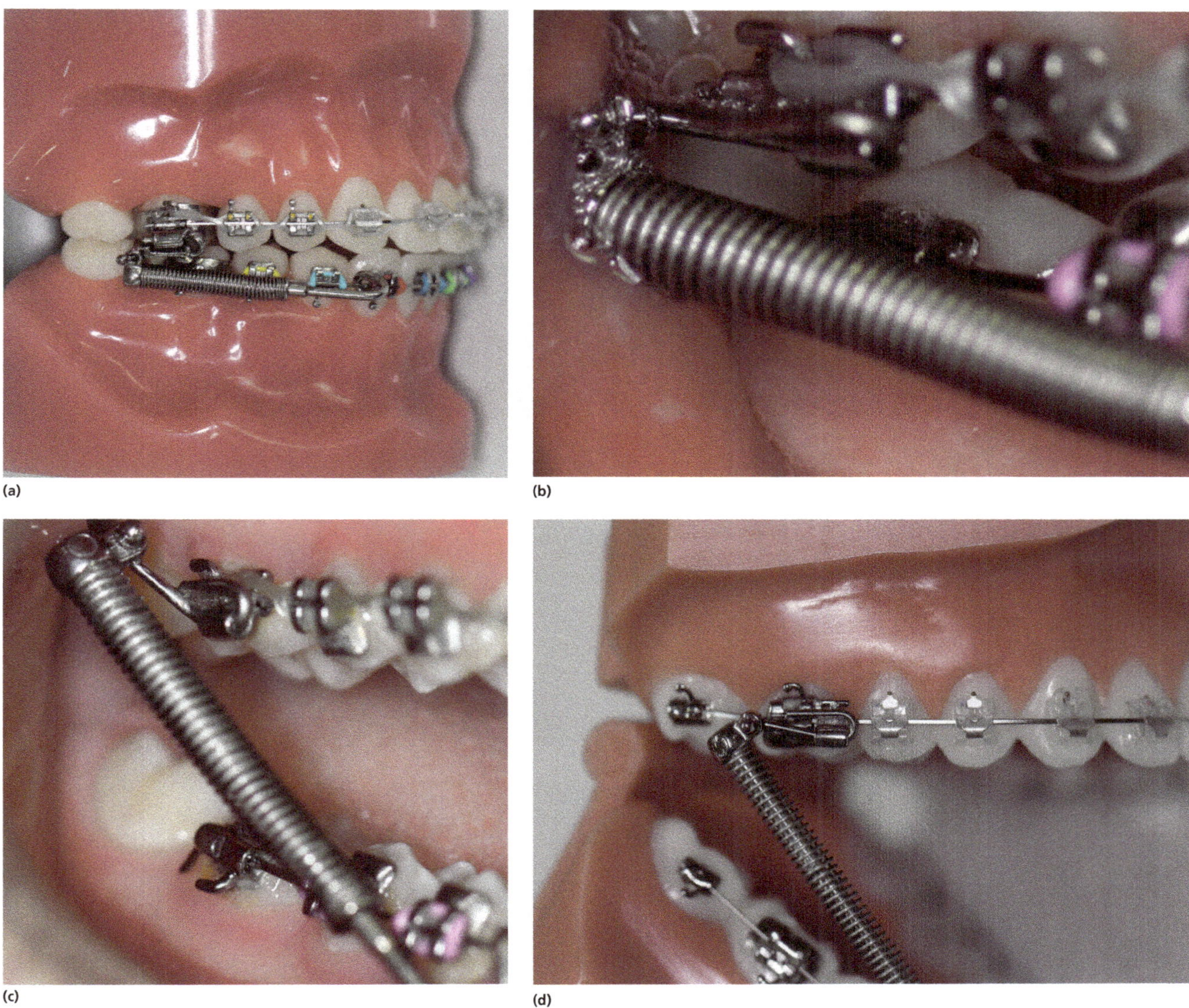

Figure 7.1 The Forsus FRD is attached to the maxillary molar tube and in the lower arch either to a bypass wire or directly to the lower archwire, as pictured. When the patient closes the spring is compressed, but the mandible is not forced forward as with the rigid FFAs, although the patient may posture forward in some cases.

Not surprisingly, the effects of the Jasper Jumper and Forsus FRD are similar and a consistent degree of lower incisor proclination (approximately 6 degrees) has been noted. However, patient comfort and technical problems such as breakages or ulcerations/trauma from the fixed functional appliance (Figure 7.3) and their cost, which may have an impact on a clinician's choice of appliance, are rarely considered within these studies.

Twin Force

A more recent study examined the Twin Force appliance in conjunction with fixed pre-adjusted Edgewise appliances.[17] When used in both pre-pubertal (mean = 12.4 years) and post-pubertal (mean = 13.8 years) subjects as assessed by the cervical vertebral method, there was no difference in the overall dento-skeletal correction achieved, with the overjet correction being approximately 4 mm in both groups. However, the pre-pubertal group had significantly greater skeletal correction than the post-pubertal group, similar to that identified with the Forsus appliance.[16] No difference was found between the groups at the end of treatment. The treatment time was significantly longer in the pre-pubertal group (3.7 years) than the post-pubertal group (2.8 years), which could partly be attributed to time spent waiting for the eruption of permanent teeth. It would seem logical, therefore, that treatment is more efficient when commenced once the permanent teeth have erupted sufficiently to place brackets.

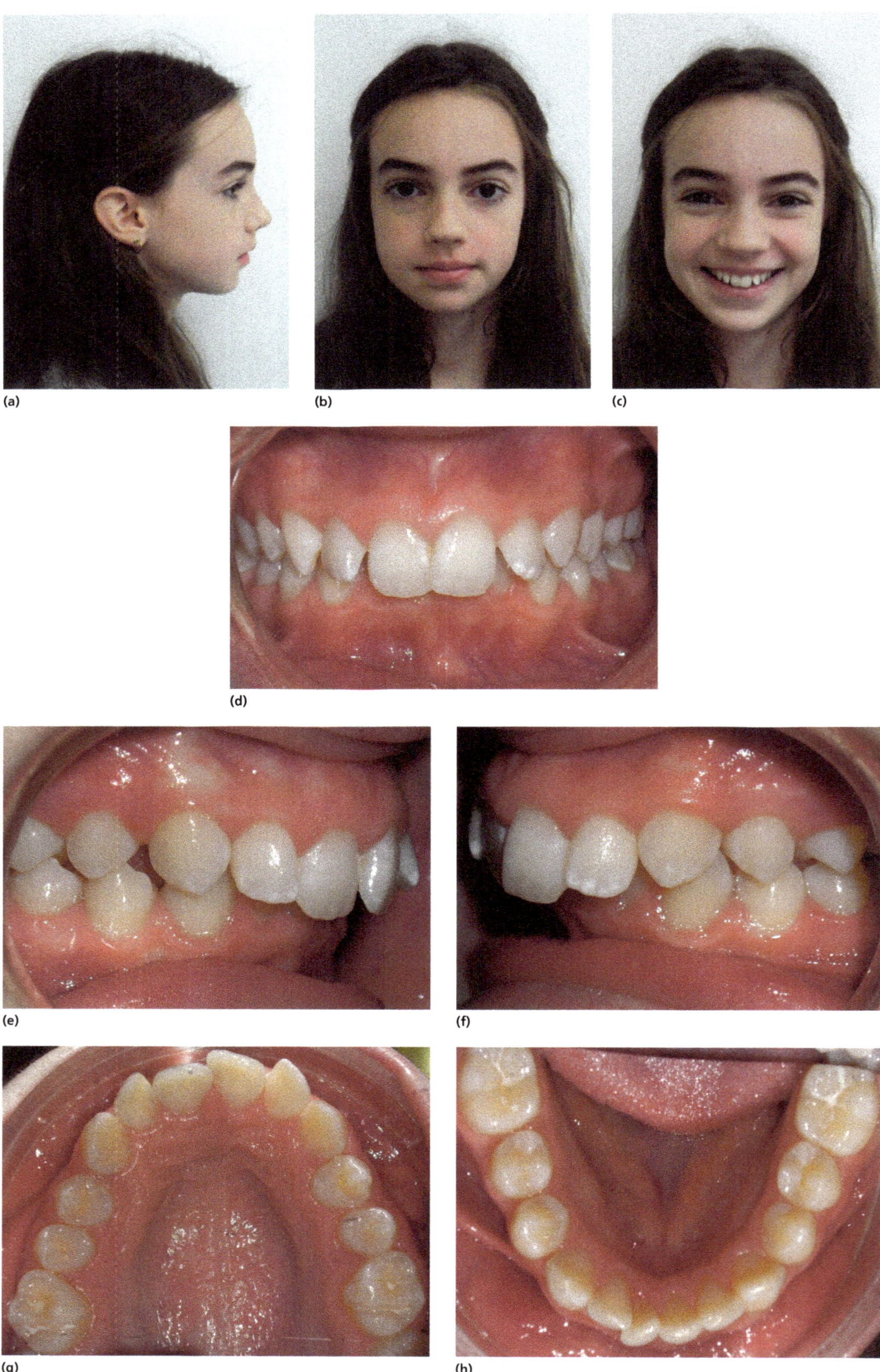

Figure 7.2 This 14-year-old female (a–h) had a ¼ unit Class II relationship on the right and ¾ unit Class II on the left side. She was treated with the Forsus FRD in conjunction with 0.018 inch pre-adjusted Edgewise appliances. The Forsus abutted against the lower canines, so rotational bends were placed to counteract the rotational moment from the rod pressing against them and tied with a stainless steel ligature to reduce the risk of breakage by the Forsus pressing against the tie. No trans-palatal arch was used, as the second molars were included with a 0.017 inch x 0.025 inch stainless steel archwire to limit maxillary posterior buccal rolling and reduce posterior bite opening. Treatment was completed in 19 months with 5 months of Forsus wear, which was more active on the left side due to the requirement for greater correction on that side (i–p).

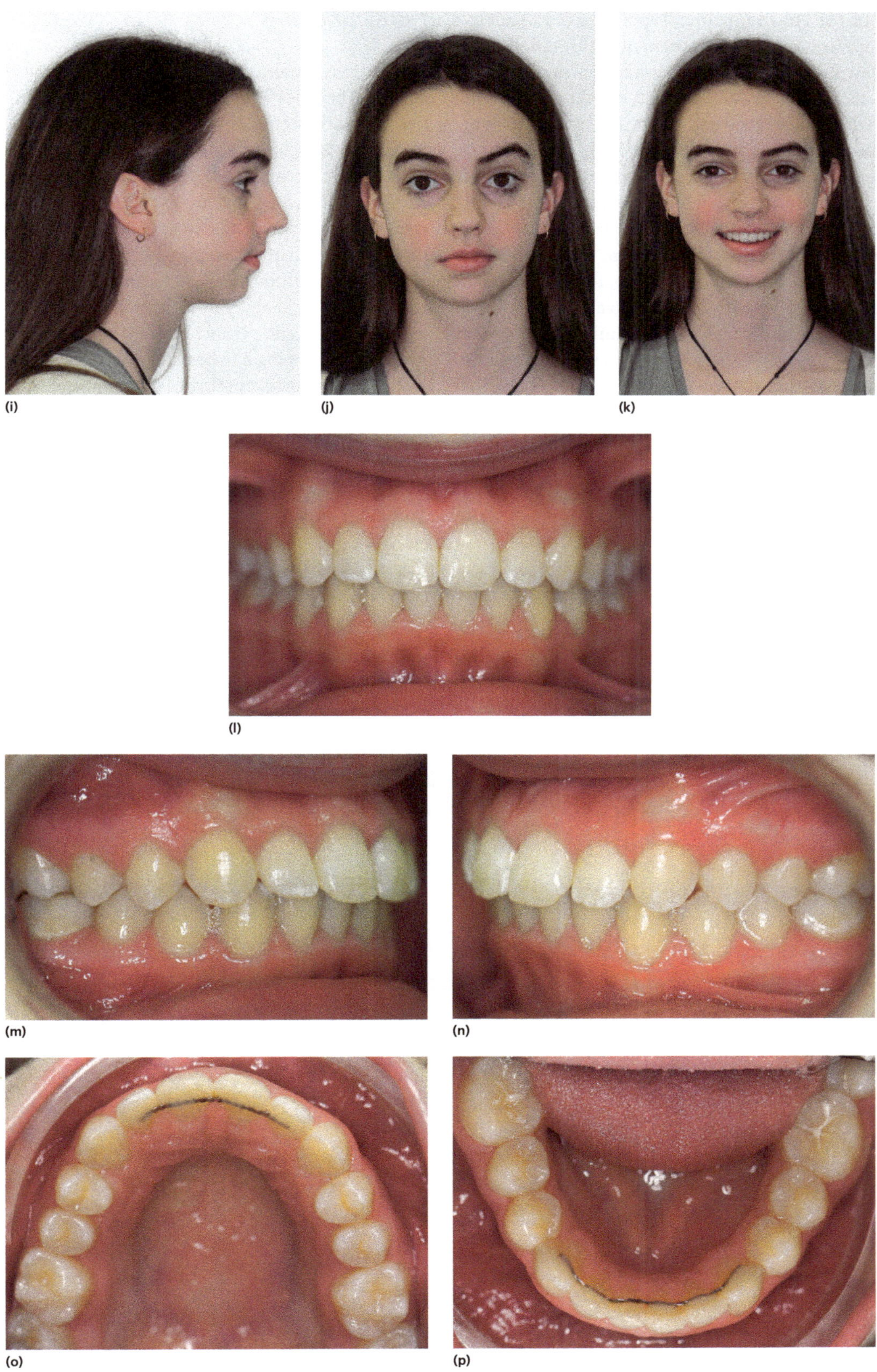

Figure 7.2 (*Continued*)

The mechanics of a fixed functional appliance (FFA) apply a vertical force upwards and distal to the centre of rotation of the maxilla and downwards and anterior to the centre of rotation of the lower arch. This would suggest that canting of the occlusal plane down anteriorly can occur due to the moments being generated. However, in an observational study,[17] despite extrusion of upper and lower molars in both groups, there was no change in the vertical parameters (similar to the Herbst studies) and minimal changes in the palatal and occlusal plane angles, suggesting that mesial movement of the molars maintains the vertical dimension. Observations were again undertaken before and after comprehensive treatment with pre-adjusted Edgewise appliances and not immediately before and after the FFA phase. Therefore, if any palatal or occlusal plane cant occurred due to the FFA, it may have reverted following the appliance's withdrawal. A similar reversion of the occlusal plane was observed once the Herbst appliance was discontinued.[18] Maintenance of the mandibular plane angle has also been observed by others with the Herbst[19, 20] as well as with other FFAs such as the Jasper Jumper[21–23], Forsus[15, 23] and Eureka Spring.[24]

Eureka Spring

DeVincenzo first described the Eureka Spring in 1997.[25] Similar in action to the other flexible FFAs, the Eureka Spring (Eureka Spring Co., San Luis Obispo, CA) is an open-wound coil spring encased in a triple-telescoping plunger assembly with flexible ball-and-socket attachments. In non-compliant subjects during pre-adjusted Edgewise appliance treatment, the Eureka Spring achieved a correction that was 90% dento-alveolar at a rate of molar correction of 0.7 mm/month.[24] Although this study did not report results through to the completion of fixed Edgewise treatment, no change in the vertical dimension including the anterior face height, palatal plane and mandibular plane angle was observed, suggesting it to be neutral vertically like other FFAs.

The molar correction (mm) and appliance efficiency (molar correction per year) are also plotted in Figures 7.4 and 7.5. It can be seen that all the appliances have some effect on molar change, but the least effective was the Twin Force appliance, which also had the longest treatment time.[17] However, there are a number of variables that may influence the outcome in a retrospective study; ideally, more research on the Twin Force is

Table 7.1 A comparison of the effects of various fixed functional appliances in conjunction with comprehensive fixed Edgewise appliances. Studies were excluded if there was a delay in treatment between the fixed functional appliance and comprehensive Edgewise appliances treatment, as this extended the overall observation period. Molar correction and overjet were either measured directly or, if that was not available, the change in relation to a vertical reference line was used.

Appliance reference	Molar correction (mm)	Overjet correction (mm)	Treatment time (years)	Molar correction/ year (mm/yr)
	Jasper Jumper			
Covell et al. 1999[9]	2.8	4.5	2.3	1.22
Oliveira et al. 2007[10]	3.0	3.9	1.95	1.54
Herrera et al. 2011[11]	3.9	3.7	2.15	1.81
	Forsus			
Jones et al. 2008[14]	3.2	3.2	2.7	1.19
Franchi et al. 2011[15]	3.4	5.4	2.4	1.42
Azizollahi 2012[28]	3.8	5.6	2.2	1.73
	MARA			
Azizollahi 2012[28]	3.1	2.6	2.8	1.1
Ghislanzoni et al. 2013[30]	3.5	3.4	2.3	1.52
Pre	2.9	2.9	2.3	1.26
Peak	2.9	2.9	2.0	1.45
Post				
Al-Jewair et al. 2012[29]	3.6	3.1	3.3	1.09
	AdvanSync			
Al-Jewair et al. 2012[29]	3.6	3.4	2.3	1.57
	Herbst			
Franchi et al. 1999[26]	3.7	4.1	2.3	1.61
Schaefer et al. 2004[27]	3.3	3.8	2.3	1.30
	Twin Force			
Chhibber et al. 2013[17]	1.2	4.0	2.8	0.43

required to evaluate this. Apart from this one study, the average molar changes ranged from 2.8 mm to 3.9 mm, equating to a half-unit molar correction. In terms of treatment efficiency measured by the amount of molar change achieved during comprehensive treatment (FFA and pre-adjusted Edgewise appliances), the change in millimetres per year ranged from 1.09 to 1.81, and so the overall molar change, treatment time and efficiency (mm/year) did not seem to be any more or less effective using a continuous two-stage approach with a Herbst[26, 27] or MARA[28] followed immediately by pre-adjusted Edgewise appliances than using a single phase of pre-adjusted Edgewise appliances with a Jasper Jumper, Forsus FRD, Herbst[29] or MARA (Table 7.1).[28, 30] This contrasts with the UNC clinical trial[31] of removable functional appliances and headgear, which found the overall treatment time to be significantly longer with the two-phase approach. One possible explanation is the delay between phases in the UNC trial, so some loss of the molar correction may have occurred that then needed to be recovered later. Another possibility could be related to the shorter treatment times using FFAs (Herbst, MARA) compared with the Bionator removable appliance used in the UNC trial. As mentioned previously, the efficiency (mm/month change) of the Bionator is reported to be less than that of the Herbst.[32]

Another study comparing the MARA, Bionator, Herbst and Twin Block followed by pre-adjusted Edgewise appliances also found treatment involving the Bionator to be slower by approximately 7 months or 17%.[33] However, when comparing the Twin Block with the Herbst appliance in a randomized study with both followed by pre-adjusted Edgewise appliances, it was found that the time saved with the Herbst was mostly lost in the pre-adjusted Edgewise appliance phase of treatment.[5] Although the treatment times and molar effects are similar in Table 7.1 and Figure 7.4, this analysis does not factor in the number of appointments, appointment duration or appliance cost, which would influence the cost effectiveness and ideally would be the subject of future research.

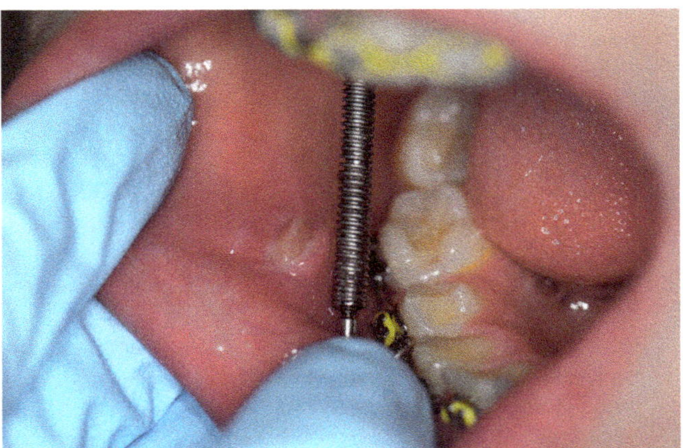

Figure 7.3 An ulcer on the cheek has resulted from the fixed functional appliance. Care kits including ulcer gels and cotton rolls to hold the cheek away from the device help to reduce the incidence of ulcers until the cheek mucosa toughens and the patient adapts to the device. However, once an ulcer has developed, the appliance may need to be removed temporarily to allow resolution.

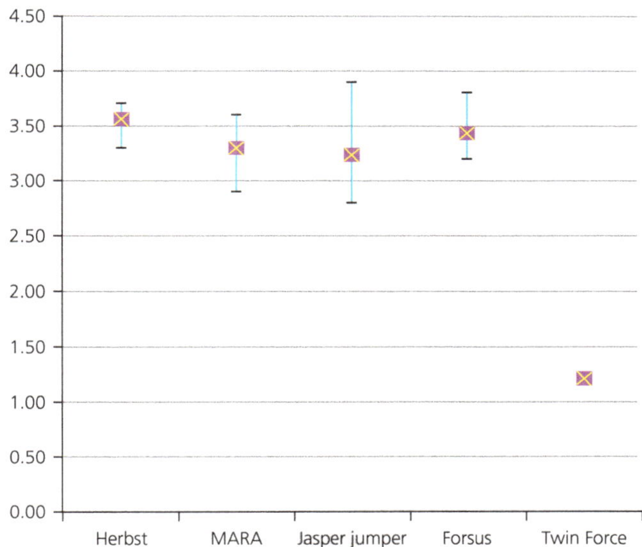

Figure 7.4 For each appliance the molar correction in millimetres was combined from Table 7.1 and the blue line represents the range of reported mean values. The purple square represents the mean molar change of the combined data weighted by the number of subjects in each group.

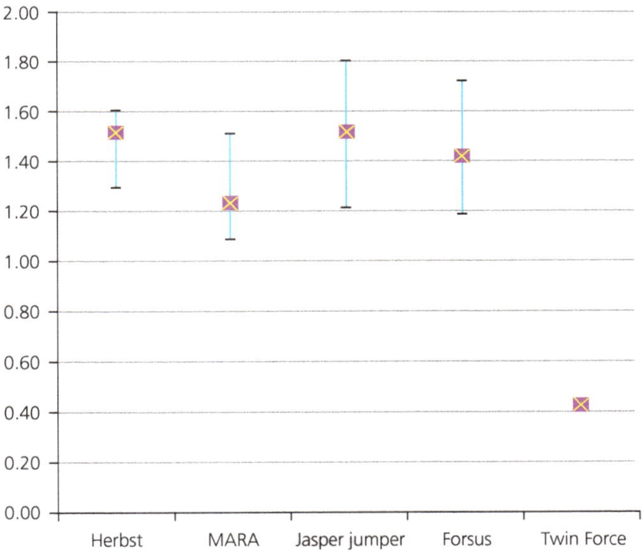

Figure 7.5 The appliance efficiency (molar change in millimetres per year) was combined from Table 7.1, with the blue line representing the range of reported mean values. The purple square represents the mean appliance efficiency of the combined data weighted by the number of subjects in each group.

Summary

Flexible functional appliances or Class II correctors have met with increasing popularity in recent years. They offer a non-compliance alternative to Class II elastics or headgear in the management of Class II malocclusion with fixed appliances. As such they are a useful adjunct, but predominantly result in dento-alveolar change, including lower incisor proclination and distal movement of maxillary molars. There are a number of limitations inherent in much of the research related to these appliances, most of which are retrospective in design, with limited description of inclusion criteria, lack of controls or use of historical control groups among other shortcomings. The current evidence suggests that the comprehensive correction of a Class II malocclusion may be just as efficient in two stages involving a Herbst or MARA appliance when followed immediately by comprehensive pre-adjusted Edgewise appliances as it is in one comprehensive phase of pre-adjusted Edgewise appliances in conjunction with a Forsus FRD or Jasper Jumper. However, prospective clinical trials are required to confirm this.

References

1. Keim RG, Gottlieb EL, Vogels DS III, Vogels PB. 2014 JCO study of orthodontic diagnosis and treatment procedures, Part 1: Results and trends. J Clin Orthod. 2014; 48: 607–30.
2. Chadwick SM, Banks P, Wright JL. The use of myofunctional appliances in the UK: A survey of British orthodontists. Dent Update. 1998; 25: 302–8.
3. Miles, P. 2013 survey of Australian Orthodontists' procedures. Aus Orthod J. 2013; 29: 170–75.
4. Tulloch JF, Phillips C, Koch G, Proffit WR. The effect of early intervention on skeletal pattern in Class II malocclusion: A randomized clinical trial. Am J Orthod Dentofacial Orthop. 1997; 111: 391–400.
5. O'Brien K, Wright J, Conboy F, Sanjie Y, Mandall N et al. Effectiveness of early orthodontic treatment with the Twin-block appliance: A multicenter, randomized, controlled trial. Part 1: Dental and skeletal effects. Am J Orthod Dentofacial Orthop. 2003: 124: 234–43.
6. Jasper JJ, McNamara JA Jr. The correction of interarch malocclusion using a fixed force module. Am J Orthod Dentofacial Orthop. 1995: 108: 641–50.
7. Weiland FJ, Ingervall B, Bantleon HP, Droacht H. Initial effects of treatment of Class II malocclusion with the Herren activator, activator-headgear combination, and Jasper Jumper. Am J Orthod Dentofacial Orthop. 1997; 112: 19–27.
8. Cope JB, Buschang PH, Cope DD, Parker J, Blackwood HO III. Quantitative evaluation of craniofacial changes with Jasper Jumper therapy. Angle Orthod. 1994; 64: 113–22.
9. Covell DA Jr, Trammell DW, Boero RP, West R. A cephalometric study of class II Division 1 malocclusions treated with the Jasper Jumper appliance. Angle Orthod. 1999; 69: 311–20.
10. Oliveira J Jr, Rodrigues de Almeida R, Rodrigues de Almeida M, de Oliveira JN. Dentoskeletal changes induced by the Jasper Jumper and cervical headgear appliances followed by fixed orthodontic treatment. Am J Orthod Dentofacial Orthop. 2007; 132: 54–62.
11. Herrera F, Henriques JF, Janson G, Francisconi MF, de Freitas KM. Cephalometric evaluation in different phases of Jasper Jumper therapy. Am J Orthod Dentofacial Orthop. 2011; 140: e77–e84.
12. Karacay S, Akin E, Olmez H, Gurton AU, Sagdic D. Forsus Nitinol flat spring and Jasper Jumper corrections of Class II division 1 malocclusions. Angle Orthod. 2006; 76: 666–72.
13. Vogt W. The Forsus fatigue resistant device. J Clin Orth. 2006; 40: 368–77.
14. Jones G, Buschang PH, Kim KB, Oliver DR. Class II non-extraction patients treated with the Forsus fatigue resistant device versus intermaxillary elastics. Angle Orthod. 2008; 78: 332–8.
15. Franchi L, Alvetro L, Giuntini V, Masucci C, Defraia E, Baccetti T. Effectiveness of comprehensive fixed appliance treatment used with the Forsus fatigue resistant device in Class II patients. Angle Orthod. 2011; 81: 678–83.
16. Aras A, Ada E, Saracoğlu H, Gezer NS, Aras I. Comparison of treatments with the Forsus fatigue resistant device in relation to skeletal maturity: A cephalometric and magnetic resonance imaging study. Am J Orthod Dentofacial Orthop. 2011; 140: 616–25.
17. Chhibber A, Upadhyay M, Uribe F, Nanda R. Mechanism of Class II correction in prepubertal and postpubertal patients with Twin Force bite corrector. Angle Orthod. 2013; 83: 718–27.
18. Pancherz H, Anehus-Pancherz M. The headgear effect of the Herbst appliance: A long-term cephalometric study. Am J Orthod Dentofac Orthop. 1993; 103: 510–20.
19. VanLaecken R, Martin CA, Dischinger T, Razmus T, Ngan P. Treatment effects of the Edgewise Herbst appliance: A cephalometric and tomographic investigation. Am J Orthod Dentofac Orthop. 2006; 130: 582–93.
20. Ruf S, Pancherz H. The effect of Herbst appliance treatment on the mandibular plane angle: A cephalometric roentgenographic study. Am J Orthod Dentofac Orthop. 1996; 110: 225–9.
21. Nalbantgil D, Arun T, Sayinsu K, Fulya I. Skeletal, dental and soft-tissue changes induced by the Jasper Jumper in late adolescence. Angle Orthod. 2005; 75: 382–92.
22. Stucki N, Ingervall B. The use of Jasper Jumper for the correction of Class II malocclusion in the young permanent dentition. Eur J Orthod. 1998; 20: 271–81.
23. Karacay S, Akin E, Olmez H, Gurton AU, Sagdic D. Forsus Nitinol flat spring and Jasper Jumper corrections of Class II division 1 malocclusions. Angle Orthod. 2006; 76: 666–72.
24. Stromeyer EL, Caruso MJ, Devincenzo JP. A cephalometric study of the Class II correction effects of the Eureka Spring. Angle Orthod. 2002; 72: 203–10.
25. DeVincenzo J. The Eureka Spring: A new interarch force delivery system. J Clin Orth 1997; 31: 454–67.
26. Franchi L, Baccetti T, McNamara JA Jr. Treatment and posttreatment effects of acrylic splint Herbst appliance therapy. Am J Orthod Dentofacial Orthop. 1999; 115: 429–38.
27. Schaefer AT, McNamara JA, Franchi L, Baccetti T. A cephalometric comparison of treatment with the Twin-block and stainless steel crown Herbst appliances followed by fixed appliance therapy. Am J Orthod Dentofac Orthop. 2004; 126: 7–15.
28. Azizollahi S. Comparison of skeletal and dentoalveolar effects of the Forsus and MARA in treatment of Class II malocclusions. Doctoral dissertation, Saint Louis University, 2012.

29. Al-Jewair T, Preston CB, Moll EM, Dischinger T. A comparison of the MARA and the AdvanSync functional appliances in the treatment of Class II malocclusion. Angle Orthod. 2012; 82: 907–14.
30. Ghislanzoni LT, Toll DE, Defraia E, Baccetti T, Franchi L. Treatment and posttreatment outcomes induced by the Mandibular Advancement Repositioning Appliance: A controlled clinical study. Angle Orthod. 2011; 81: 684–91.
31. Tulloch JF, Proffit WR, Phillips C. Outcomes in a 2-phase randomized clinical trial of early Class II treatment. Am J Orthod Dentofacial Orthop. 2004; 125: 657–67.
32. Cozza P, Baccetti T, Franchi L, De Toffol L, McNamara JA. Mandibular changes produced by functional appliances in Class II malocclusion: A systematic review. Am J Orthod Dentofac Orthop. 2006; 129: 599.e1–e12.
33. Siara-Olds N, Pangrazio-Kulbersh V, Berger J, Bayirli B. Long-term dentoskeletal changes with the Bionator, Herbst, Twin Block, and MARA functional appliances. Angle Orthod. 2010; 80: 18–29.

CHAPTER 8

Transferring from functional to fixed appliances

While the mode of action of functional appliances has long been disputed and debated, there is certainly a significant dento-alveolar component to the resultant occlusal change. As such, both pre-existing crowding, malalignment and other occlusal problems, combined with certain dental changes related to appliance therapy, ensure that functional appliance therapy is now rarely considered as a standalone treatment. Fixed appliances usually follow relatively soon after the functional phase. Occasionally, however, where early treatment has been instigated, there is a delay prior to progression to fixed appliances to allow further maturation to occur. Sometimes fixed appliances are not required following the functional phase; however, more typically, fixed appliance treatment is undertaken to address any residual malocclusion, including concurrent crowding, and to allow optimal occlusal interdigitation while preserving the favourable changes induced by the functional appliance treatment.

Dento-alveolar changes occurring with functional appliances relate to Class II effects in both the upper and lower arches. Specific dental changes induced with therapy include uprighting or retroclination of the upper anteriors, proclination of the lower labial segment allied to distal tipping of the maxillary posterior teeth and mesial tipping of mandibular posteriors; effectively a Class II effect to the upper and lower arches (Figure 8.1). While the magnitude of incisor inclination changes is quantifiable cephalometrically, less is known regarding angulation and inclination changes posteriorly. Nevertheless, these changes should be retained to address the malocclusion definitively, preserving the Class II correction and allowing maximum inter-cuspation.

Fixed appliances may either be used in conjunction with functional appliances or as a separate stage of treatment involving a seamless transition or following an interval. However, when removable functional appliances are used, fixed appliance therapy typically follows the functional phase in a two-stage treatment approach. The key decisions involved in overseeing transfer to fixed appliances relate to timing of the transition and selection of the most suitable approach to consolidate Class II correction.

Planning the transition

While early functional appliance therapy is followed by a prolonged phase of consolidation or retention (Figure 8.2), fixed appliances are normally planned a relatively short interval after functional appliance therapy in most cases. Contraindications to a fixed appliance phase, however, include manifestations of poor compliance such as poor oral hygiene, active caries, repeated failed appointments and multiple breakages.

A further reason to postpone progression to fixed appliances is delayed dental development, particularly with insufficient eruption of the posterior dentition or poor compliance. Generally, however, seamless progression to the fixed phase is preferable, limiting overall treatment time and the associated burdens.[1]

Post-functional records including study models, photographs and a lateral cephalogram are recommended following functional appliance therapy. The relative influence of skeletal and dento-alveolar effects on overjet reduction and molar correction may be evaluated using cephalometric analysis.

Cephalometric superimposition

The magnitude of dental and skeletal contributions to overjet reduction or molar correction can be assessed via overall and regional cephalometric superimpositions. Commonly used cephalometric analyses focus primarily on diagnosis and treatment planning. While orthopaedic and orthodontic effects can be assessed using superimposition, each evaluation is performed independently of the other, using different reference lines and structures. This complicates assessment of interrelationships between skeletal and dental components that contribute to occlusal changes. Therefore, to highlight treatment-related changes over an extended period, while excluding the influence of growth and maturation, superimposition on stable reference structures is preferable.[2]

Overall superimposition on a stable structure has the potential to highlight skeletal changes during appliance

Orthodontic Functional Appliances: Theory and Practice, First Edition. Padhraig Fleming and Robert Lee.

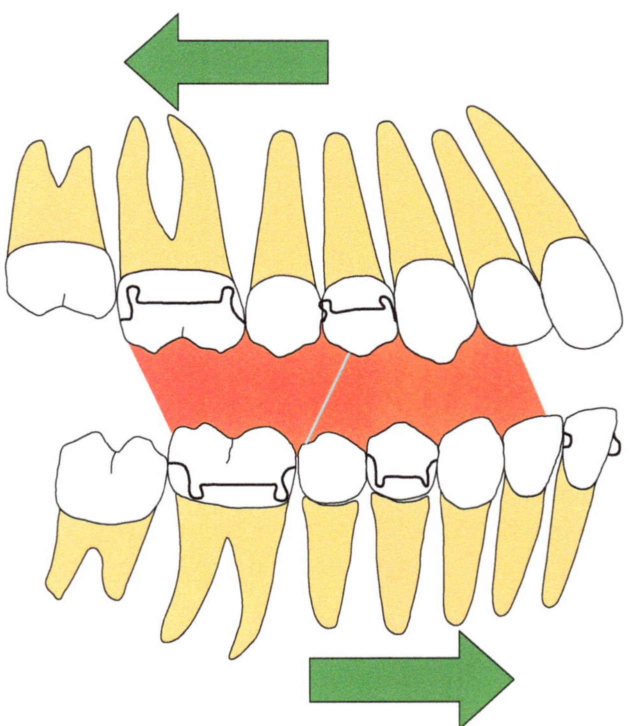

Figure 8.1 Class II effect on maxillary and mandibular arches with distal tipping of upper buccal segments and mesial tipping of the lower arch associated with a Twin Block appliance.

therapy. Typically, the cranial base or Sella-Nasion line is used to represent an area of relative stability. Regional superimpositions are particularly useful in highlighting the magnitude of dental inclination change during the functional phase. No single cephalometric superimposition technique has gained widespread acceptance and a wide variety are in use. In relation to the mandibular dentition, Björk's structures for assessment of growth and treatment changes are commonly used. However, superimposition on the mandibular outline has also been shown to be reliable, particularly where the interval between serial radiographs is less than 12 months.[3,4] Regional superimposition of the maxillary arch has been accomplished using various structures, planes and registration points, including ANS–PNS, Bjork's key ridge, palatal vault, Pancherz analysis[5,6] and Johnston's pitchfork analysis. Repeated cephalograms are also reliant on ionizing radiation and superimposition is prone to introduce further inaccuracy.[7]

Ideally, a degree of overcorrection of the excessive overjet may be produced during the functional phase to compensate for expected relapse. A Class III incisor relationship with edge-to-edge incisors or reverse overjet may be obtained with a ¼–½ unit Class III molar relationship (Figure 8.3). Typically, this overcorrection gradually dissipates during the fixed appliance phase.

Timing

The transition to fixed appliances may be immediate, gradual or delayed.[8] Gradual transition involves a period of part-time appliance wear, typically on a night-time basis. While complete withdrawal of a functional appliance or other mode of Class II maintenance during the transition to the fixed appliance phase may be an efficient approach, it risks relapse of Class II correction. Unwanted manifestations of relapse are likely to include increased overjet, proclination of the upper labial segment, uprighting of the lower labial segment, loss of molar correction and mesial tipping of the maxillary buccal segments. The relative merits of each approach to managing the transition to fixed appliances are shown in Table 8.1.

Methods of consolidating Class II correction

Reinforced anchorage

The use of extra-oral anchorage has been advocated as a technique in facilitating the transfer to fixed appliances. While mandibular retrognathia and reduced mandibular length usually accompany a Class II division 1 incisor relationship, maxillary protrusion occasionally contributes to the malocclusion.[9] Headgear is particularly useful where the malocclusion has arisen from a degree of maxillary protrusion[10] or in the presence of an increased vertical dimension. Advantages of headgear use include the following:

- Versatility: A high vector is of additional value in patients with a high maxillo-mandibular plane angle (MMPA) and increased lower anterior facial height. Functional appliance therapy has consistently been shown to result in an increase in the vertical dimension.[11–14]
- Maintenance of molar correction and overjet reduction.
- Allows immediate transition to fixed appliance phase.
- Facility to use adjunctive Class III traction. Class III elastics may be useful in uprighting the lower labial segment, which is likely to have proclined during the functional phase, possibly into a zone of instability. By applying headgear in conjunction with the elastics, loss of anchorage is prevented (Figure 8.4).

The major drawback of this approach is compliance 'burnout'. Sub-optimal compliance among patients wearing headgear as an adjunct to fixed appliances is well documented.[15,16] A prolonged functional phase followed by introduction of headgear may well be very demanding in terms of cooperation.

Maintaining postured bite

Part-time functional appliance wear

Maintenance of the functional appliance during the transition to fixed appliances keeps the mandible in a protruded position and even if worn only at night maintains the neuromuscular response and growth stimulatory effect.[17] Part-time wear is generally advocated at night rather than during the day for

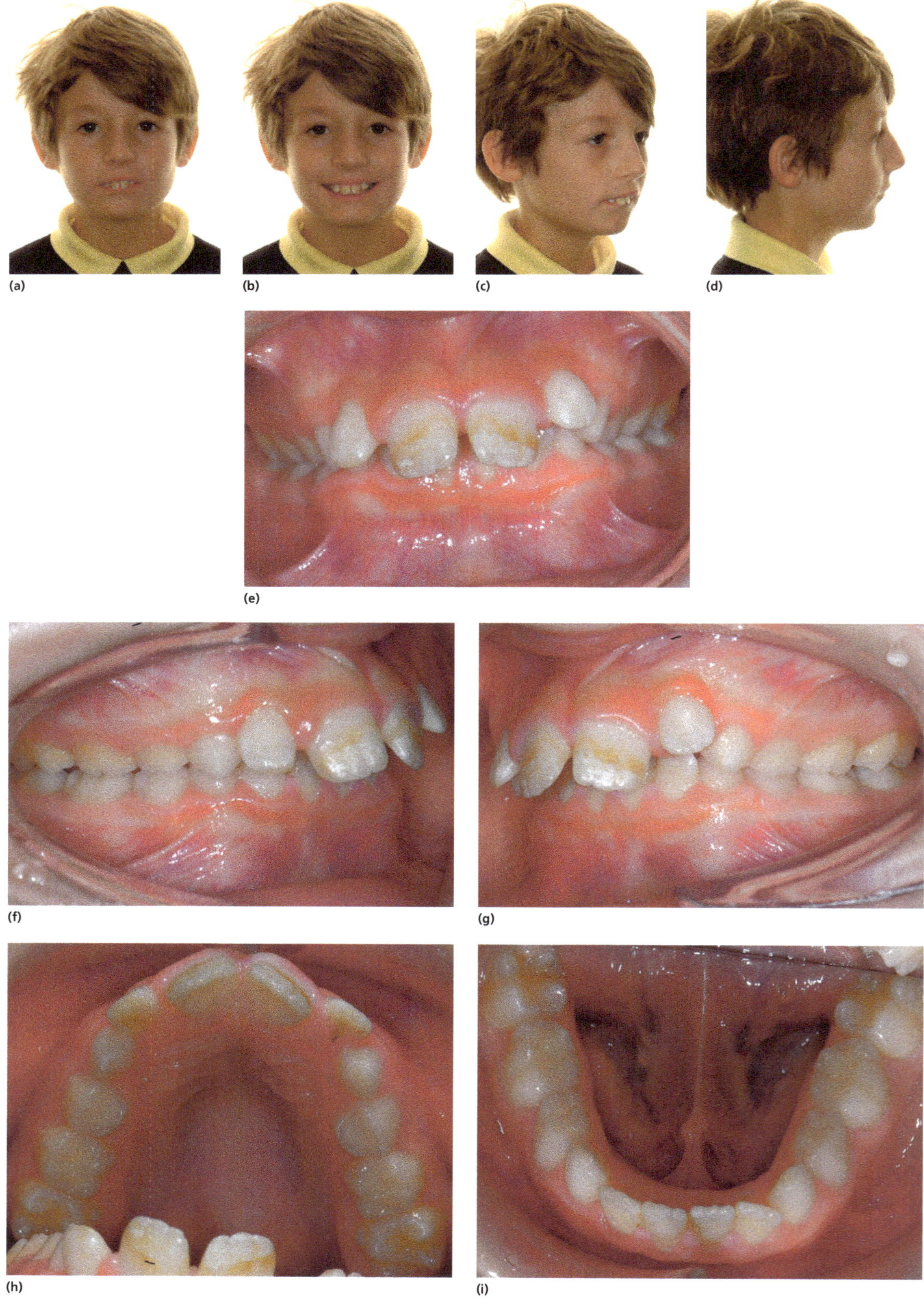

Figure 8.2 This 8-year-old male presented with concerns in relation to his dentofacial appearance with reports of associated teasing (a–i). A decision was, therefore, made to carry out interceptive treatment to reduce the overjet at least partially during the first treatment phase. A further objective of the initial phase was to achieve lip competence. A modified Twin Block was worn for a period of 9 months on a full-time basis resulting in antero-posterior correction and lip competence (j–l). In view of the stage of dental development with multiple retained primary teeth, definitive correction was delayed (m–q). The functional appliance was therefore maintained on a nights-only basis for a further 12-month period before being withdrawn for a further 12 months. Thereafter, a second treatment phase was instituted involving fixed appliances on a non-extraction basis. In this instance, sagittal relapse of the Class II did not arise during the intervening period, ensuring that a second phase of functional appliance therapy or other form of Class II correction was not required during Phase 2 (r–z).

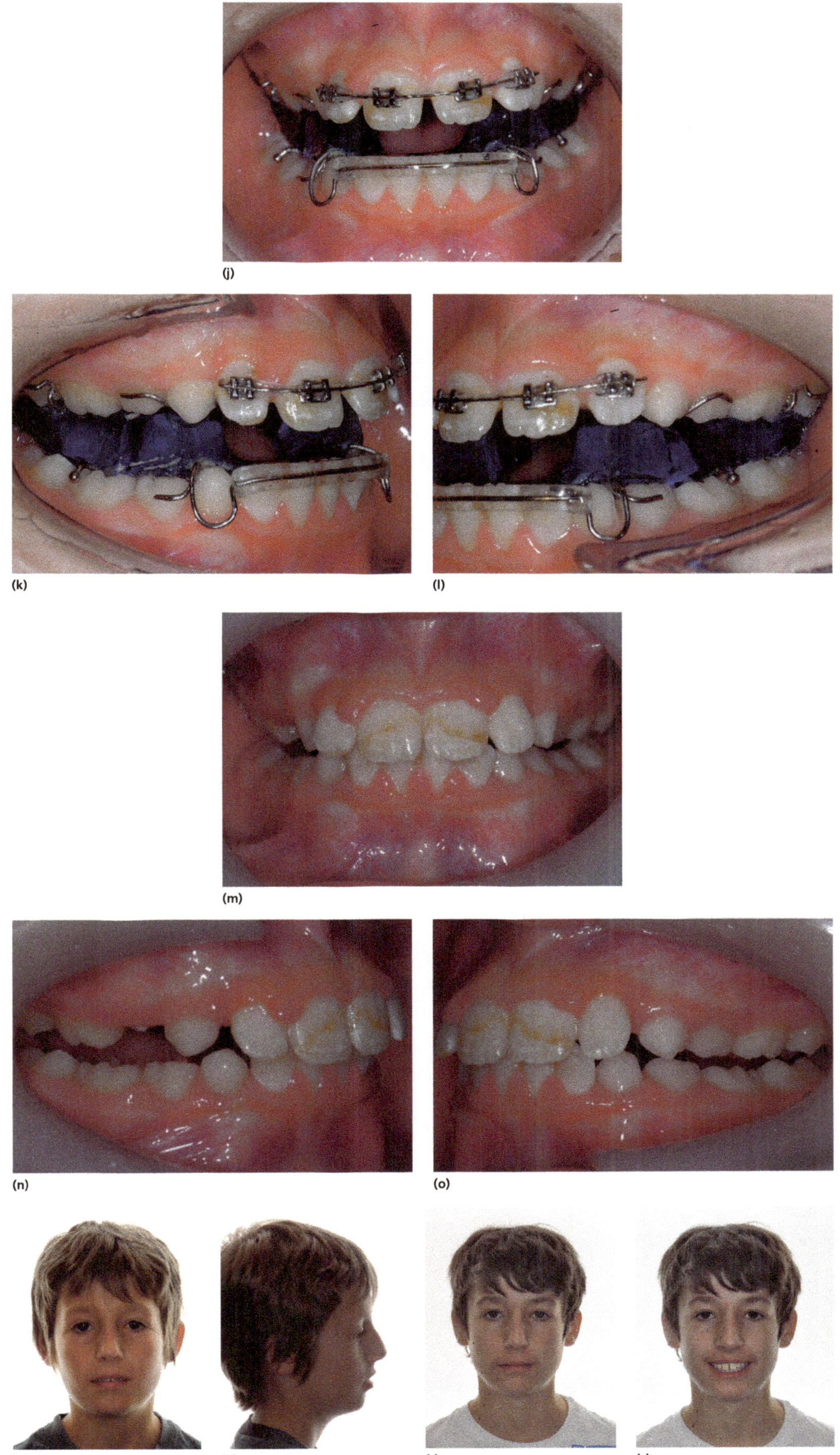

Figure 8.2 (*Continued*)

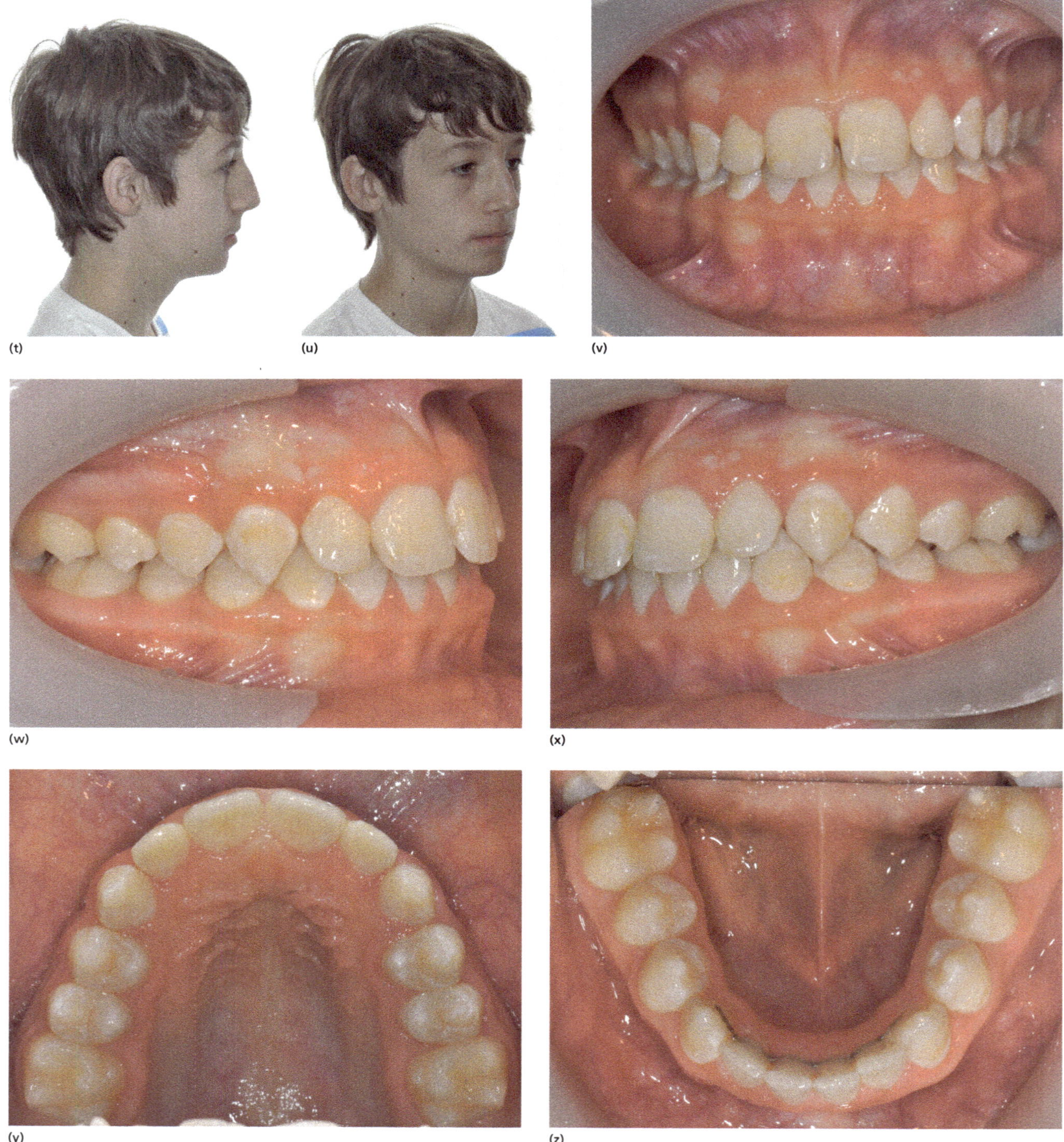

Figure 8.2 (*Continued*)

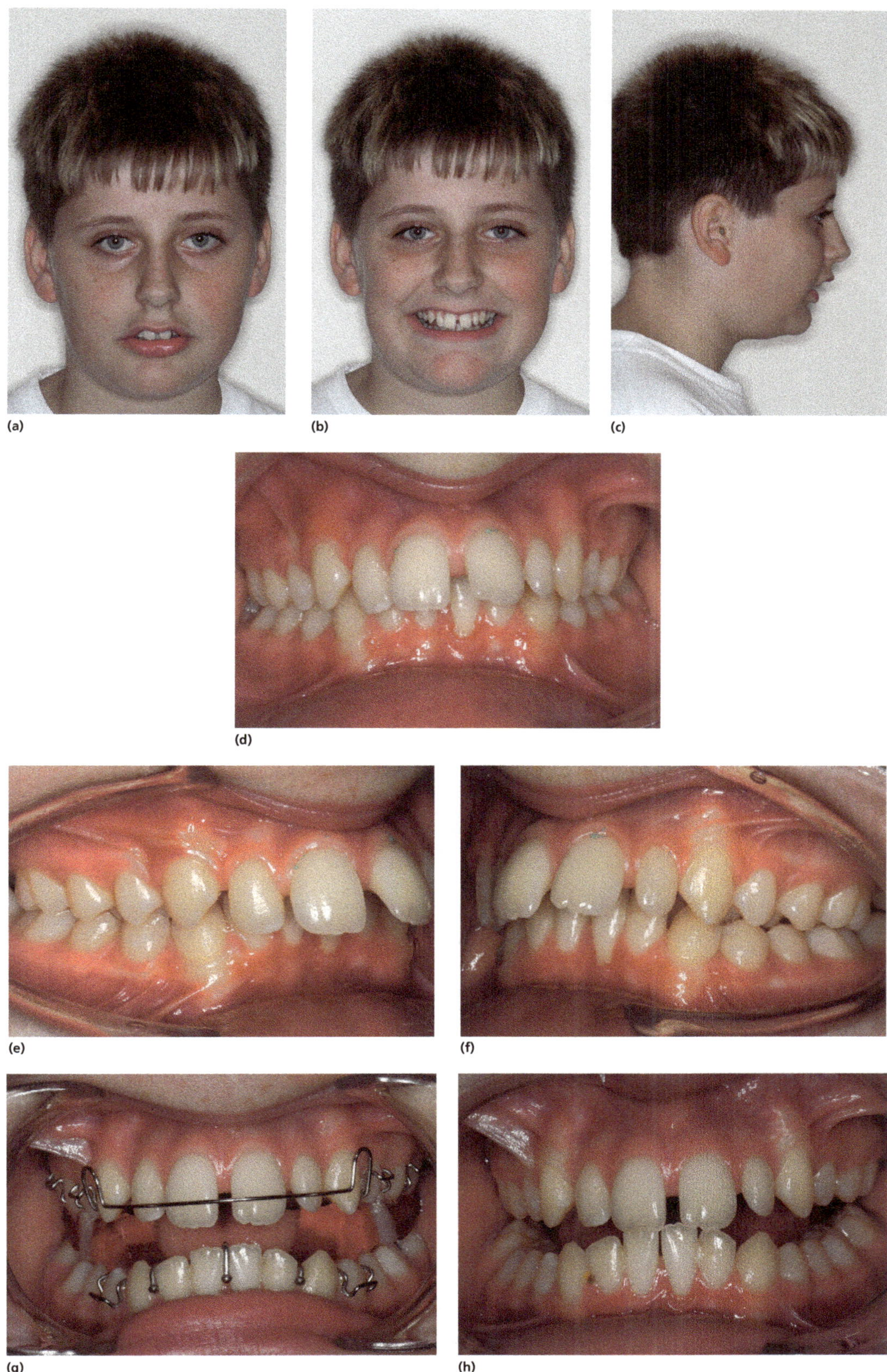

Figure 8.3 This 12-year-old male presented with a very significant overjet (15 mm) on a moderate skeletal II pattern with mandibular retrognathia and spaced arches. He reported teasing in relation to his dentofacial appearance (a–f). He was treated with a modified Twin Block for a period of 12 months. He was very compliant; the appliance was reactivated with light-cured acrylic after 8 months (g). The malocclusion was significantly overcorrected with the overjet fully eliminated and molar relationships overcorrected to Class III (h–j). Significant lateral open bites also reflect the excellent wear of the appliance. Subsequently, upper and lower fixed appliances were placed with restorative build-up of the maxillary lateral incisors to consolidate the spacing and seat the buccal occlusion. The overcorrection resolved during the fixed phase with a resultant Class I, well-interdigitated buccal occlusion (k–s).

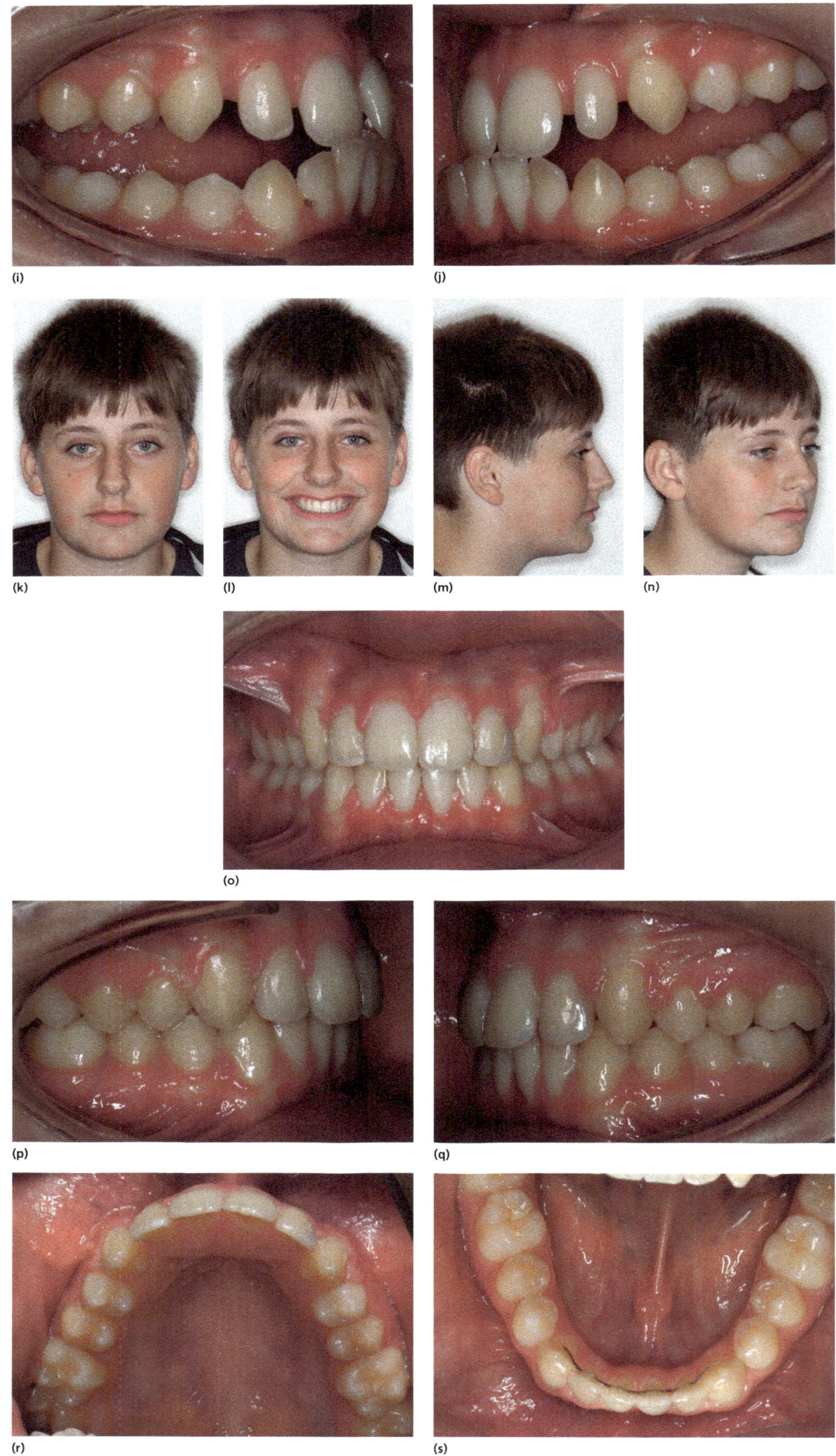

Figure 8.3 (*Continued*)

Table 8.1 Relative merits of options to manage the transition from functional to fixed appliances.

	Immediate	Period of night-time retention	Period of no appliance wear
Overall treatment length	Reduced	No effect	No effect/may be increased
Maintenance of Class II correction	Variable	Good	Poor
Prediction of relapse/anchorage demands	Poor	Poor	Good
Spontaneous occlusal settling	Poor	Moderate	Good
Allows condylar adaptation	No	Yes	No

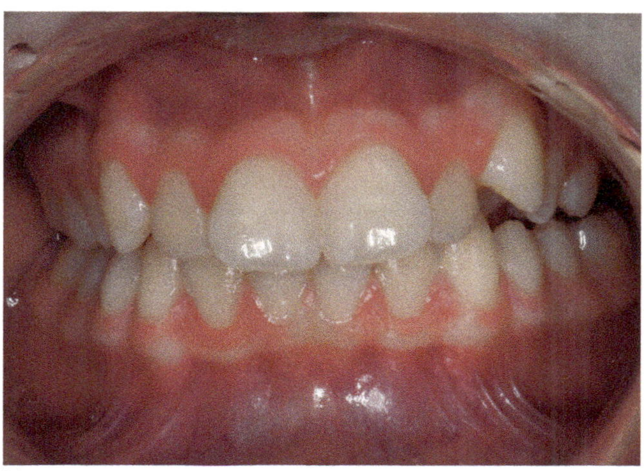

(a)

(b)

(c)

(d)

(e)

Figure 8.4 This 11-year-old female presented with a Class II division 1 incisor relationship with an increased overjet of 10 mm. There was crowding of both dental arches (a–e). She was treated with a modified Twin Block to address the skeletal II pattern. Incisor and molar relationships were overcorrected during the functional phase (f–h). In view of the pre-existing crowding allied to proclination of the mandibular incisors during the functional phase, a space requirement existed to align the lower incisors in a stable position. Consequently, bands were fitted to the maxillary first molars to permit night-time headgear wear, while Class III elastics were used to upright the mandibular incisors. An acceptable final occlusal outcome was achieved (o–s).

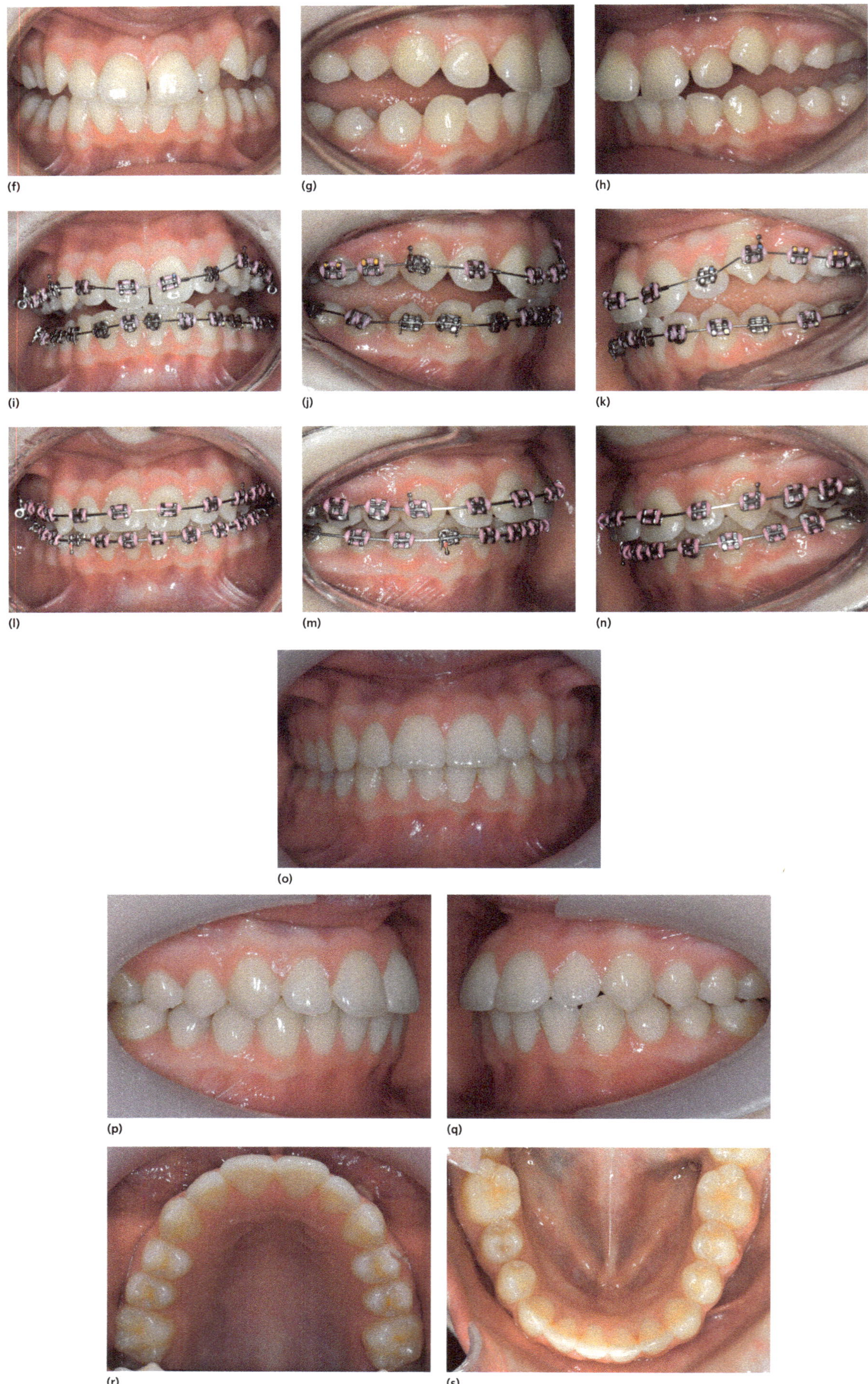

Figure 8.4 (*Continued*)

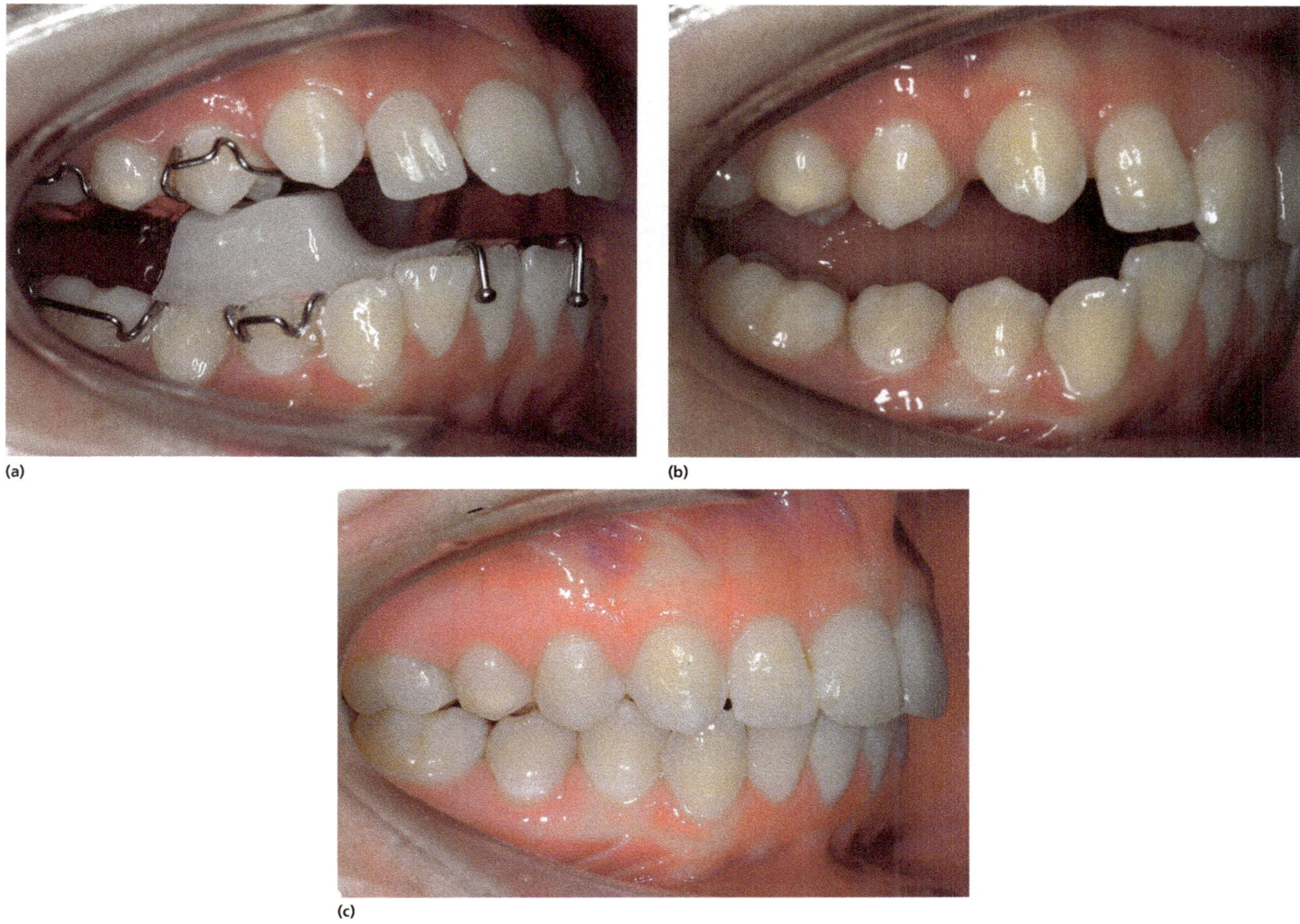

Figure 8.5 Typical lateral open bites arising following Twin Block therapy (a, b) due to impeded vertical development of the posterior teeth related to the acrylic coverage, while continued eruption of the anteriors proceeds during the functional phase. These resolve rather easily during or prior to the fixed appliance phase (c).

convenience; however, there is also evidence that tooth eruption occurs preferentially during the evening[18] and orthodontic tooth movement also appears to be more rapid at night rather than during the day.[19] However, similar research pertaining to the influence of circadian rhythm on mandibular growth has not been undertaken. A part-time appliance has the following advantages:

- Allows resolution of lateral open bites and eruption of teeth that may arise with certain functional appliances. Lateral open bites tend to be a common finding following Twin Block therapy in particular. These may be prevented or limited by judicious trimming of the upper blocks to encourage eruption during the functional phase. This does, however, risk weakening the appliance, leading to fracture. Irrespective of how these open bites are managed, they do tend to resolve very easily either during or prior to the fixed phase (Figure 8.5).
- Reduced compliance demand.
- Simple approach not requiring additional appliances or expense (Figure 8.6).

Maintenance of removable functional appliance during early fixed phase

Certain functional appliances may be streamlined to allow integration with fixed appliances. For example, the Twin Block may be adjusted to incorporate fixed appliances in the anterior segments and worn nightly to retain Class II correction. To facilitate integration of fixed appliances, retentive clasps may be removed from the first molars and premolars. Ball-ended clasps may be used in the premolar region to preserve retention without compromising bracket positioning. Similarly, use of hybrid functional appliances, such as the Dynamax, permits placement of a lower fixed appliance in concert with the functional phase. Moreover, the upper appliance may be modified to allow placement of a sectional upper appliance simultaneously (Figure 8.7).

The advantages of this approach include resolution of lateral open bites while maintaining the decrease in overjet and preservation of molar correction. Inevitably, however, streamlining the appliances means that they may be weakened and retention

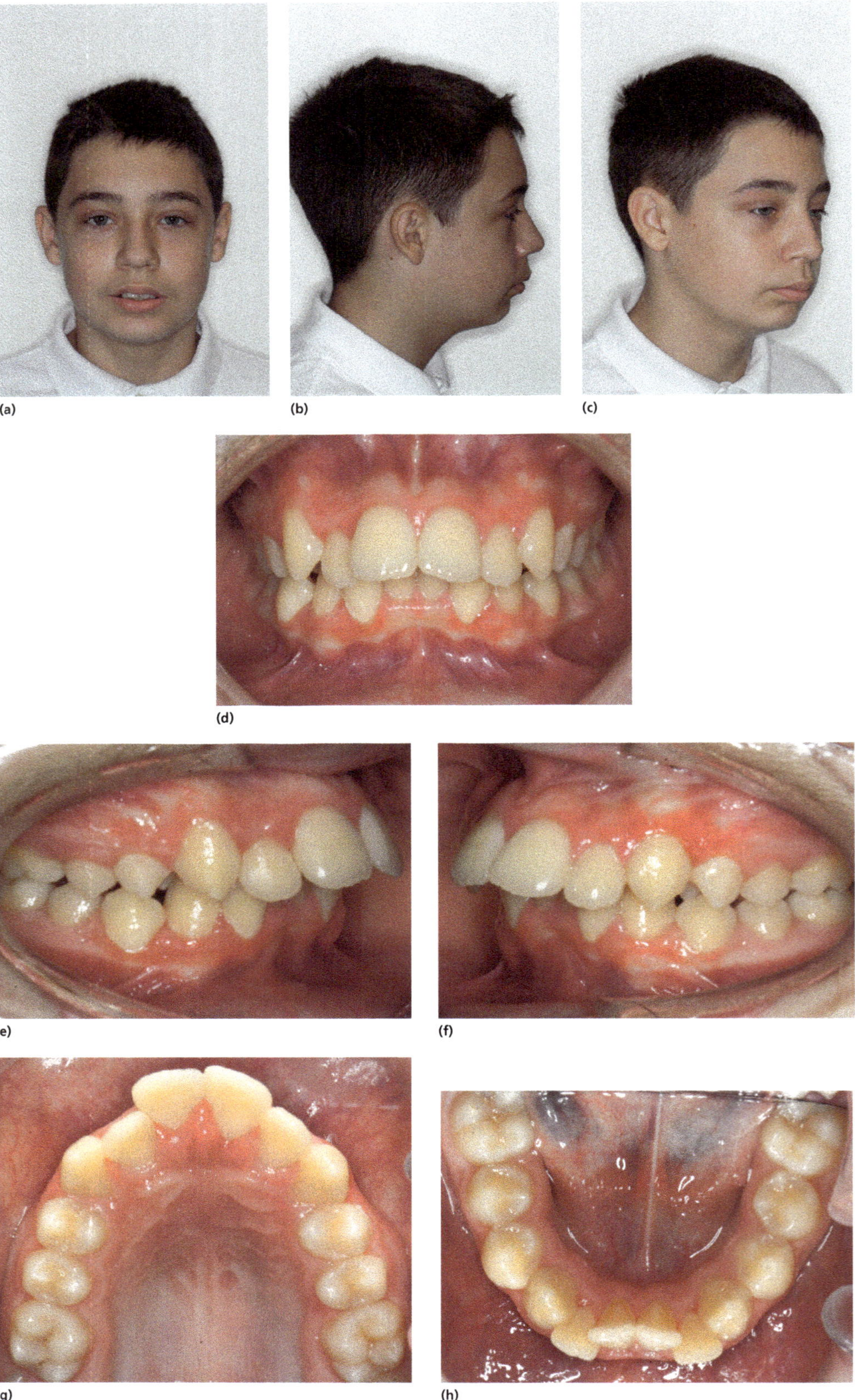

Figure 8.6 This 12-year-old male presented with a large overjet (12 mm) on a moderate skeletal II pattern with mandibular retrognathia, crowding of both dental arches and proclined maxillary incisors with a lower lip trap (a–h). He was treated with a modified Twin Block over a 10-month period (i, j) before withdrawing the appliance for a period of 6 weeks. The molar relationships were overcorrected to ½ unit Class III with bilaterally and lateral open bites developed (k–n). Following withdrawal of the appliance, slight antero-posterior relapse occurred and the lateral open bites began to close (o–q). A decision was made to remove four second premolar units to facilitate relief of crowding and further retraction of the maxillary incisors (r–t).

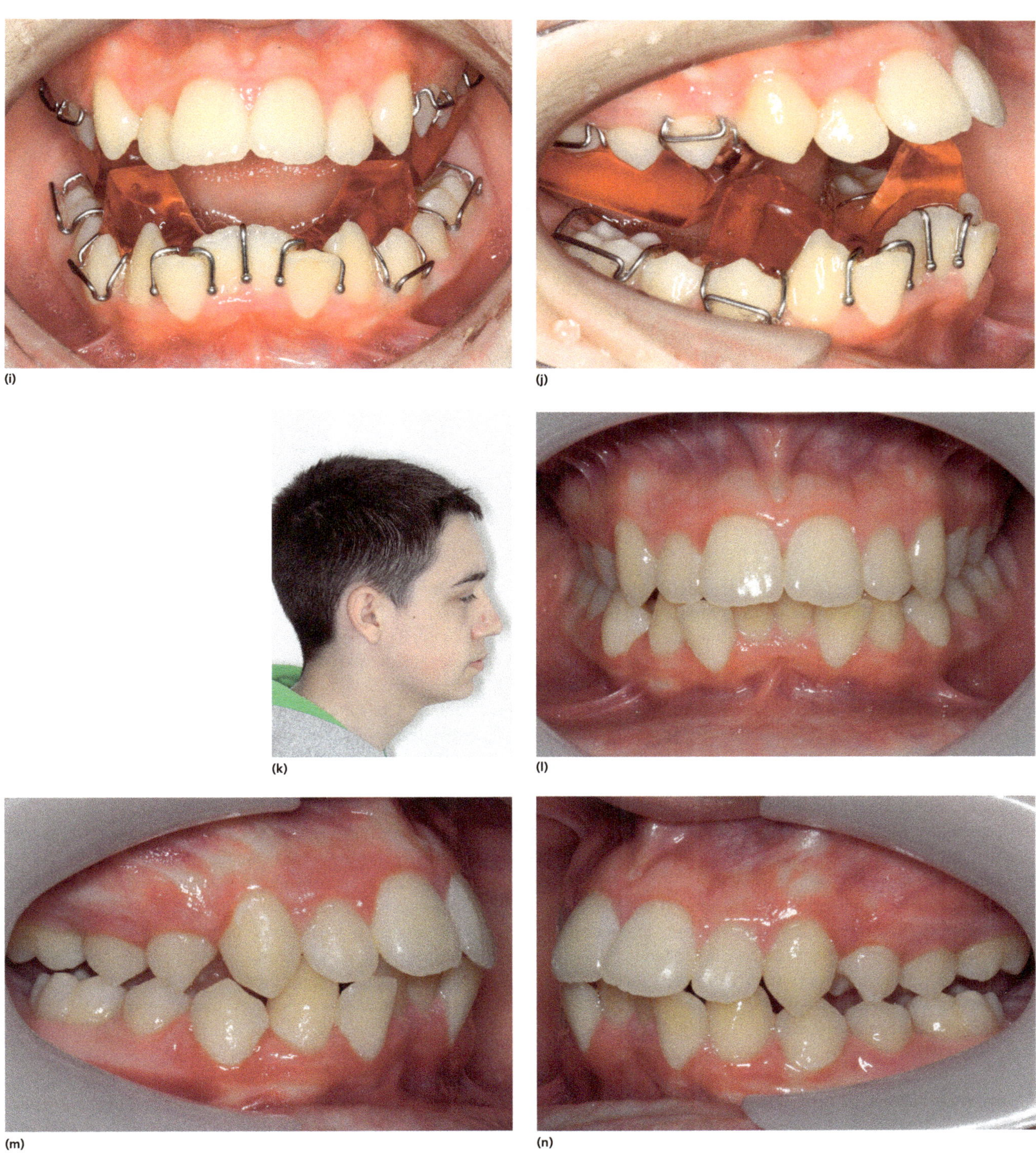

(i) (j) (k) (l) (m) (n)

Figure 8.6 *(Continued)*

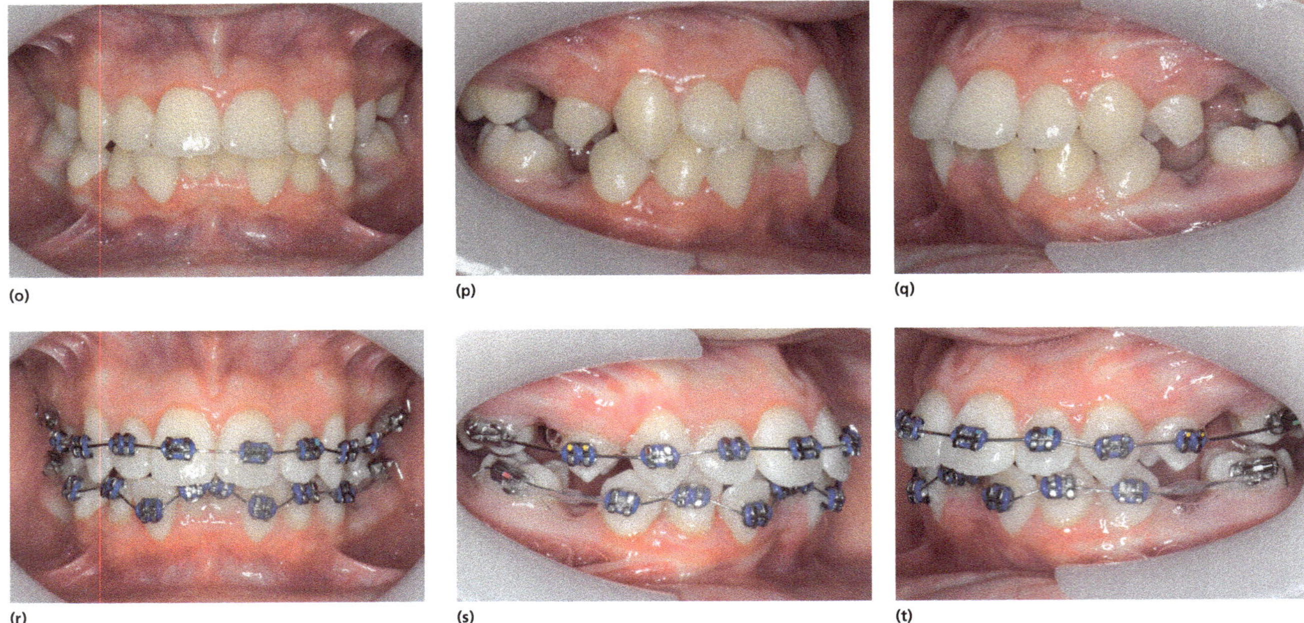

Figure 8.6 (*Continued*)

compromised to a degree. At this late stage of functional therapy, however, appliance retention tends to be less important, as patients usually develop an ability to withstand shortcomings in terms of retention and comfort.

Fixed functional appliance

The possibility of placing fixed appliances concurrent with the functional appliance permits simultaneous Class II correction in conjunction with achievement of other unrelated occlusal objectives, including alignment and relief of crowding. Therefore, use of fixed functional appliances may avoid the problem of maintaining the Class II correction, with the potential to result in more efficient treatment.

Fixed functional appliances were considered in greater detail in Chapter 6. However, potential advantages of their use in terms of treatment progression include the following:

- Molar correction and overjet reduction preserved.
- Rapid and seamless treatment sequence.
- Reduced compliance demand.
- Reduced likelihood of non-completion of treatment.[20–25]

Upper removable appliance with inclined bite plane

A steep anterior inclined bite plane as part of an upper retainer represents a simple method of retention of Class II correction.[26] The precise type of retainer used relates to the treatment goals. Begg-type retainers are favoured if occlusal settling and closure of lateral open bites are necessitated. In cases where molar positions are acceptable and retention of the appliance is a priority, a Hawley-type retainer may be used. If the plan is to transfer immediately to fixed appliances, a 'clip-over' bite plane is recommended. Potential benefits of this approach include the following:

- May be worn in conjunction with fixed appliances, integrating phases.
- Fixed appliance placement unimpeded.
- Allows closure of lateral open bites.
- Time efficient.
- Maintains Class II effect.

Potential disadvantages, however, include these:

- Proclination of the lower labial segment, although this can be controlled and can be rectified if necessary during the fixed appliance phase with a variety of mechanics.
- Insufficient depth of the plane may allow relapse of overjet, particularly due to postural changes during sleep.
- Can allow differential eruption of second molars, introducing anterior open bites in cases with a high Frankfurt-mandibular planes angle. In such cases, inclusion of terminal molars within the appliance is recommended to limit vertical development of posterior teeth, which may otherwise culminate in unwanted decrease in the anterior overbite.

Early use of Class II elastics

Light Class II elastics used in round wires may reinforce dento-alveolar changes achieved during functional treatment. Elastics may favour retroclination of upper incisors and proclination of lower incisors, leading to further reduction of the overjet. Elastic wear may lead to extrusion of mandibular molars, which may be favourable in low-angle cases, further reducing the overbite. Extrusion of the maxillary incisors is also possible with elastics on light aligning wires. This may counteract the impact of elastic wear on the overbite; however, the net effect is likely to be a reduction in overbite overall due to the proximity of the posterior teeth to the terminal hinge axis of the mandible.

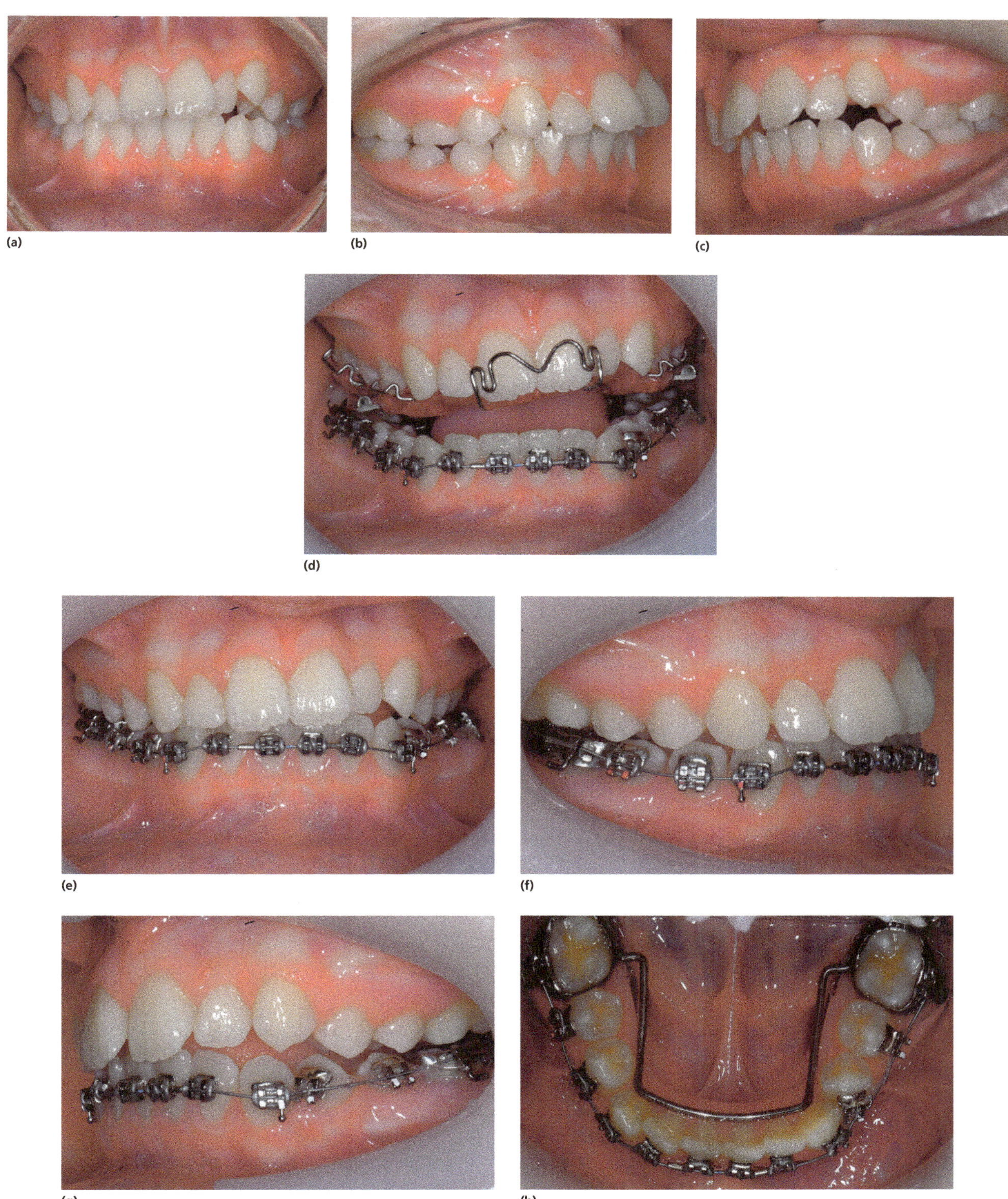
(a) (b) (c) (d) (e) (f) (g) (h)

Figure 8.7 This Class II malocclusion was treated with a Dynamax in the first instance to address the antero-posterior discrepancy (a–d). The Dynamax was maintained during the fixed phase to facilitate maintenance of the Class II correction as lower arch alignment proceeded (e–h).

In high-angle cases and in patients with vertical maxillary excess, an unfavourable downward–backward mandibular rotation will occur unless the patient has some vertical growth during treatment with elastic wear. Moreover, extrusion of the maxillary incisors may be unfavourable in high-angle cases, increasing the maxillary incisal display and potential, leading to unwanted uprighting of the maxillary incisors and compromising the anterior aesthetics.[27,28] A further unwanted effect may be lingual tipping of lower molars with excessive force when non-rigid wires are in place. Consequently, early use of Class II elastics should be undertaken judiciously and may be confined to nights-only use.

Extraction pattern

Extractions may be necessitated in the post-functional phase. In the study by Tulloch et al., extractions were carried out in 30% of patients after the functional appliance phase.[29] Similarly, O'Brien et al.[13] reported a 27% extraction rate in an early functional appliance group, with 37% of subjects undergoing later functional therapy also having extractions. The decision to remove teeth in this situation should be based on an assessment of space requirements and availability.[30] The chosen extraction pattern depends on a number of factors, including the following:

- Presence of teeth
- Health of teeth
- Degree and location of crowding
- Soft tissue profile
- Overbite
- Vertical growth pattern
- Lower incisor inclination

Significant proclination of the lower labial segment has been shown with Twin Block[31] and Herbst[32] appliances and indeed is common to all functional appliance systems. Space is therefore required to upright the lower labial segment in this situation, as lower incisors proclined during orthodontic treatment are known to be unstable.[33] The effect of functional therapy in some patients is to induce a requirement for lower extractions where an uncrowded or mildly crowded arch is inadvertently advanced by the appliance.[29] While some degree of incisor uprighting will arise spontaneously following withdrawal of the appliance, it may be desirable to return the incisors towards the original position. For this reason most functional therapy is devised to limit lower arch advancement, other than in patients where the lower incisors would be beneficially advanced, perhaps being considered artificially upright.

Maxillary arch extractions in isolation or extraction of upper first premolars and lower second premolars facilitates molar correction in Class II cases, and simplifies the mechanics needed for differential space closure, although successful functional appliance therapy is rarely followed by maxillary extractions, in isolation.

Fixed appliance prescription

Fixed appliance prescription may be tailored to reinforce the effects of functional appliance therapy, particularly by limiting antero-posterior anchorage strain in the upper arch, while counteracting significant dento-alveolar changes induced during the functional phase. For example, the MBT prescription, incorporating enhanced palatal root torque to the maxillary incisors, labial root torque to the lower incisor limited mesial tip in the maxillary canines and supplementary buccal root torque in the maxillary molars, may theoretically reinforce favourable effects produced by the functional phase, promoting conservation of molar correction and overjet reduction.

In terms of torque values, increased palatal root torque (17 degrees) of the upper incisors and labial root torque (6 degrees) in the lower incisors counteracts the dento-alveolar effects produced by the functional phase. The potency of these torque alterations, however, may be limited in view of the play within the pre-adjusted Edgewise system.[34] Moreover, the anchorage value provided by the lower incisor roots is likely to be minimal, given their short length and narrow shape. Buccal root torque (14 degrees) of the upper molars corrects buccal flaring caused by expansion with the functional appliance.

As far as tip values are concerned, in the upper arch mesial tip is reduced, limiting anchorage requirements and the tendency for overjet relapse. In the mandibular arch mesial tip in the premolars is maintained, favouring molar correction. Functional appliances do tend to exert a potent Class II effect on the maxillary posterior segments with distal tipping of the maxillary premolars and molars (Figure 8.8). By reducing mesial tip in the fixed appliance in these areas, anchorage loss may be controlled.

Local bracket variations may also be useful to limit relapse of Class II correction by, for example, limiting mesial tip in the maxillary canines via the use of premolar brackets with negligible or zero mesial tip. Similarly, artistic positioning of brackets can be undertaken to promote uprighting of maxillary canine crowns, which are normally programmed to position the roots of these teeth distally, with a consequent anchorage demand.

Conclusions

The aim of transfer to the fixed appliance phase is to retain the beneficial dento-alveolar and skeletal changes introduced in the functional appliance phase, while allowing treatment to proceed in a time-efficient manner. The use of functional appliances to which fixed appliances can be fitted concurrently facilitates a smooth transition.

In non-extraction cases, with a high Frankfurt–mandibular angle and vertical maxillary excess, high-pull headgear may be used, and the use of Class II elastics is best avoided. In patients with a low Frankfurt–mandibular angle, reduced lower anterior facial height and deep overbite, inclined bite planes or early use of Class II elastics may be preferable. Tailored fixed appliance bracket prescription and differential extractions where indicated can reinforce the favourable changes introduced during the functional phase.

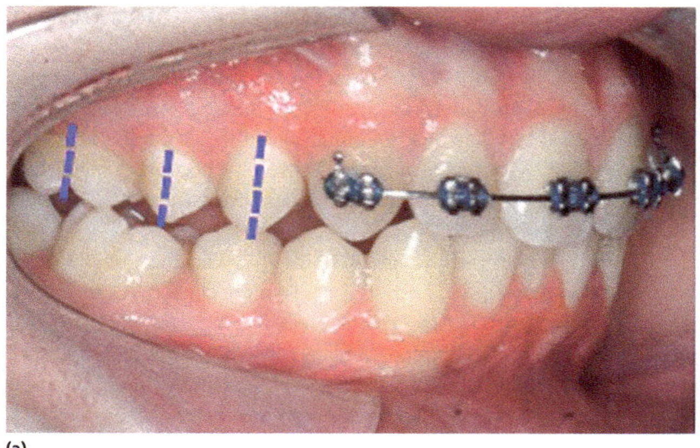
(a)

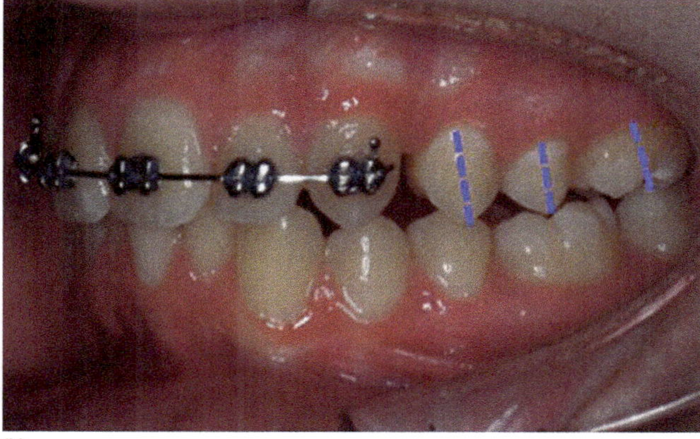
(b)

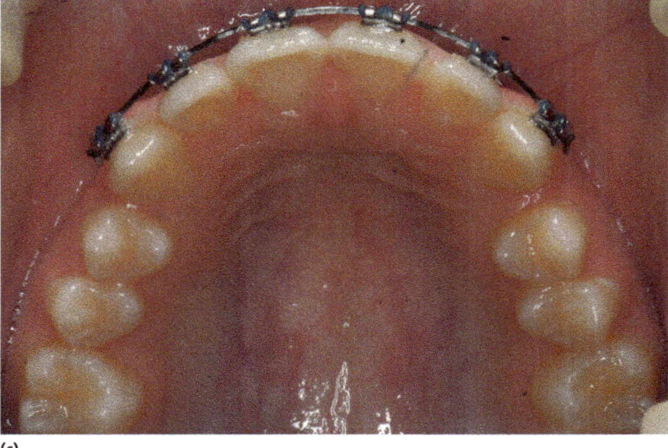
(c)

Figure 8.8 Pronounced distal tipping of the maxillary posterior teeth has occurred, manifesting as space posterior to the maxillary canines allied to the distal angulation of the maxillary premolars and first molars (a–c).

References

1. Proffit WR. The timing of early treatment: An overview. Am J Orthod Dentofacial Orthop. 2006; 129: S47–S49.
2. Efstratiadis S, Baumrind S, Shofer F, Jacobsson-Hunt U, Laster L, Ghafari J. Evaluation of Class II treatment by cephalometric regional superpositions versus conventional measurements. Am J Orthod Dentofacial Orthop. 2005; 128: 607–18.
3. Björk A, Skieller V. Normal and abnormal growth of the mandible: A synthesis of longitudinal cephalometric implant studies over a period of 25 years. Eur J Orthod. 1983; 5: 1–46.
4. Cook PA, Southall PJ. The reliability of mandibular radiographic superimposition. Br J Orthod. 1989; 16: 25–30.
5. Pancherz H. The mechanism of Class II correction in Herbst appliance treatment: A cephalometric investigation. Am J Orthod. 1982; 82: 104–13.
6. Feldmann I, Bondemark L. Anchorage capacity of osseointegrated and conventional anchorage systems: A randomized controlled trial. Am J Orthod Dentofacial Orthop. 2008; 133: 339. e19–e28.
7. Houston WJ, Lee RT. Accuracy of different methods of radiographic superimposition on cranial base structures. Eur J Orthod. 1985; 7: 127–35.
8. Fleming PS, Scott P, DiBiase AT. Managing the transition from functional to fixed appliances. J Orthod. 2007; 34: 252–9.
9. McNamara JA Jr. Components of Class II malocclusion in children 8–10 years of age. Angle Orthod. 1981; 51:177–202.
10. Ozturk Y, Tankuter N. Class II: A comparison of activator and activator headgear combination appliances. Eur J Orthod. 1994; 16: 149–57.
11. Mills CM, McCullough KJ. Posttreatment changes after successful correction of Class II malocclusions with the twin block appliance. Am J Orthod Dentofacial Orthop. 2000; 118: 24–33.
12. Cozza P, Baccetti T, Franchi L, De Toffol L, McNamara JA. Mandibular changes produced by functional appliances in Class II malocclusion: A systematic review. Am J Orthod Dentofacial Orthop. 2006; 129: 599.e1–e12.
13. O'Brien K, Macfarlane T, Wright J, Conboy F, Appelbe P et al. Early treatment for Class II malocclusion and perceived improvements in facial profile. Am J Orthod Dentofacial Orthop. 2009; 135: 580–85.
14. Ruf S, Pancherz H. The mechanism of Class II correction during Herbst therapy in relation to the vertical jaw base relationship: A cephalometric roentgenographic study. Angle Orthod. 1997; 67: 271–6.
15. Cureton SL, Regennitter FJ, Yancey JM. Clinical versus quantitative assessment of headgear compliance. Am J Orthod Dentofacial Orthop. 1993; 104: 277–84.

16. Brandao M, Pinho HS, Urias D. Clinical and quantitative assessment of headgear compliance: A pilot study. Am J Orthod Dentofacial Orthop. 2006; 129: 239–44.
17. Wiltshire WA, Tsang S. A modern rationale for orthopedics and orthodontic retention. Semin Orthod. 2006; 12: 60–66.
18. Proffit WR, Frazier-Bowers SA. Mechanism and control of tooth eruption: Overview and clinical implications. Orthod Craniofac Res. 2009; 12: 59–66.
19. Igarishi K, Miyoshi K, Shinoda H, Saeki S, Mitani H. Diurnal variation in tooth movement in response to orthodontic force in rats. Am J Orthod Dentofacial Orthop. 1998; 114: 8–14.
20. Read MJ, Deacon S, O'Brien K. A prospective cohort study of a clip-on fixed functional appliance. Am J Orthod Dentofacial Orthop. 2004; 125: 444–9.
21. Read MJF. The integration of functional and fixed appliance treatment. J Orthod. 2001; 28: 13–18.
22. Pancherz H. Treatment of class II malocclusions by jumping the bite with the Herbst appliance: A cephalometric investigation. Am J Orthod. 1979; 76: 423–42.
23. Bass NM, Bass A. The Dynamax system: A new orthopedic appliance. J Clin Orthod. 2003; 37: 268–77.
24. Weiland FJ, Ingervall B, Bantleon HP, Droacht H. Initial effects of treatment of Class II malocclusion with the Herren activator, activator-headgear combination, and Jasper Jumper. Am J Orthod Dentofacial Orthop. 1997; 112: 19–27.
25. Coelho Filho CM. Mandibular protraction appliances for Class II treatment. J Clin Orthod. 1995; 29: 319–36.
26. Sandler J, DiBiase D. The inclined biteplane: A useful tool. Am J Orthod Dentofacial Orthop. 1996; 110: 339–50.
27. Ross VA, Isaacson RJ, Germane N, Rubenstein LK. Influence of vertical growth pattern on faciolingual inclinations and treatment mechanics. Am J Orthod Dentofacial Orthop. 1990; 98: 422–9.
28. Knosel M, Kubein-Meesenburg D, Sadat-Khonsari R. The third-order angle and the maxillary incisor's inclination to the NA line. Angle Orthod. 2007; 77: 82–7.
29. Tulloch JF, Phillips C, Koch G, Proffit WR. The effect of early intervention on skeletal pattern in Class II malocclusion: A randomized clinical trial. Am J Orthod Dentofacial Orthop. 1997; 111: 391–400.
30. Kirschen RH, O'Higgins EA, Lee RT. The Royal London space planning: An integration of space analysis and treatment planning: Part I: Assessing the space required to meet treatment objectives. Am J Orthod Dentofacial Orthop. 2000; 118: 448–55.
31. Lund DJ, Sandler PJ. The effects of Twin Block: A prospective controlled study. Am J Orthod Dentofacial Orthop. 1988; 113: 104–10.
32. Pancherz H, Malmgren O, Hagg U, Omblus J, Hansen K. Class II correction in Herbst and Bass therapy. Eur J Orthod. 1989; 11: 17–30.
33. Mills JR. The long-term results of the proclination of lower incisors. Br Dent J. 1966; 120: 355–63.
34. Mittal M, Thiruvenkatachari B, Sandler PJ, Benson PE. A three-dimensional comparison of torque achieved with a preadjusted Edgewise appliance using a Roth or MBT prescription. Angle Orthod. 2015; 85: 292–7.

CHAPTER 9

The use of functional appliances in the correction of Class III malocclusion

Andrew DiBiase

The use of functional appliances is synonymous with the treatment of an increased overjet and a Class II malocclusion. This, however, does not mean that they have not been used in the treatment of Class III malocclusion. Indeed, for every functional appliance for Class II correction, there is usually a version for the treatment of Class III malocclusion. Many have been described, but few are routinely used. There are many reasons for this that will be explored in this chapter.

In Western societies, Class III malocclusion has a much lower prevalence than Class II, making up less than 5% of the population.[1, 2] This means that generally there is less demand and experience of treatment for this type of malocclusion. However, in East Asian societies such as China, Japan and Korea, Class III is far more prevalent.[3] Consequently, numerous modalities of Class III correction have emanated from this region or have been popularized by researchers there, with varying degrees of short- and long-term success.

Aetiology of Class III malocclusion

The majority of Class II malocclusions have a degree of mandibular retrognathia and are therefore amenable to correction with a functional appliance.[4] However, Class III malocclusion is not a single entity, but rather a range with significant variation in patterns of skeletal presentation in both the antero-posterior and vertical planes. Comparing a sample of 144 Class III malocclusions to a Class I sample matched for age and gender from the Bolton–Brush Growth study, Guyer and co-workers[5] found considerable skeletal variability in the Class III group, with the following features being exhibited on cephalometric analysis:

- Mandibular prognathism alone 18.7%
- Maxillary retrusion alone 25%
- Maxillary retrusion/mandibular protrusion 22%
- Increased lower anterior face height 41%

The Class III sample also had longer cranial bases, larger gonial angles, longer mandibles, maxillary incisor protrusion and mandibular incisor retrusion compared to the Class I sample.[5] Clearly, children and adolescents with Class III malocclusion do not have a typical skeletal phenotype.[6, 7]

The treatment of Class III malocclusion in growing patients is further complicated by growth potential, which is usually unfavourable. Unlike Class II malocclusions, which tend to improve skeletally with growth, a Class III malocclusion if allowed to develop will become worse with age, with the growth of the mandible exceeding the growth of the maxilla.[8, 9] This growth can also occur late in adolescence or even in early adulthood, particularly in relation to mandibular prognathism.[10] Therefore, there is the risk that even in cases that are successfully treated, the Class III growth pattern may re-establish itself.[11]

Early treatment

The chosen treatment modality for any orthodontic problem should be primarily based on the aetiology of the presenting malocclusion; this principle also applies to Class III malocclusion. Therefore, in a case with maxillary hypoplasia, treatment should ideally be geared at advancing the maxilla. In a case with mandibular prognathism, treatment should be directed at controlling mandibular growth and ideally even setting the mandible back. Of course, effecting skeletal change with orthodontic treatment is very difficult, and there is little or no evidence that any modality of treatment will have a long-term effect on growth. There is also the added problem in Class III cases with mandibular prognathism that the growth will often continue into late adolescence and even early adulthood. Unlike Class II cases where any mandibular growth is welcome and indeed implicit in the correction, in Class III cases it can mean that patients will outgrow early treatment. Collectively, these factors make the decision in terms of whether and when to address a Class III malocclusion with an underlying skeletal base discrepancy very difficult. There have been attempts to define skeletal and cephalometric parameters as possible limits of orthodontic correction.[12–14] However, while forming a useful guide, treatment decisions cannot be based on arbitrary

Orthodontic Functional Appliances: Theory and Practice, First Edition. Padhraig Fleming and Robert Lee.

cephalometric values alone, due to the variability and unpredictability of growth in Class III malocclusion and other parameters that may affect the prognosis for successful outcome.

If early treatment is attempted, it is advisable for this to take place in late childhood before adolescent growth. This is to take advantage of the greater pre-adolescent growth of the maxilla compared to the mandible and to correct any anterior crossbites, particularly if there is associated functional displacement. Compliance with treatment at this age is usually good if clear instructions and short-term goals are given.

Mechanisms of Class III correction

Numerous techniques have been described for early Class III correction, including the use of functional appliances, which is indicative of the uncertainty and problems associated with the treatment of Class III malocclusions. Other techniques include:

- Protraction headgear
- Chin caps
- Bone anchored maxillary protraction (BAMP)

Theoretically, in cases with mandibular prognathism, treatment should be directed at restriction or redirection of any further mandibular growth. While there is some weak evidence that chin caps can have some skeletal effect, mandibular growth occurs throughout adolescence and beyond, particularly in cases of mandibular prognathism.[15] Therefore, to be truly effective the chin cap would ideally need to be worn throughout this period, which is not practical or realistic. In cases of maxillary hypoplasia, treatment aimed at protracting the maxilla should be prescribed. This includes the use of protraction headgear, which in the short to medium term has been demonstrated to have a skeletal effect on the maxilla.[16, 17] More recently, BAMP has shown very promising results, with greater protraction of the maxilla than with protraction headgear alone.[18] Advocates of certain functional appliance systems have similarly claimed a skeletal effect on the maxilla, as will be discussed, but there is a lack of evidence for this.[19] Moreover, there is also a lack of high-quality research to demonstrate a meaningful skeletal effect on the mandible, with just seven cohort studies identified in a recent meta-analysis relating to the Fränkel 3 appliance, suggesting a reduction in SNB of up to 1.5 degrees in the long term.[19] In view of the absence of randomized studies with a lower risk of bias and matched contemporaneous controls, it is likely that this difference is somewhat inflated. The effects of functional appliances in Class III correction, therefore, appear to be primarily dento-alveolar, namely:

- Proclination of the upper incisors
- Retroclination of the lower incisors
- Downward and backward rotation of the mandible
- Increase in lower anterior face height

The advantage of treatment with a functional appliance is less social compromise compared with any form of headgear or chin cap, although appreciable levels of compliance are still needed. While the use of BAMP offers the possibility of more significant maxillary protraction, with forward movement of 3.7 mm recorded in an analysis of 25 consecutive cases,[20] it usually requires two episodes of surgery to place and remove the plates, with the associated morbidity and risk. Therefore, the use of a functional appliance is relatively simple, cost effective and has relatively low risk and morbidity.

Case selection

Assuming that the effects of Class III functional appliances are predominantly dento-alveolar with negligible capacity to alter growth in the medium to long term, the aim of functional appliance treatment is to create a positive overjet at the end of the treatment. The stability of crossbite correction will also be helped by the presence of a positive overbite at the end of treatment. Therefore, the ideal Class III case for correction with a functional appliance will have the following features:

- Mild to moderate skeletal III relationship
- Average to reduced lower face height and Frankfurt–mandibular planes angle
- Anterior crossbite with displacement from centric relation to centric occlusion
- Average or increased overbite
- Upright or retroclined maxillary incisors
- Upright or proclined mandibular incisors

A case like this is often described as 'pseudo-Class III' because it essentially has a skeletal I relationship, which becomes skeletal III as the mandible displaces forwards on occluding from a centric relationship to centric occlusion. Such cases are usually amenable to correction, by elimination of the crossbite and functional displacement.

Treatment is usually undertaken in the early mixed dentition following the establishment of a Class III incisor relationship secondary to the eruption of the permanent incisors. This theoretically takes advantage of the potential for greater growth of the maxilla than the mandible during the pre-pubertal period, while also eliminating any functional displacements before they become established.

Functional appliances for Class III correction

Fränkel functional regulator 3 (FR3)

This is probably the most easily recognized and commonly used functional appliance for Class III correction. It is a soft tissue–borne appliance that consists of a wire framework to which are attached acrylic pads and shields designed to displace the soft tissues and muscles that restrict maxillary development (Figure 9.1). The vestibular shields in the FR3 appliance, as with the FR2, are positioned buccally, extending from the depth of the sulci to displace the force of the buccinators and the perioral muscles away from the dentition. The labial pads are situated in

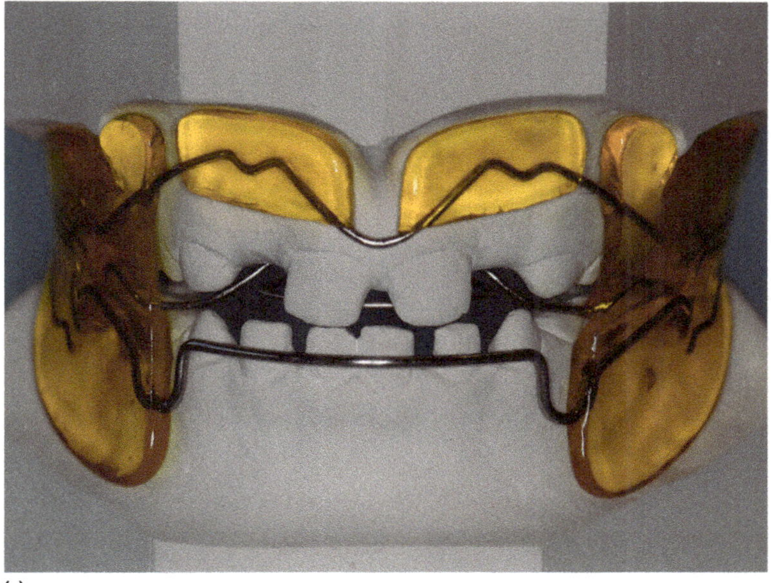

(a)

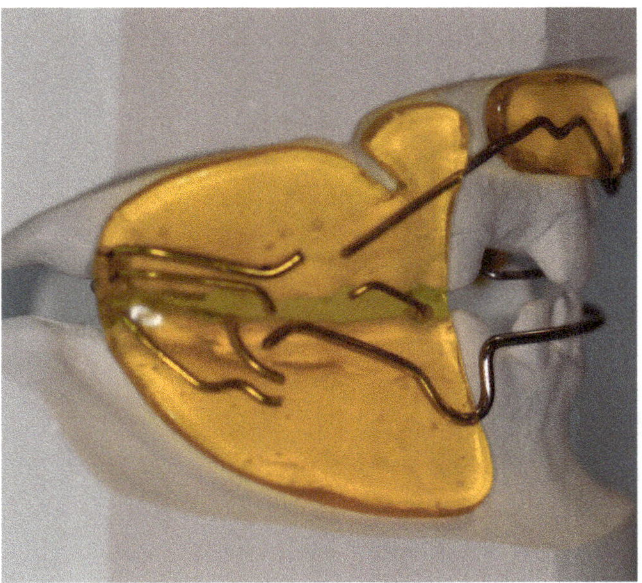

(b)

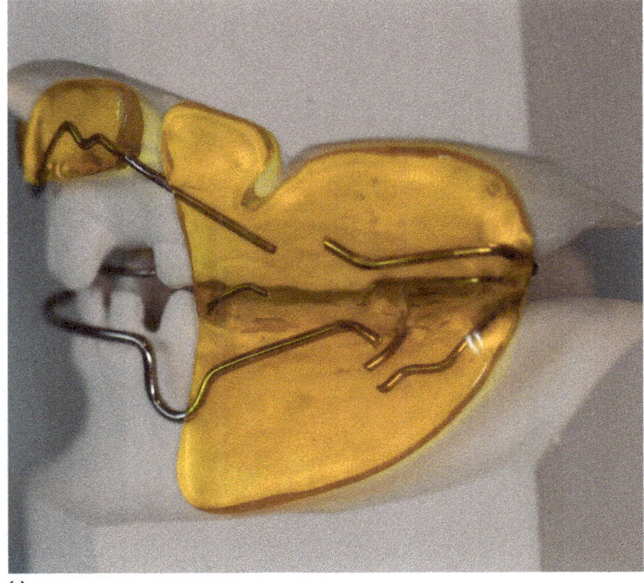

(c)

Figure 9.1 Fränkel functional regulator (a–g). The FR3 complemented Fränkel's other designs, with the underlying principles including the centrality of the soft tissues to malocclusion and the importance of ensuring normal soft tissue behaviour. The upper labial pad is designed to act in a similar way to the lower labial palots, with periosteal stretching and modulation of the influence of the upper lip on the maxillary incisors. Moreover, the forces from the upper lip were designed to be transmitted through the appliance to the lower arch and dentition, as Fränkel aimed to limit the contact between the appliance and the upper arch. The anterior trans-palatal wire rests on the cingulum of the maxillary incisors with U-loops; it should lie below the maxillary occlusal plane as it crosses the upper arch, so as not to interfere with downward and forward development of the maxillary arch. It is made in 0.8 mm spring hard stainless steel. The posterior trans-palatal wire is made in 1.2 mm wire to afford sufficient rigidity. Its distal extension is posterior to the terminal molar to limit interference with forward maxillary development and finishes in the buccal shields. There are maxillary molar occlusal rests in 1 mm spring hard stainless steel, which also enter the plate distally. There is a labial arch in 0.9 mm spring hard stainless steel, which carries the two labial palots. It is important that the wire is kept straight in the tag portion for ease of re-activation of the appliance. The lower half incorporates a 1.2 mm spring hard stainless steel labial bow and occlusal rests on the lower first molars in 1 mm spring hard stainless steel. There is 3 mm relief for the upper half of the buccal shields, while no relief is built into the lower shields to lock the lower arch both transversely and in the antero-posterior dimension. The relief for the upper labial palots is also 3 mm.

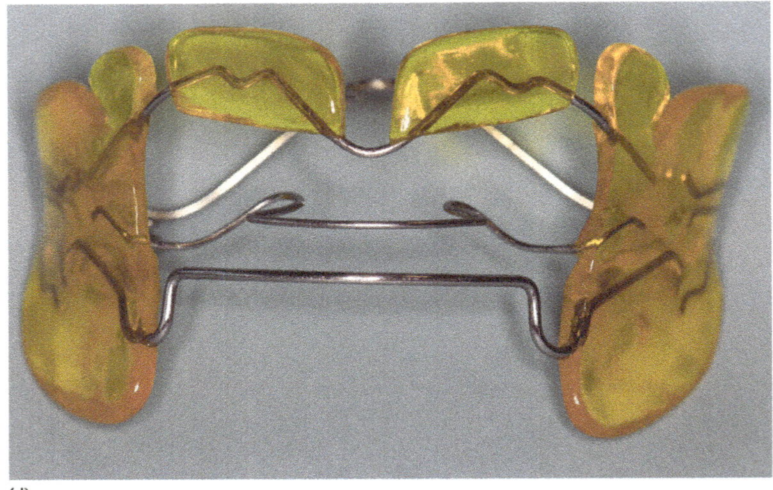

(d)

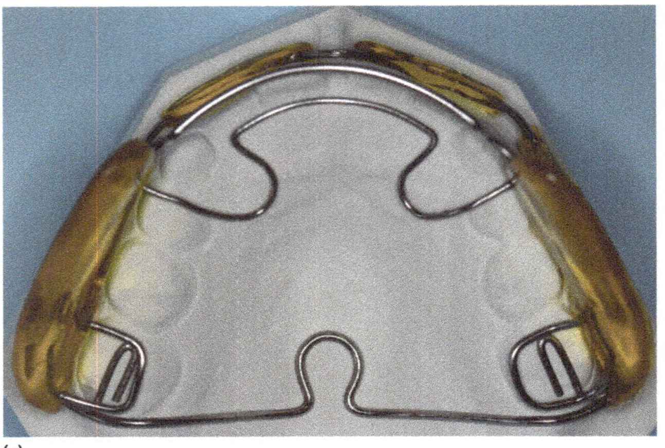

(e)

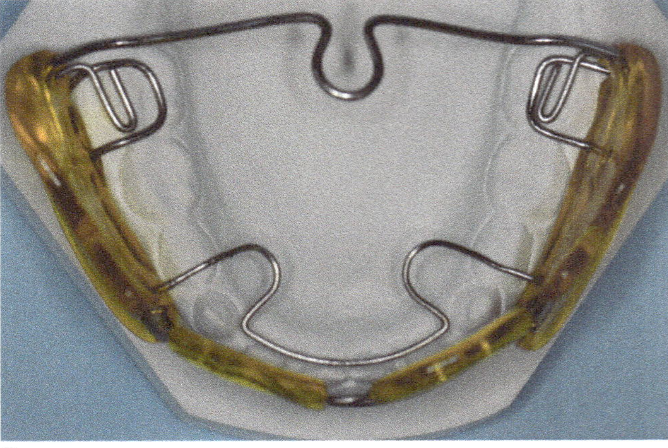

(f)

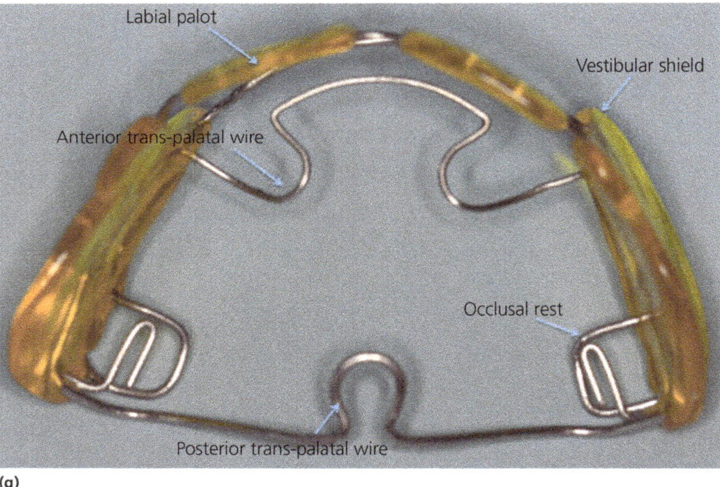

(g)

Figure 9.1 (*Continued*)

the upper labial vestibule above the teeth and extended to remove the force of the upper lip from the maxilla.

The appliance is constructed such that the sulci are extended to theoretically stretch the periosteum, stimulating bony apposition on the labial surface of the maxillary alveolus. The labial pads are connected to the vestibular shields by either a single wire or three separate wires. In this way the force from the upper lip is transferred to the vestibular shield and in turn to the mandible, potentially restricting its growth while encouraging that of the maxilla. A lower labial wire rests against the labial surfaces of the lower incisors while an upper lingual wire rests behind the upper incisors. The vestibular shields are also connected by a palatal wire passing behind the terminal upper molar. There are either one or two occlusal rests present on both sides: a lower one that extends from the vestibular shield onto the occlusal surface of the lower first permanent molar, and an upper one that extends onto the upper first permanent molar. These are included to prevent overeruption of the molars. The lower wire is recommended in the treatment of all Class III cases, while the upper wire is recommended for cases with an anterior open bite.

Construction and clinical management

The appliance is made on plaster models from impressions capturing the full sulcus depth buccally and in the upper labial segment to accommodate the vestibular shields and labial pads. The bite registration is taken with the mandible in the most retruded position achievable without causing discomfort. This can be reached by the orthodontist placing their thumb on the mandible with the patient's mouth partially open, and applying gentle pressure. The bite should be taken with a minimal opening of 1–2 mm. The models are trimmed and mounted on a simple hinge articulator.

The position of the vestibular shields and labial pads is marked on the models and wax relief applied. The wire components are then fabricated. The lower labial and palatal wires are constructed in 0.40 inch wire, while the lower arch labial wire is typically 0.28–0.32 inches in dimension. The lower occlusal wire is fabricated from 0.30 inch steel. The acrylic components are then constructed and the appliance trimmed.

The appliance should ultimately be worn on a full-time basis, but most patients will require a gradual period of wear to adjust (Figure 9.2). It should not be worn for eating, sports, language lessons, playing musical instruments or oral hygiene measures. After a few months of full-time wear, the distance between the labial pads and the underlying alveolus will decrease and the appliance will require re-activation. This is undertaken by removing the acrylic from around the wire supporting the labial pads so that it can be slid forwards until the pads sit 3 mm labial to the alveolus. This degree of clearance should be maintained throughout treatment.

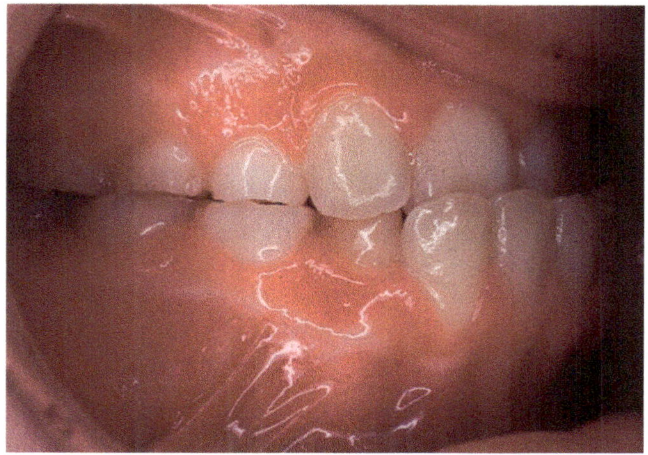
(a)

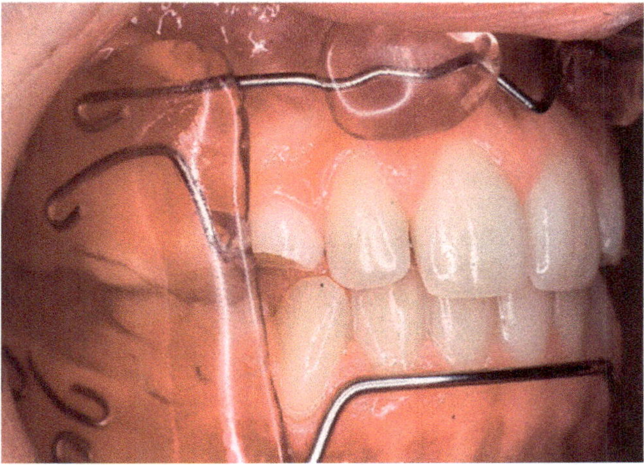
(b)

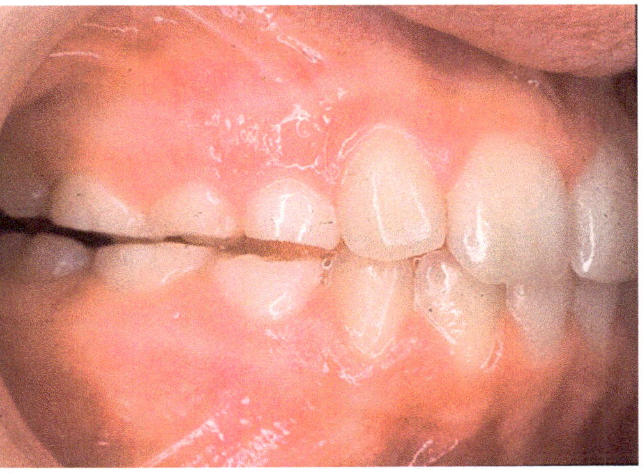
(c)

Figure 9.2 Correction of Class III malocclusion with Fränkel functional regulator 3.

Effects of the FR3 appliance

Fränkel published the results of a case series of patients treated with the FR3 appliance. He found that there was forward movement of the A point, from which he concluded that the appliance had a skeletal effect on the maxilla.[21] This was supported by a later series of cases he treated that were compared to untreated Class III malocclusions selected from two growth studies.[22] Other work has, however, shown little or no lasting skeletal effect. Indeed, it appears that the effect of the appliance is essentially dento-alveolar, proclining the upper incisors and leading to retroclination of the lower (Figure 9.3). Following correction of the anterior crossbite and elimination of any associated functional anterior displacement, a downward and backward rotation of the mandible may occur.[19,23,24] This in turn results in a reduction in cephalometric values indicative of mandibular prognathism, such as the Sella-Nasion-B point (SNB); these changes can be misinterpreted as an appliance-related effect on the growth of the mandible. However, like much research in the area of functional appliance therapy and growth modifications, the published research on the FR3 appliance is primarily retrospective in nature, consisting of cohort studies that lack matched or indeed contemporaneous controls. Therefore, this research is typically open to significant confounding related to differences in prospective growth, age and degree of maturation and vertical relationships, allied to a lack of consistency in terms of treatment protocols.

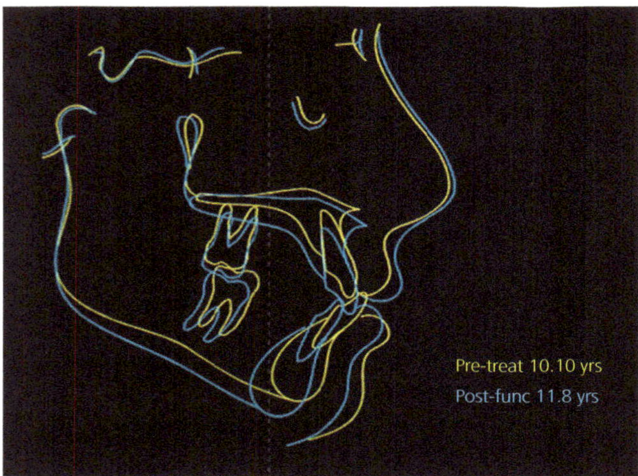

Figure 9.3 Superimposition of pre- and post-treatment lateral cephalograms for case shown in Figure 9.2.

Reverse Twin Block appliance

The Twin Block appliance was originally described by William Clark and has proved a very popular functional appliance for Class II correction, particularly in the United Kingdom. This popularity relates to its simple design and underlying concept. It also tends to be robust and well tolerated, and can be worn in function without precluding speech or eating. It also has a very potent and efficient Class II effect, resulting in significant dento-alveolar results. Clark also described a version of the appliance for Class III correction, the basic premise of which is reversing the blocks so that the lower block occludes distal to the upper block (Figure 9.4).[25,26]

Construction and management

Impressions are taken in alginate from which the working models are cast. The functional bite is taken in maximum mandibular retrusion. At least 5 mm clearance is required buccally to allow for the vertical height of the blocks. Adams clasps are placed on the first molars and ball-ended clasps between the primary first and second molars. The retention of the lower appliance can be reinforced by the use of an acrylated lower labial bow. If activated, this will also help to retrocline the lower incisors. Cantilever or recurved springs can be placed behind the upper incisors to procline them. However, care should be taken not to overactivate these, as this will tend to displace the upper appliance. Alternatively, a split plate can be used with a screw behind the upper incisors. The upper appliance can also incorporate a midline screw, which can be turned twice a week

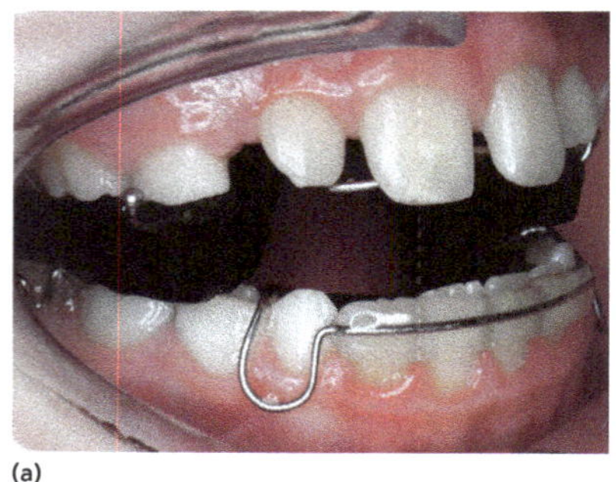
(a)

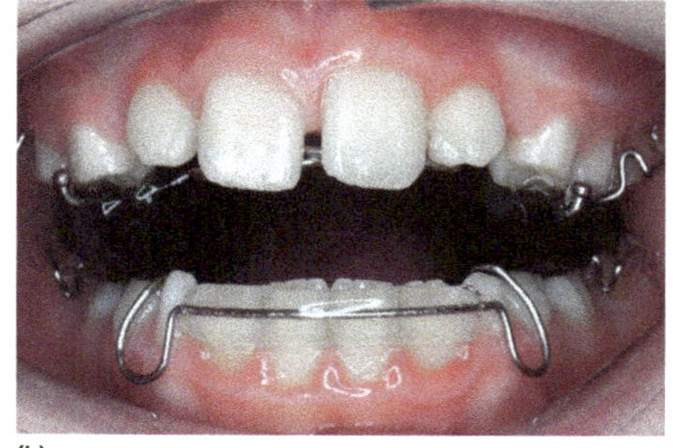
(b)

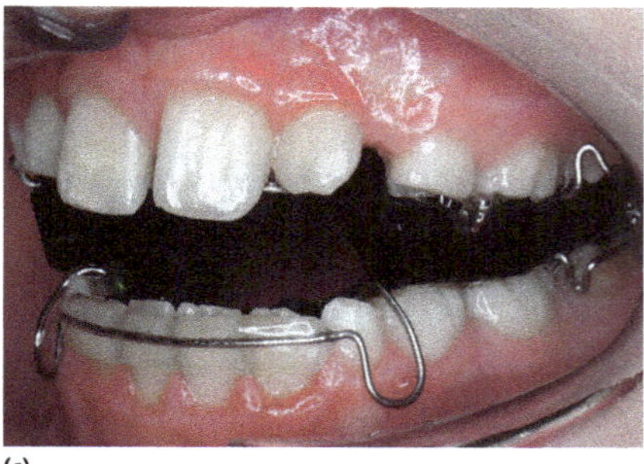
(c)

Figure 9.4 Reverse Twin Block appliance. Note that the lower block occludes distally to the upper block. A lower labial bow aids in retention of the lower appliance and springs have been placed palatal to the upper incisors to procline them.

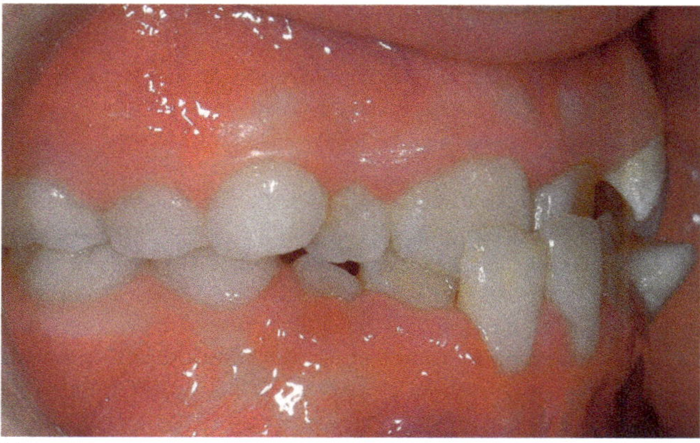

(a)

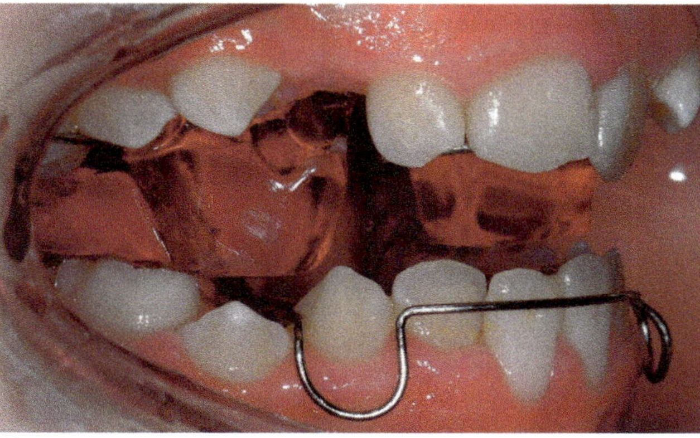

(b)

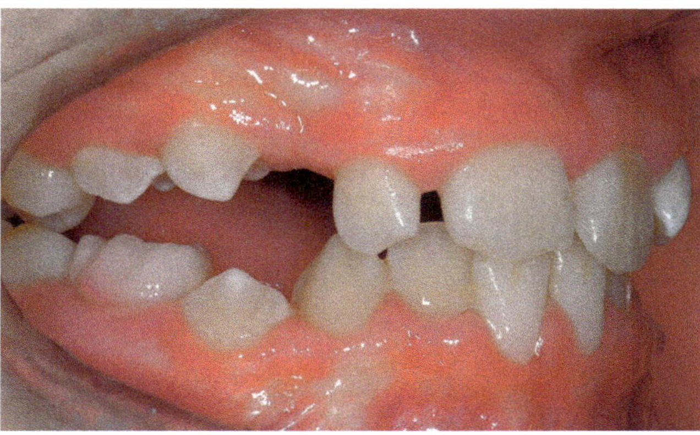

(c)

Figure 9.5 Correction of a Class III malocclusion with a reverse Twin Block appliance showing lateral open bites.

for arch coordination if necessary. The blocks themselves should be at least 5 mm high and inclined at 70 degrees to the occlusal plane, to encourage the patient to bite with the lower blocks behind the uppers.

The appliance is worn full time until a positive overjet and overbite are achieved. The patient can then wear the appliance at night to allow occlusal setting of the lateral open bites in the buccal segments (Figure 9.5).

Effects of reverse Twin Block

Like other functional appliances designed for Class III correction, the effects are primarily dento-alveolar and stability is dependent on obtaining a positive overjet and overbite as well as future growth. In a retrospective case series, Kidner et al.[27] showed that full-time wear of the appliance resulted in proclination of the upper incisors and retroclination of the lower, as well as a downward and backward rotation of the mandible. This resulted in an increase in lower anterior face height and a relative reduction in mandibular prognathism. These changes were achieved in just over 6 months, which is considerably faster than that reported with the FR3 appliance. However, the nature of the observed changes was largely in keeping with those seen with the FR3.

A further retrospective study involved comparison of the reverse Twin Block appliance and protraction headgear combined with rapid maxillary expansion (RME).[28] Both were effective treatment modalities for early correction of Class III malocclusion but, compared to the protraction headgear, the reverse Twin Block resulted chiefly in dento-alevolar changes, with greater proclination of the upper incisors and retroclination of the lower. Compared to an untreated control, the reverse Twin Block appliance was found to exert no skeletal effect on the maxilla in this study.

Summary

The effect of functional appliances in Class III correction appears to be dento-alveolar. In carefully selected cases this makes them very effective appliances. However, in Class III malocclusions with a significant skeletal component, especially mandibular prognathism, a hyperdivergent growth pattern and a reduced overbite, their use should be avoided. Moreover, if there is also already a significant degree of dento-alveolar compensation, with retroclination of the lower incisors and proclination of the upper, the use of a functional appliance will exacerbate this. A further risk associated with excessive proclination of the maxillary incisors, even if a positive overjet is achieved, is non-axial loading of the teeth with the associated risk of fremitus.

If there is any doubt, a different treatment modality with greater skeletal effect should be considered, such as protraction headgear or BAMP. Alternatively, treatment decisions should be delayed until adolescence, when the direction of growth is better understood.

References

1. Thilander B, Myrberg N. The prevalence of malocclusion in Swedish schoolchildren. Scand J Dental Res. 1973; 81: 12–21.
2. Foster TD, Day AJ. A survey of malocclusion and the need for orthodontic treatment in a Shropshire school population. Br J Orthod. 1974; 1: 73–8.

3. Tang EL. The prevalence of malocclusion amongst Hong Kong male dental students. Br J Orthod. 1994; 21: 57–63.
4. McNamara JA Jr. Components of Class II malocclusion in children 8–10 years of age. Angle Orthod. 1981; 51: 177–202.
5. Guyer EC, Ellis EC, McNamara JA, Behrents RG. Components of a Class II malocclusion in juveniles and adolescents. Angle Orthod. 1986; 56: 7–30.
6. Björk A, Skieller V. Normal and abnormal growth of the mandible: A synthesis of longitudinal cephalometric implant studies over a period of 25 years. Eur J Orthod. 1983; 5: 1–46.
7. Battagel JM. The aetiological factors in Class III malocclusion. Eur J Orthod. 1993; 15: 347–70.
8. Baccetti T, Reyes BC, McNamara JA Jr. Craniofacial changes in Class III malocclusion as related to skeletal and dental maturation. Am J Orthod Dentofac Orthop. 2007; 132: 171.e1–e12.
9. Wolfe SM, Araujo E, Behrents RG, Buschang PH. Craniofacial growth of Class III subjects six to sixteen years of age. Angle Orthod. 2011; 81: 211–16.
10. Reyes BC, Baccetti T, McNamara JA. An estimate of craniofacial growth in Class III malocclusion. Angle Orthod. 2006; 76: 577–84.
11. Wendell PD, Nanda R. The effects of chin cup therapy on the mandible: A longitudinal study. Am J Orthod Dentofac Orthop. 1985; 87: 265–74.
12. Burns NR, Musich DR, Martin C, Razmus T, Ngan P. Class III camouflage: What are the limits? Am J Orthod Dentofacial Orthop. 2010; 137: 9.e1–e13.
13. Schuster G, Lux CJ, Stellzig-Eisenhauer A. Children with Class III malocclusion: Development of multivariate statistical models to predict future needs for orthognathic surgery. Angle Orthod. 2003; 73: 135–45.
14. Kerr WJ, Miller S, Dawber JE. Class III malocclusion: Surgery or orthodontic? Br J Orthod. 1992; 19: 21–4.
15. Zurfluh MA, Kloukos D, Patcas R, Eliades T. Effect of chin-cup treatment on the temporomandibular joint: A systematic review. Eur J Orthod. 2015; 37: 314–24.
16. Mandall N, DiBiase A, Littlewood S, Nute S, Stivaros N et al. Is early Class III protraction facemask treatment effective? A multicentre, randomized, controlled trial: 15-month follow-up. J Orthod. 2010; 37: 149–61.
17. Mandall N, Cousley R, Dyer F, Littlewood S, Mattick R et al. Is early Class III protraction facemesk treatment effective? A multicentre, randomized, controlled trial: 3-year follow-up. J Orthod. 2012; 39: 176–85.
18. De Clerck H, Cevidanes L, Baccetti T. Dentofacial effects of bone-anchored maxillary protraction: A controlled study of consecutively treated Class III patients. Am J Orthod Dentofacial Orthop. 2010; 138: 577–81.
19. Yang X, Li C, Bai D, Su N, Chen T et al. Treatment effectiveness of Fränkel function regulator on Class III malocclusion: A systematic review and meta-analysis. Am J Orthod Dentofacial Orthop. 2014; 146: 143–54.
20. Nguyen T, Cevidanes L, Cornelis MA, Heymann G, de Paula LK, De Clerck H. Three-dimensional assessment of maxillary changes associated with bone anchored maxillary protraction. Am J Orthod Dentofacial Orthop. 2011; 140: 790–98.
21. Fränkel R. Maxillary retrusion in Class III and treatment with function corrector III. Trans Eur Orthod Soc. 1970; 46: 249–59.
22. Levin AS, McNamara JA, Franchi L, Baccetti T, Fränkel C. Short-term and long-term treatment outcomes with the FR-3 appliance of Fränkel. Am J Orthod Dentofacial Orthop. 2008; 134: 513–24.
23. Loh MK, Kerr WJS. The function regulator III: Effects and indications for use. Br J Orthod. 1985; 12: 153–7.
24. Ülgen M, Firatli S. The effects of Fränkel's function regulator on the Class III malocclusion. Am J Orthod Dentofac Orthop. 1994; 105: 561–7.
25. Clark WJ. Treatment of Class III Malocclusion: Twin Block Functional Therapy Application in Dentofacial Orthopaedics, 2nd ed. London: Mosby; 2002: 217–30.
26. Seehra J, Fleming PS, DiBiase AT. Reverse Twin Block appliance for early dental Class III correction. J Clin Orthod. 2010:44; 44: 602–10.
27. Kidner G, DiBiase AT, DiBiase DD. Class III Twin Blocks: A case series. J Orthod. 2003; 30: 197–201.
28. Seehra J, Fleming PS, Mandall N, DiBiase AT. A comparison of two different techniques for early correction of Class III malocclusion. Angle Orthod. 2012; 82: 96–101.

CHAPTER 10

Functional appliances: A focused review of the clinical evidence

There is a widespread consensus that orthodontic practice should be underpinned by best available evidence, providing patients with up-to-date treatment proven to be safe, effective and efficient. While evidence-based approaches are increasingly accepted, a limited knowledge of evidence sources, including the Cochrane database, and the low utility of established evidence portals have constrained their uptake.[1] The use of functional appliances is established among orthodontic practitioners.[2] However, as is typical of many aspects of dentistry and orthodontics, clinical processes and appliance design and modification have outpaced the underlying research base, with debate surrounding a range of aspects, including the effectiveness and timing of treatment in addition to the relative merits of various appliances.

Evidence-based care is ingrained within medicine and dentistry; research is now a fundamental pillar underpinning clinical decisions. Clinical research can be categorized into either non-randomized or randomized studies. Non-randomized studies include observational designs such as controlled clinical trials, cohort and case-control studies, case series and reports, cross-sectional and ecological studies (Table 10.1).[3] The key distinction between these designs is the random and unpredictable allocation of interventions by the investigator in randomized controlled trials (RCTs). The relative merits of both approaches have been contested; however, RCTs are accepted as the optimal design in the assessment of the efficacy and safety of a clinical intervention. Randomization allows for a 'fair' comparison, facilitating more assured deduction of causal inferences than is the case with non-randomized designs. For example, a comparison of the efficacy and safety of competing functional appliances may be undertaken within a randomized design, limiting the potential for selection bias, whereby compliant participants with favourable skeletal patterns might otherwise subconsciously be allocated to the preferred appliance in a non-randomized study. However, much of the debate concerning RCTs has surrounded their ability to produce lasting skeletal change. To investigate this question fully necessitates prolonged follow-up and may involve depriving patients of a potentially valuable intervention. The emergence of high-level evidence to address this and other questions was initially not forthcoming, therefore. However, over the past 20 years a body of prospective evidence concerning the effectiveness of functional appliances has begun to emerge.

The popularity of functional appliances has fluctuated over the past 100 years. In particular, they were initially espoused in Europe and had relatively little usage in the United States. However, over the past 20 years functional appliances have gained more traction in America.[2] Ironically, this change has arisen despite the emergence of evidence alluding to constraints in terms of growth modification with early treatment. A greater number of fixed functional appliances appear to be in use in the United States than is the case in the United Kingdom.[4] It is difficult to attribute these trends to the available evidence, although early cephalometric studies certainly indicated a limited capacity to modify growth in Class II malocclusion.[5]

These issues will be considered in this chapter in an evidence-based manner, with particular emphasis on high-level studies, including systematic reviews, randomized controlled trials and other prospective research studies based on an electronic database search (OVID via MEDLINE, see Appendix).

Levels of evidence and evidence-based dentistry

Evidence-based dentistry (EBD) has been described as an 'unbiased approach to oral health care that follows a process of systematically collecting and analyzing scientific evidence with the objective of gaining useful decision making information with minimal bias'.[6] Current principles of evidence-based practice require an expert for quick and correct identification of the underlying condition; the use of the best available evidence; and consideration of patient choice and preference. High-quality meta-analyses and systematic reviews (SRs), or RCTs with very low risk of bias, constitute the higher levels of evidence. Conversely, while expert opinion is important in shaping clinical practice, it is afforded a low level of evidence. A number of SRs relating to the potential of functional appliance therapy to modify mandibular growth have been published. As is common in most studies, even those with higher levels of

Orthodontic Functional Appliances: Theory and Practice, First Edition. Padhraig Fleming and Robert Lee.

Table 10.1 Uses, advantages and disadvantages of case-control and cohort studies.

Characteristic	Cohort studies	Case-control studies
Outcome	Common outcome Multiple outcomes for one exposure	Rare outcome and outcomes with long latent periods
Exposure	Efficient for rare exposures Good information on exposures	Can evaluate multiple exposures for a single outcome
Bias	Less vulnerable to bias Selection and information bias*	More vulnerable to bias Selection and information bias
Types of bias	Attrition bias Confounding Easier to establish sequence of events (i.e. exposure may be the result of the outcome)	No attrition bias Confounding Harder to establish sequence of events (i.e. exposure may be the result of the outcome)
Duration	Long	Quicker
Cost	Expensive	Less expensive

* Information bias refers to information collected on exposures and/or outcomes, and includes detection and recall bias.

evidence, these have had methodological limitations.[7] Notwithstanding this, the consistent message has been that these appliances are capable of short-term elongation of the mandible and limited maxillary growth restraint.

While the results of low-quality evidence have often led to important developments and discoveries, the results from high-quality studies are afforded greater weight in respect of decision making, as there are fewer associated risks.[8] Systematic reviews aim to assimilate the available evidence in a systematic, transparent and unbiased manner and, where applicable, to pool results from individual studies. High-quality RCTs should form the basis for systematic reviews of treatment interventions.

Primary study design (randomized and non-randomized studies)

RCTs involve a control group and randomization to assign participants to treatment arms, and aim to create similar treatment groups in all respects (known and unknown factors) other than the intervention. The use of a control group ensures that the treatment outcome is unrelated to natural improvement, selection of patients expected to do well (selection bias) or biased follow-up (performance bias) and outcome recording (observer bias) by the investigator and/or the participant (Table 10.2).

While RCTs constitute the highest level of evidence for assessing causality, it is not always possible or ethical to conduct such a trial. For example, if we wish to compare the effects of a functional appliance to no active treatment in age- and gender-matched groups in adolescence, an RCT would be considered unethical, as it would likely involve depriving deserving patients of a beneficial treatment. Alternatives, involving historical control groups or contemporary controls undergoing some other form of active treatment, may therefore be considered. Non-randomized studies are typically observational in nature. Observational studies are divided into three main categories: cross-sectional, case-control and cohort studies. In general, observational studies are more prone to bias and confounding compared to RCTs, with causality harder to assert. Observational studies are used extensively to describe the distribution of disease and exposure in populations and for hypothesis generation; where possible, hypotheses may be further assessed within randomized controlled trials. Conversely, although highly controlled and likely to be less biased due to performance in highly selected settings, RCTs may yield less pragmatic results that are of lower external validity (generalizability) to other populations and settings. Cohort studies generally include a wider, more heterogeneous population and are more representative of real life. Large clinical trials, however, can provide a high-quality data source that may be relevant if the prognostic model is applied to the patient population specified by the trial. In the context of functional appliance therapy, it is noteworthy that early observational studies may have led to exaggerated estimates of the potency of these appliances in terms of skeletal change.[9]

Research concerning the effectiveness of functional appliance therapy is complicated by a number of factors:

- Ethical concerns: The relative value of functional appliance therapy may be difficult to compare to alternatives, in view of the importance of growth to the achievement of a successful outcome. Randomly allocating subjects either to receive or not receive a functional appliance may result in a subset of participants missing an opportunity to have non-surgical correction of a malocclusion with a skeletal element. Consequently, non-randomized studies of participants treated during the pre-pubertal growth spurt may be required from an ethical viewpoint. Alternatively, assessment of the effectiveness of early interceptive correction of Class II malocclusion may be undertaken, given the safety net of offering later treatment in the pre-pubertal period should the control group be deprived of initial therapy.
- Need for long-term follow-up: Evaluation of the prolonged effects of functional appliance therapy on the skeletal pattern

Table 10.2 Types of bias encountered in randomized controlled trials.

Type of bias	Explanation	Remedies
Selection bias	Assigning patients in a way that proves preconceived beliefs	Appropriate randomization
Performance bias	Closer follow-up of patients in the treatment group favoured by the investigator	Standardization of procedures Personnel training Blinding, if feasible
Detection bias	Recording outcomes in a way that proves investigator's and/or participant's beliefs	Standardization of procedures Personnel training Blinding, if feasible
Attrition bias	Large and unequal loss to follow-up associated with intervention/outcome	Measures to reduce losses Blinding, if feasible Intention to treat (ITT) analysis
Publication bias	Selective reporting of only statistically significant or 'interesting' results	Trial registration Publication of trial protocol and reporting in accordance with protocol
Other biases	Associated with certain designs such as cluster randomized and cross-over (or split-mouth) trials	Avoid contact of cluster members Avoid carry-over effects

in particular necessitates prolonged follow-up. Consequently, RCTs may be onerous, time consuming and expensive. In addition, attrition of participants is problematic, necessitating large sample sizes and rigorous methodology in order to reduce losses to follow-up leading to attrition bias. Therefore, functional appliance research should include sample size estimation that makes provision for dropouts and analysis on an intention-to-treat basis to account for attrition bias. A further issue in relation to skeletal assessment is the ethical issue concerning radiographic assessment of patients who are no longer undergoing active treatment. Research investigating soft tissue changes using non-ionizing approaches is therefore optimal.

- Assessment of effectiveness of removable functional appliance therapy: The success of removable functional appliance therapy is dependent on patient compliance. Inclusion of objective measures to assess compliance is therefore important; unfortunately, doing this reliably may be costly and laborious. Differential loss to follow-up may result from differences in appliance design and be associated with lack of improvement, side effects or burden. Depending on the reasons for missing data, an intention-to-treat analysis is an accepted method for reducing the risk of associated bias stemming from attrition of participants. This approach may provide an indication of the effectiveness of the appliance, accounting for the propensity for unsuccessful treatment.

What are the short-term effects of functional appliances on the skeletal pattern?

The advent of cephalometry tempered earlier beliefs that orthodontics was capable of significant alteration to the skeletal pattern. Indeed, on the basis of research by Broadbent[5] and Brodie et al.,[10] it was concluded that the skeletal pattern was unalterable.[11] While debate continues in relation to the degree to which skeletal change persists following functional appliance therapy, prospective research has consistently alluded to a meaningful skeletal contribution to short-term changes. Johnston[12] has speculated that functional appliance therapy induces a temporary acceleration in mandibular growth rate allied to artificial forward positioning of the condyles in the glenoid fossae; these tendencies subside, meaning that the pre-ordained mandibular growth potential is ultimately not exceeded. Overall, the short-term effects of either fixed or removable functional appliances are both dento-alveolar and skeletal, with the relative contribution being greater in terms of dento-alveolar change with respect to overjet than is the case with molar correction. Broadly speaking, changes can be categorized as skeletal, encompassing maxillary restraint, mandibular growth acceleration and increased lower anterior facial height, and dento-alveolar.

Nelson and Harkness,[13] in a comparison of the Harvold appliance, the FR2 and an untreated control group, observed increases in both mandibular length (Ar-Pog) and gonial angle in the treated groups. Both appliances also resulted in significant increases in the lower anterior facial height, with vertical eruption of the molars. Overall, the authors were unable to prove that an increase in the size of the mandible was associated with treatment. They speculate, however, that changes occurring in the position of the condyle arose with treatment, although this assumption was based purely on cephalograms in the closed position. They could find no evidence that either appliance was capable of altering the size of the mandible, although detailed imaging of the temporo-mandibular joints was not undertaken. The radiographs were also taken in the closed position, further complicating accurate assessment.

O'Brien et al.[14] found that maxillary restraint accounted for just 13% (0.88 mm) of overjet reduction overall. Moreover, assessment of maxillary position is complex and usually relies on the A point, which is sensitive to dento-alveolar changes. It is therefore difficult to isolate the precise contribution of

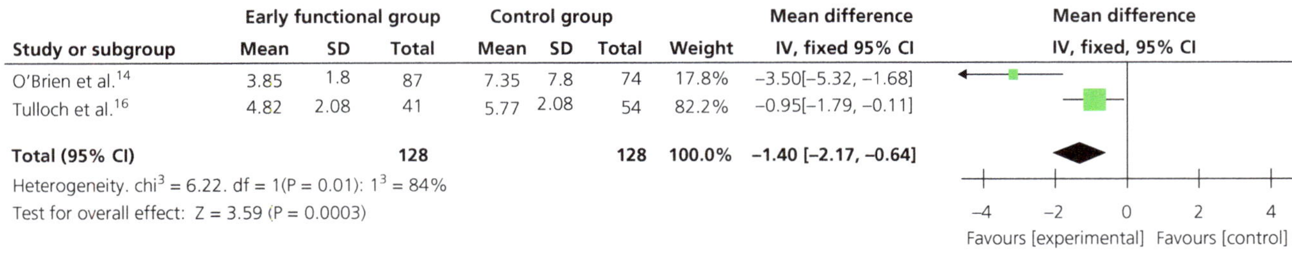

Figure 10.1 Change in ANB with early functional appliance treatment and untreated control group.

	Early headgear group			Control group				Mean difference
Study or subgroup	Mean	SD	Total	Mean	SD	Total	Weight	IV, fixed 95% CI
Mäntysaari et al.[18]	2.6	1.53	25	4.2	2.34	29	29.4%	−1.60[−2.64, −0.56]
Tulloch et al.[16]	4.83	1.5	52	5.7	2	54	70.6%	−0.87[−1.54, −0.20]
Total (95% CI)			77			83	100.0%	−1.08 [−1.65, −0.52]

Heterogeneity. chi^3 = 1.33. df = 1(P = 0.25): 1^3 = 25%
Test for overall effect: Z = 3.77 (P = 0.0002)

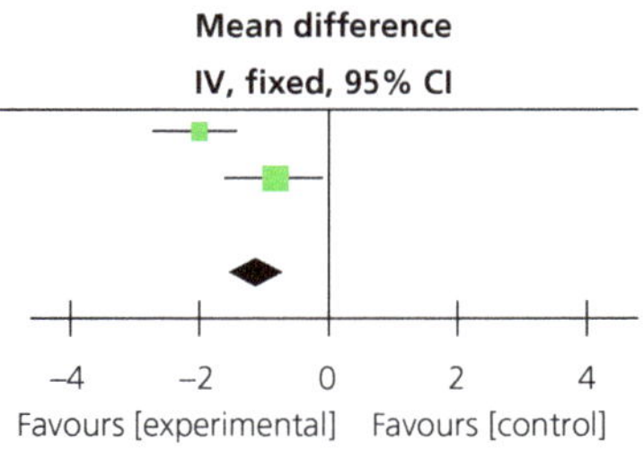

Mean difference IV, fixed, 95% CI: −4 −2 0 2 4; Favours [experimental] Favours [control]

Figure 10.2 Change in ANB with early headgear appliance treatment and untreated control group.

maxillary restraint to the overall correction of Class II malocclusion, although it does appear to be limited. Moreover, while efforts are made to improve skeletal II discrepancy with both sagittal and vertical restraint,[15] there remains limited prospective evidence that adjunctive use of extra-oral anchorage exerts a significant additive effect.

With respect to mandibular growth, early retrospective studies appear to have overstated the degree of additional growth engendered by functional appliance therapy. For example, Mills and McCulloch[9] reported an increase in mandibular growth of the order of 4.2 mm over a 14-month treatment period. In this study the treatment group was compared with an age- and gender-matched historical control group from the Burlington Growth Study. Prolonged follow-up for up to 3 years demonstrated that the majority of this additional growth was preserved in the treated group. Well-conducted prospective studies involving pre-adolescents have pointed to additional change of the order of just 1 mm with appliance therapy.[14, 16, 17] O'Brien et al.[14] therefore alluded to a cumulative antero-posterior skeletal contribution of 1.88 mm. While this is a limited degree of change, this additional growth does appear to be instrumental in producing occlusal change with functional appliance therapy.

Lower anterior facial height is known to increase with functional appliance therapy; in particular, facial height has typically been shown to increase in the region of 2–4 mm more than in untreated controls during adolescent therapy. This increase relates to the inclination of the occlusal plane, which is orientated inferiorly and anteriorly; consequently, with antero-posterior advancement of the lower arch related to postural changes and accelerated condylar growth, the lower facial height tends to increase.

Based on the literature search (Appendix), three studies considering the short-term effects of growth modification treatment with either early headgear or functional appliances for skeletal II correction[14, 16, 18] could be identified. A statistically significant decrease in ANB with functional appliance therapy compared to the control can be seen in the meta-analysis, with a mean reduction of 1.4 degrees (weighted mean difference [WMD]: -1.4, 95% confidence interval [CI]: -2.17, -0.64; Figure 10.1). The results were heavily weighted towards the Tulloch et al.[16] study (82.2%). The heterogeneity between the studies was high (I^2 =84%); therefore, the meta-analysis should be interpreted with caution. It does however confirm that functional appliance therapy is associated with at least a transitory degree of improvement in the skeletal pattern. When comparing the effects of functional therapy to intervention with headgear in a similar age group (prior to 11 years), a statistically significant mean reduction in the SNA of -1.33 degrees (WMD: -1.33, 95% CI: -1.68, -0.97) was found. Similarly, a reduction in the ANB was seen in both studies and the result was statistically significant (WMD: -1.08, 95% CI: -1.65, -0.52; Figure 10.2); however, there was a significant degree of statistical heterogeneity (I^2 =88%) given the relatively small sample size and limited number of studies.

What are the short-term effects of functional appliances on the dentition?

Functional appliances are proven to produce meaningful occlusal change, predominantly due to dento-alveolar change. In particular, the effect of postural change is to introduce a Class II effect on the dentition, resulting in maxillary incisor retroclination allied to distal tipping of the maxillary posteriors. In the mandibular arch, the reverse is true, with proclination of mandibular incisors and mesial tipping of the lower dentition.

Table 10.3 Maxillary incisor retroclination with functional appliances.

Author	Incisor modification	Incisor retroclination (degrees)
Illing et al.[22]	None	5.7
Mills and McCulloch[15]	None	5.6
Lund and Sandler[20]	Labial bow	10.8
Trenouth[23]	Labial bow	7.2
Harradine and Gale[19]	Labial bow	8.4
Gill et al.[24]	None	8

While the magnitude of dento-alveolar changes in the buccal segments has been difficult to quantify due to limitations in research techniques, including radiographic measurement techniques, the effects on the incisors are well known. O'Brien et al.[14] apportioned 44% of overjet reduction (3.03 mm) to maxillary incisor retroclination. Similarly, lower incisor proclination accounted for 2.03 mm (29%) of the overall change. Modifications to various appliances including torquing spurs[19] and labial bows[20, 21] have been introduced in an effort to modulate the relative proportion of dento-alveolar to skeletal change. Maxillary incisor retroclination of the order of 5–11 degrees, however, may be considered representative (Table 10.3). In terms of lower incisor proclination, modifications have been introduced to limit advancement of the incisors, as proclination is considered unstable. Moreover, if the duration of appliance wear is titrated against overjet and significant proclination occurs, dental changes may restrict the resultant amount of skeletal change.

Combining the results from primary studies identified in the literature search, a statistically significant reduction in overjet was found with appliance therapy (WMD: -5.80, 95% CI: -6.36, -5.24). These results therefore confirm the propensity of functional appliances to reduce overjets very effectively in growing patients. Comparing these dento-alveolar changes with functional therapy to dental changes with early use of headgear, functional appliances appear to be considerably more effective, with Mäntysaari et al.[18] failing to identify a significant difference in overjet reduction at 2-year follow-up with use of headgear. Similarly, Tulloch et al.[16] found a relatively limited degree of overjet reduction with headgear in comparison to an untreated control group. Overall, a mean decrease in overjet of just 0.48 mm was attributable to early headgear (CI 95%: -1.07, -0.12). Clearly, therefore, functional appliance therapy is proven to reduce overjets very effectively in growing patients in the short term.

What are the effects of functional appliances on the soft tissues?

Soft tissue changes commensurate with functional appliance therapy typically reflect underlying skeletal and dento-alveolar changes. In particular, overjet reduction is likely to enhance lip competence, while increases in lower anterior facial height typically result in unfurling of the lower lip, with a decrease in the depth of the labio-mental fold. In terms of transverse changes, widening of the lower face is usual with functional appliance therapy.[25] In terms of antero-posterior lip position, little effect has been shown in terms of the upper lip, although some studies have alluded to a small degree of upper lip retraction commensurate with overjet reduction and maxillary restraint with the Herbst appliance.[26, 27] Limited advancement of the lower lip has also been demonstrated,[22] although other studies have not highlighted a change in this respect.[26, 27]

In an analysis of a subset of participants from a larger clinical trial, O'Brien et al.[28] demonstrated an improvement the attractiveness of the facial profile among subjects undergoing an initial phase of early Class II correction. This study involved assessment of profile views with removal of lip traps; reduction in the overjet was associated with improved profile appearance, confirming that dental and limited skeletal changes related to functional appliance therapy may translate into improved facial appearance in a significant percentage of patients. These results differ from a similar investigation that compared attractiveness following treatment with either Harvold activators or functional regulators,[29] although the latter study had a slightly smaller sample size. The authors attributed the lack of between-group difference to growth-related changes, whereby attractiveness was found to improve in two-thirds of the untreated control group over the 18-month period.

What are the long-term effects of functional appliances on the dentition, supporting structures and soft tissues?

The ability of functional appliance therapy to produce lasting skeletal change has long been disputed. This controversy and debate have spawned a significant body of prospective research, with prolonged follow-up to delineate the long-term effects of appliance therapy. The prolonged skeletal effects appear to be minimal in the antero-posterior plane, and there is a growing consensus that mandibular length is genetically pre-ordained, with only limited capacity to alter it.

Ten-year follow-up of randomized trials involving untreated control groups has been undertaken in the United States[30, 31] and the United Kingdom.[28] Due to ethical concerns pertaining to not harnessing available growth potential during adolescence, the 'control' groups were in receipt of subsequent treatment in these trials. The long-term effect of growth modification in both groups was to reduce overall facial convexity; however, normative data has highlighted that some degree of straightening of a skeletal II profile is expected during adolescence.[32] Two-dimensional measurement of mandibular length changes has attested to sustained increases of less than 2 mm compared to untreated groups. These studies, however, could be criticized, as cephalometric assessment lacks sensitivity to condylar changes and glenoid fossa remodeling. Moreover, cephalometric measurements are confounded by errors in projection of non-midline structures and two-dimensional measurement of mandibular length based on midline and non-midline structures.[33]

What is the optimal timing for functional appliance therapy?

There is relatively little evidence-based foundation for this decision. The majority of functional appliance therapy is undertaken prior to or during the pre-pubertal growth spurt. However, as mentioned, ethical concerns preclude direct comparison of treatment versus untreated control during this period, as such a design risks depriving patients of beneficial therapy. In a non-randomized study, however, Baccetti et al.[34] demonstrated a more favourable response in subjects at or after the pre-pubertal growth spurt (12 years 11 months +/- 14 months). The authors concluded that a later Twin Block resulted in a greater skeletal contribution to molar correction, and greater increases in both mandibular length and ramus height. Randomized studies undertaken in younger subjects appear to corroborate these findings, with supplementary mandibular projection below 2 mm.[14]

Are fixed or removable functional appliances more effective?

In a randomized study comparing the Twin Block with the Herbst in subjects with a mean age of 12.5 years, no differences in skeletal and dental changes were found.[35] However, failure to complete treatment was considerably higher (2.4-fold) among Twin Block subjects than was the case with the Herbst appliance. In terms of the impact of the appliance, speech seemed to be less affected with the Herbst and sleep patterns were worse with the Twin Block. Although the functional appliance phase of treatment was shorter with the Herbst by 1.5–2.2 months, there was no significant difference in the overall treatment time, as the second phase in the Herbst group was longer. The Herbst was more expensive, being 4.4 times the cost of the Twin Block to fabricate in this study, although the cost varies based on the design. A major shortcoming with the Herbst design was the high breakage rate of the cast Co-Cr Herbst, with an associated increase in repair time and number of emergency appointments. It should be borne in mind, however, that both operators and technicians involved were more experienced in the use and fabrication of the Twin Block than with the Herbst appliance. Simpler pre-fabricated designs such as those using crowns on the lower premolars or cantilevered off the lower molars may have reduced breakage rates or be less prone to debonding, although this has not yet been subject to randomized assessment.

A further trial has involved comparison of the Herbst and Twin Block focusing on cephalometric changes. Slightly greater degrees of mandibular skeletal change were observed with the Twin Block, with a more profound upper arch distalization effect in the Herbst group. Overall, the proportion of skeletal change contributing to incisor correction was found to be as high as 70% with the Twin Block, but just 30% with the Herbst; this discrepancy is inconsistent with the majority of similar research studies, suggesting that the dental contribution to overjet reduction with the Twin Block may have been underestimated.[36]

Research in context

This summary is primarily based on prospective research, most typically randomized studies. Critics of studies assessing growth modification, however, highlight a number of limitations of these studies.[10, 37] Some of these issues are discussed in this section.

Limitations of cephalometric assessment

Two-dimensional cephalometric assessment of mandibular growth is problematic, as the mandible is not a straight bone, while linear assessments (e.g. Go-Me, Ar-Gn, Go-Gn or Co-Pog) are commonly undertaken. Moreover, condylar growth occurs in both sagittal and vertical directions.[38] It has been estimated that linear assessment may underestimate the magnitude of condylar growth by up to 3.9 mm.[39] Notwithstanding this, many studies have incorporated clinically relevant cephalometric parameters focusing on the position of the chin point, and have revealed little difference in sagittal projection, irrespective of appliance type. A further problem with cephalometrics is the ability to locate relevant points (particularly Condylion) and the use of a non-anatomical alternative (Articulare). Preliminary retrospective analysis incorporating three-dimensional imaging with cone beam computed tomography scanning has highlighted condylar enlargement immediately following Twin Block treatment. Moreover, inter-condylar distances were greater due to posterior-superior growth allied to transverse increases.[40] However, more prolonged and indeed prospective three-dimensional analysis has not been undertaken.

Compliance

Significant differences in compliance with functional appliances have been shown, with O'Brien et al.,[14] for example, finding a discontinuation rate of 33% with the Twin Block and 13% with the Herbst. Depending on the reasons for missing data, intention-to-treat (ITT) analysis is considered most appropriate in investigation of the primary outcome in RCTs. In ITT analysis, all the participants in a trial are analysed according to the intervention to which they were allocated, irrespective of whether they received it. From a research design perspective, ITT preserves the aims of randomization, reducing selection bias and confounding. It is also appropriate for the assessment of effectiveness, reflecting the 'real-world' non-compliance and treatment changes that are likely to occur when the method of Class II correction is used.

However, ITT does have limitations, with those interested in gauging the potential of functional appliances often concerned with the efficacy (the performance under ideal conditions) of the technique. It is also difficult to apply an ITT analysis adequately when there are early dropouts, because this approach requires all randomized participants to be analysed irrespective of whether they received the prescribed intervention or completed the study. Therefore, the specific method of analysis may actually deviate from the reported ITT method. For instance, in an attempt to apply ITT analysis, some trials mishandle missing outcome data by including missing participants in the randomized sample without imputing their outcomes. This approach may dilute or exaggerate the effect of the interventions, as it represents an extreme and highly unlikely scenario where dropouts were either all successes or all failures. Nevertheless, by considering only successful outcomes responding particularly well to treatment, we risk 'cherry-picking' the best responders and perhaps those who were destined for favourable facial growth irrespective of appliance therapy.

Inter-individual growth variation

A general reduction in facial convexity during childhood and adolescence is accepted, with ample evidence from cephalometric studies attesting to this.[32] However, significant differences in the growth pattern have been demonstrated on an individual basis.[10] This pattern has been highlighted further by Darendeliler,[37] who has highlighted the perils of analysing mean responses within RCTs, as this approach tends to obscure the outcomes of those who fare particularly well. Moreover, he has also drawn attention to the variability of Class II presentation, with selection criteria within studies concerning functional appliances often encompassing heterogeneous presentations, including varying degrees of skeletal discrepancy with differing levels of maxillary or mandibular contribution, ranges of overjet and a spectrum of vertical discrepancies. These variations are often dictated by a necessity to recruit a significant sample size to provide sufficient statistical power to afford the research findings credibility and the ability to identify positive results when they do exist. Darendeliler[37] has suggested, for example, that the highest 25% of responders within the UNC study are likely to have experienced ANB reductions of 4.48 degrees, as opposed to changes of just 0.97 degrees in the poorest responders. He argues that this variation may be attributed to unique growth patterns and emphasizes that functional appliance treatment may harness this potential at least in a subset of individuals, even if the reported mean changes within a study are limited.

Summary

Functional appliance therapy has grown in popularity and become more widespread in recent years, in spite of contemporary evidence pointing to a limited capacity to effect skeletal change, particularly in the long term. Increasingly, it is becoming accepted that skeletal proportions and configuration are predominantly pre-ordained genetically, and that orthodontists are incapable of prompting meaningful change. Nevertheless, there is plentiful evidence that functional appliances are adept at Class II correction, offering a versatile and effective solution in growing patients. Further research with an emphasis on patient-centred outcomes is needed to inform clinical decisions further in respect of appliance design and timing.

Appendix

Ovid MEDLINE® in-process and other non-indexed citations and Ovid MEDLINE® (1946–October 2014) search strategy

1. RANDOMIZED CONTROLLED TRIAL.pt.
2. CONTROLLED CLINICAL TRIAL.pt.
3. RANDOMIZED CONTROLLED TRIALS.sh.
4. RANDOM ALLOCATION.sh.
5. DOUBLE BLIND METHOD.sh.
6. SINGLE BLIND METHOD.sh.
7. or/1-6
8. (ANIMALS not HUMANS).sh.
9. CLINICAL TRIAL.pt.
10. exp Clinical Trial/
11. (clin$ adj25 trial$).ti,ab.
12. ((singl$ or doubl$ or trebl$ or tripl$) adj25 (blind$ or mask$)).ti,ab.
13. PLACEBOS.sh.
14. placebo$.ti,ab.
15. random$.ti,ab.
16. RESEARCH DESIGN.sh.
17. or/10-16
18. 17 not 8
19. 18 not 9
20. 9 or 19
21. exp ORTHODONTICS/
22. orthod$.mp.
23. 21 or 22
24. (functional app$).mp.
25. (Class II or Herbst or Twin Block or Forsus or Jasper Jumper or Bionator or Fraenkel).mp.
26. 23 and 24 and 25
27. 26 and 20

References

1. Madhavji A, Araujo EA, Kim KB, Buschang PH. Attitudes, awareness, and barriers toward evidence-based practice in orthodontics. Am J Orthod Dentofacial Orthop. 2011; 140: 309–16.
2. Keim RG, Gottlieb EL, Vogels DS III, Vogels PB. 2014 JCO study of orthodontic diagnosis and treatment procedures, Part 1: Results and trends. J Clin Orthod. 2014; 48: 607–30.
3. Pandis N, Tu YK, Fleming PS, Polychronopoulou A. Randomized and nonrandomized studies: Complementary or competing? Am J Orthod Dentofacial Orthop. 2014; 146: 633–40

4. Banks P, Elton V, Jones Y, Rice P, Derwent S, Odondi L. The use of fixed appliances in the UK: A survey of specialist orthodontists. J Orthod. 2010; 37: 43–55.
5. Broadbent BH. The face of the normal child. Angle Orthod. 1937; 7: 183–208.
6. Ismail AI, Bader JD. Practical science: Evidence-based dentistry in clinical practice. J Amer Dent Assoc. 2004; 135: 78–83.
7. D'Anto V, Bucci R, Franchi L, Rongo R, Michelotti A, Martina R. Class II functional orthopaedic treatment: A systematic review of systematic reviews. J Oral Rehabil. 2015; 42: 624–42.
8. Straus S, Haynes R, Glasziou P, Dickersin K, Guyatt G. Misunderstandings, misperceptions and mistakes. ACP JC. 2007; 146: A8.
9. Mills CM, McCulloch KJ. Treatment effects of the Twin Block appliance: A cephalometric study. Am J Orthod Dentofacial Orthop. 1998; 114: 15–24.
10. Brodie AG, Downs WB, Goldstein A, Myer E. Cephalometric appraisal of orthodontic results: A preliminary report. Angle Orthod. 1938; 8: 261–5.
11. Meikle MC. Guest editorial: What do prospective randomized clinical trials tell us about the treatment of class II malocclusions? A personal viewpoint. Eur J Orthod. 2005; 27: 105–14.
12. Johnston LE Jr. A comparative analysis of Class II treatments: Science and clinical judgment in orthodontics. In: Vig PS, Ribbens KA, eds., Science and clinical judgement in orthodontics. Craniofacial Growth Series, vol. 19. Ann Arbor, MI: Center for Human Growth and Development, University of Michigan; 1986: 103–48.
13. Nelson CN, Harkness M. Mandibular changes during functional appliance treatment. Am J Orthod Dentofacial Orthop. 1993; 104: 153–61.
14. O'Brien K, Wright J, Conboy F, Sanjie Y, Mandall N et al. Effectiveness of early orthodontic treatment with the Twin-block appliance: A multicenter, randomized, controlled trial. Part 1: Dental and skeletal effects. Am J Orthod Dentofacial Orthop. 2003: 124: 234–43.
15. Bass NM. The Dynamax system: A new orthopaedic appliance and case report. J Orthod. 2006; 33: 78–89.
16. Tulloch JF, Phillips C, Koch G, Proffit WR. The effect of early intervention on skeletal pattern in Class II malocclusion: A randomized clinical trial. Am J Orthod Dentofacial Orthop. 1997; 111: 391–400.
17. Keeling SD, Wheeler TT, King GJ, Garvan CW, Cohen DA et al. Anteroposterior skeletal and dental changes after early Class II treatment with bionators and headgear. Am J Orthod Dentofacial Orthop. 1998; 113: 40–50.
18. Mäntysaari R, Kantomaa T, Pirttiniemi P, Pykäläinen A. The effects of early headgear treatment on dental arches and craniofacial morphology: A report of a 2 year randomized study. Eur J Orthod. 2004; 26: 59–64.
19. Harradine NWT, Gale D. The effects of torque control spurs in twinblock appliances. Clin Orthod Res. 1998; 3: 202–9.
20. Lund DI, Sandler PJ. The effects of Twin Blocks: A prospective controlled study. Am J Orthod Dentofacial Orthop. 1998; 113: 104–10.
21. Yaqoob O, DiBiase AT, Fleming PS, Cobourne MT. Use of the Clark Twin Block functional appliance with and without an upper labial bow: A randomized controlled trial. Angle Orthod. 2011; 82: 363–9.
22. Illing HM, Morris DO, Lee RT. A prospective evaluation of Bass, Bionator and Twin Block appliances. Part 1: The hard tissues. Eur J Orthod. 1998; 20: 501–16.
23. Trenouth MJ. Cephalometric evaluation of the Twin-block appliance in the treatment of Class II Division 1 malocclusion with matched normative growth data. Am J Orthod Dentofacial Orthop. 2000; 117: 54–9.
24. Gill DS, Lee RT. Prospective clinical trial comparing the effects of conventional Twin-block and mini-block appliances: Part 1. Hard tissue changes. Am J Orthod Dentofacial Orthop. 2005; 127: 465–72.
25. McDonagh S, Moss JP, Goodwin P, Lee RT. A prospective optical surface scanning and cephalometric assessment of the effect of functional appliances on the soft tissues. Eur J Orthod. 2001; 23: 115–26.
26. Ursi WJS, McNamara JJ, Martins DR, Ursi WJS. Evaluation of the soft tissue profile of class II patients treated with cervical headgear, Frankel's FR-2 and the Herbst appliances. Rev Dent Press Ortodon Ortoped Facial. 2000; 5: 20–46.
27. Pancherz H, Anehus-Pancherz M. The headgear effect of the Herbst appliance: A cephalometric long-term study. Am J Orthod Dentofacial Orthop. 1993; 103: 510–20.
28. O'Brien K, Wright J, Conboy F, Appelbe P, Davies L et al. Early treatment for Class II Division 1 malocclusion with the Twin-block appliance: A multi-center, randomized, controlled trial. Am J Orthod Dentofacial Orthop. 2009; 135: 573–9.
29. O'Neill K, Harkness M, Knight R. Ratings of profile attractiveness after functional appliance treatment. Am J Orthod Dentofacial Orthop. 2000; 118: 371–6.
30. Tulloch JF, Proffit WR, Phillips C. Outcomes in a 2-phase randomized clinical trial of early Class II treatment. Am J Orthod Dentofacial Orthop. 2004; 125: 657–67.
31. King GJ, McGorray SP, Wheeler TT, Taylor M. Comparison of peer assessment ratings (PAR) from 1-phase and 2-phase treatment protocols for Class II malocclusions. Am J Orthod Dentofacial Orthop. 2003; 123: 489–96.
32. Lande MJ. Growth behavior of the human bony facial profile as revealed by serial cephalometric roentgenology 1. Angle Orthod. 1952; 22: 78–90.
33. Clark WJ. New horizons in orthodontics and dentofacial orthopedics. DDS thesis, University of Dundee, 2010.
34. Baccetti T, Franchi L, Toth LR, McNamara JA Jr. Treatment timing for Twin-block therapy. Am J Orthod Dentofacial Orthop. 2000; 118: 159–70.
35. O'Brien K, Wright J, Conboy F, Sanjie Y, Mandall N et al. Effectiveness of treatment for Class II malocclusion with the Herbst or twin-block appliances: A randomized, controlled trial. Am J Orthod Dentofacial Orthop. 2003; 124: 128–37.
36. Baysal A, Uysal T. Dentoalveolar effects of Twin Block and Herbst appliances in patients with Class II division 1 mandibular retrognathy. Eur J Orthod. 2014; 36: 164–72.
37. Darendeliler MA. Validity of randomized clinical trials in evaluating the outcome of Class II treatment. Semin Orthod. 2006; 12: 67–79.
38. Björk A. Variations in the growth pattern of the human mandible: Longitudinal radiographic study by the implant method. J Dent Res. 1963; 42: 400–11.
39. Hägg U, Attström K. Mandibular growth estimated by four cephalometric measurements. Am J Orthod Dentofacial Orthop. 1992; 102: 146–52.
40. Yildirim E, Karacay S, Erkan M. Condylar response to functional therapy with Twin-Block as shown by cone-beam computed tomography. Angle Orthod. 2014; 84: 1018–25.

CHAPTER 11

Cases

QH

Diagnosis

A male patient (Figure 11.1) aged 12 years had with a skeletal II profile related to mandibular retrognathia and slightly reduced vertical dimension in the permanent dentition. Lips were incompetent at rest, with the lower lip functioning palatal to the maxillary central incisors. There was also an inverted conical supernumerary in the anterior maxilla.

The arches were generally well aligned, although there was mild lower anterior crowding and an upper median diastema with proclined maxillary central incisors. In occlusion, molar and canine relationships were Class II bilaterally with an increased overjet of 9.5 mm (a–i).

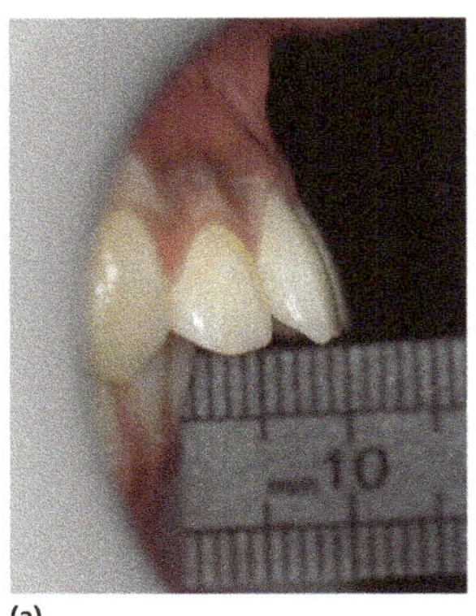

(a)

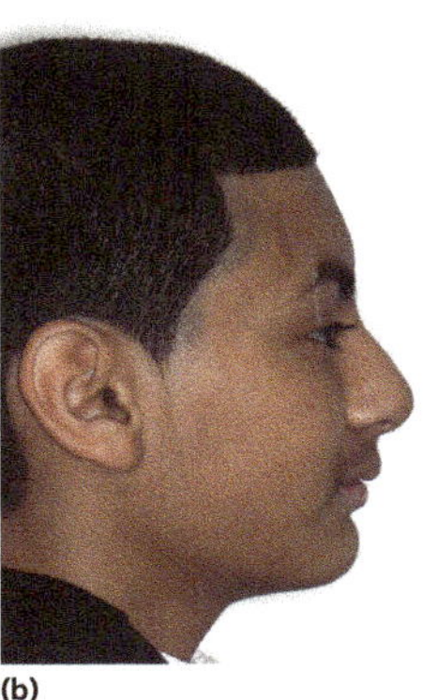
(b)

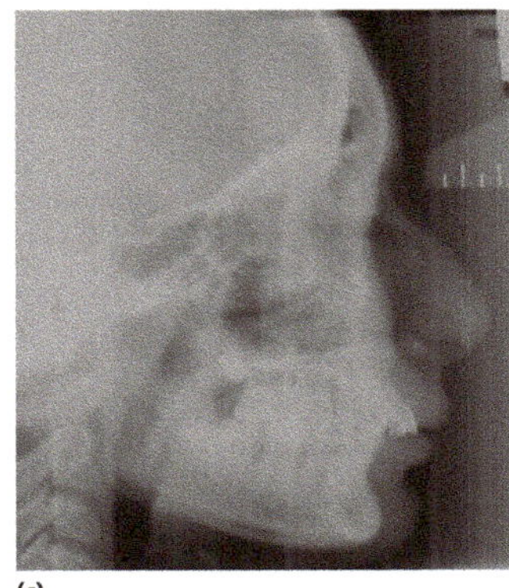
(c)

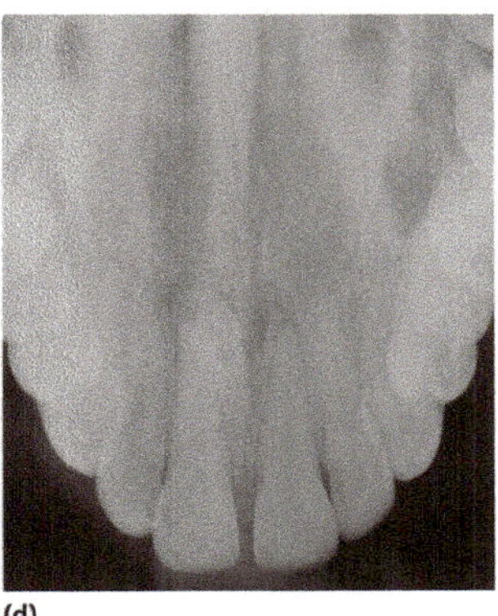
(d)

Figure 11.1 Reproduced with permission from C. Siew-Yee.

Orthodontic Functional Appliances: Theory and Practice, First Edition. Padhraig Fleming and Robert Lee.

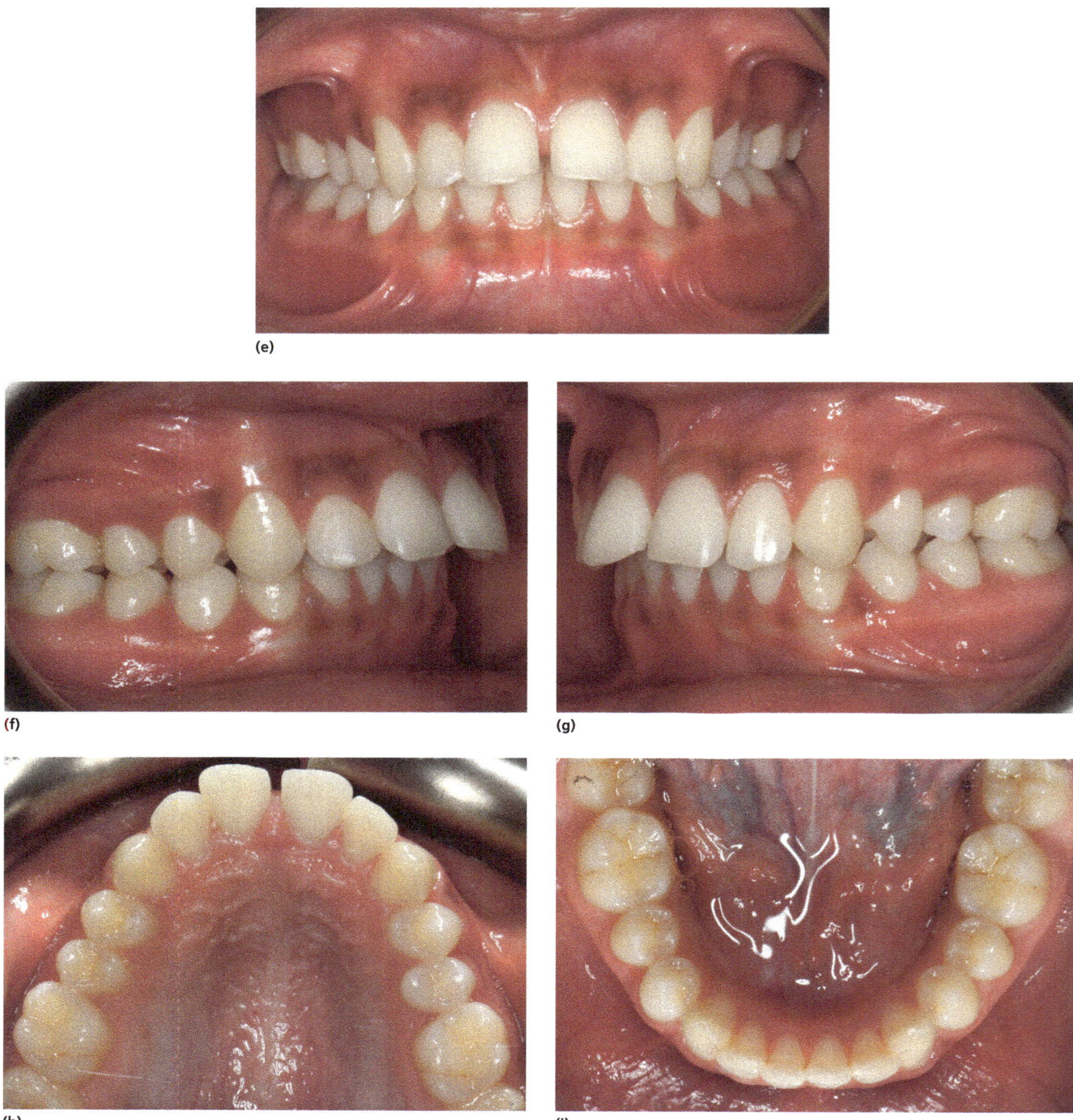

Figure 11.1 (*Continued*)

Treatment

A modified Twin Block appliance was worn on a full-time basis for 12 months (j–t), resulting in full correction of the malocclusion with overcorrection to an edge-to-edge incisor relationship. The appliance was withdrawn for a period of 3 months, allowing partial closure of the lateral open bites and slight relapse of the incisor relationship. Thereafter, fixed appliances were placed to finish and detail the occlusion (u–ac).

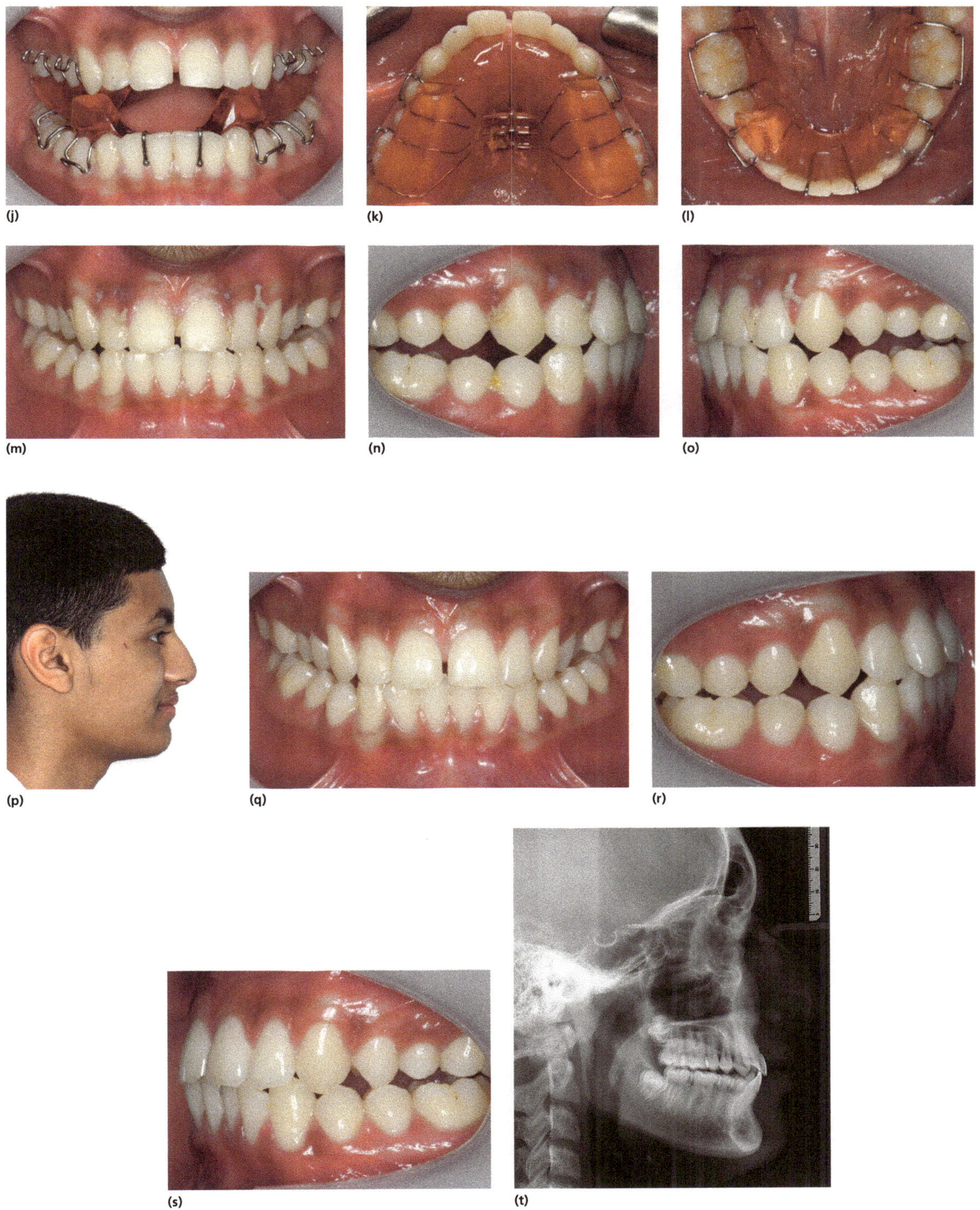

Figure 11.1 *(Continued)*

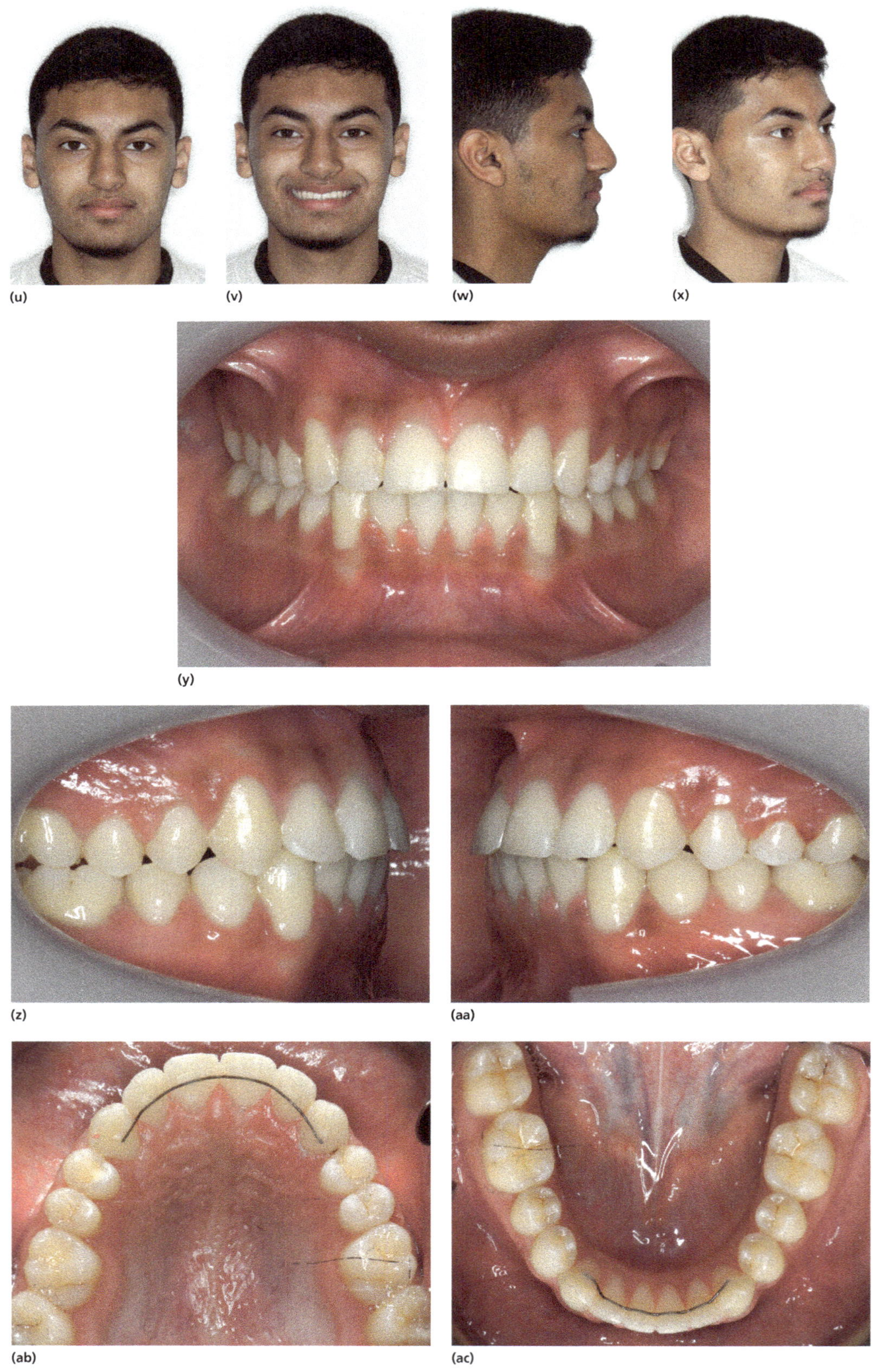

Figure 11.1 (*Continued*)

FA

Diagnosis

A male patient (Figure 11.2) aged 8 years attended with a severe skeletal II profile and increased vertical dimension in the mixed dentition. Lips were grossly incompetent with anterior vertical maxillary excess.

The arches were spaced, with proclined maxillary incisors and developmental absence of the lower central incisors. In occlusion, molar and canine relationships were Class II bilaterally with an increased overjet of 15 mm (a–i).

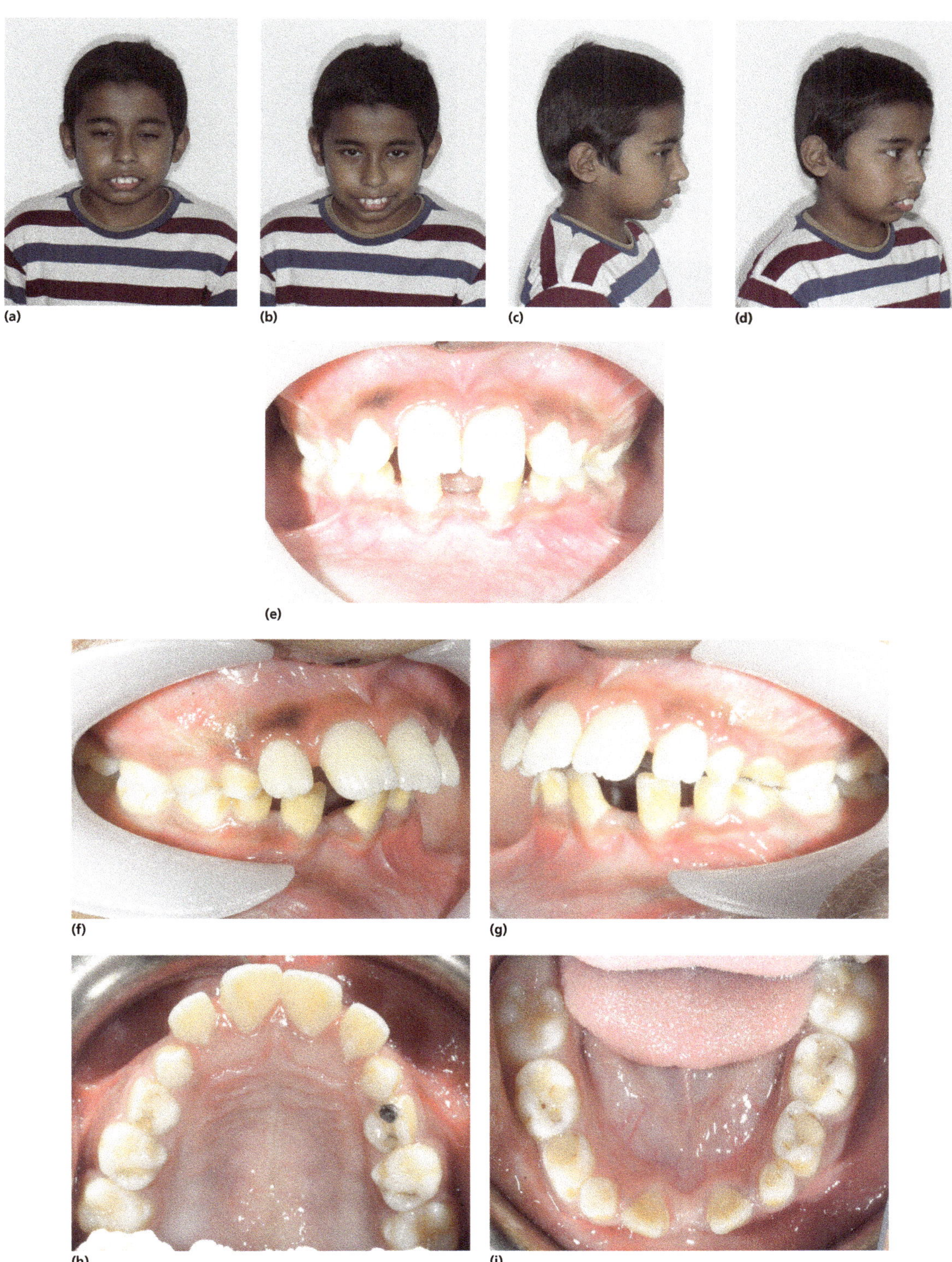

Figure 11.2

Treatment

A modified activator was worn 14 hours per day for a period of 9 months to reduce the overjet and improve lip competence. High-pull extra-oral traction was added to enhance vertical control. The activator was modified to allow placement of a sectional upper fixed appliance to consolidate the upper anterior spacing (j–s). The overjet was reduced to 5 mm, and a second phase of treatment will be required commencing in the late mixed dentition (t–ab).

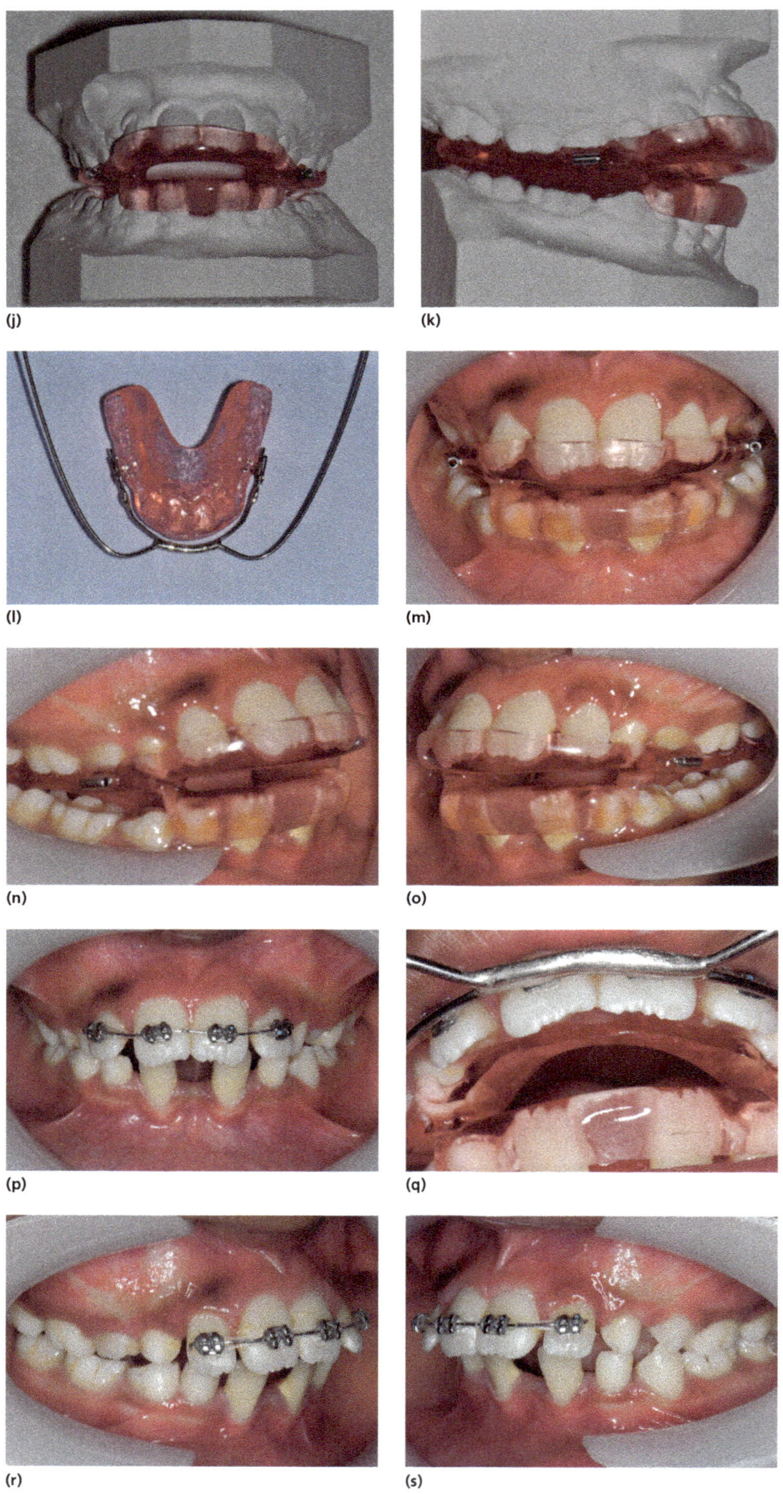

Figure 11.2 (*Continued*)

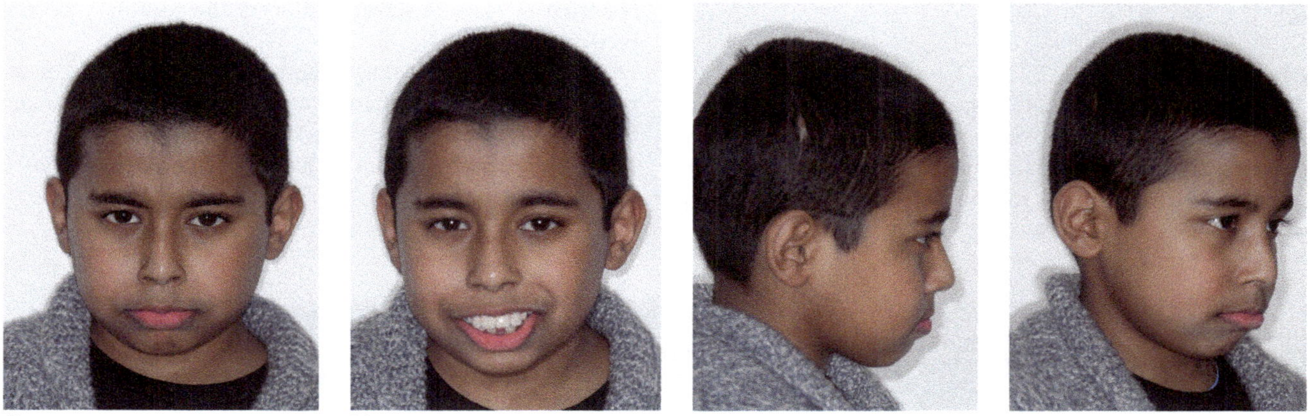

(t) (u) (v) (w)

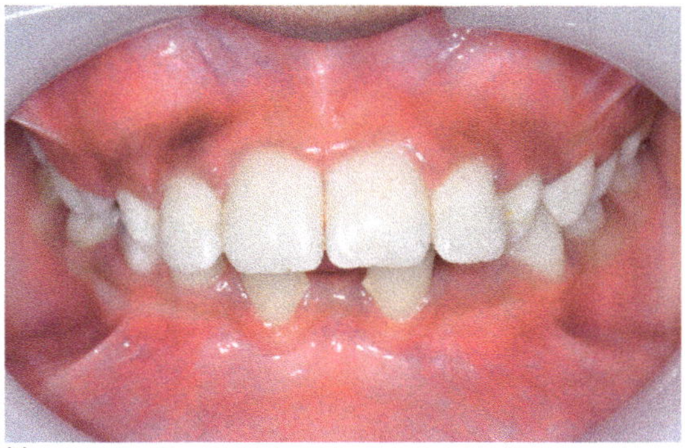

(x)

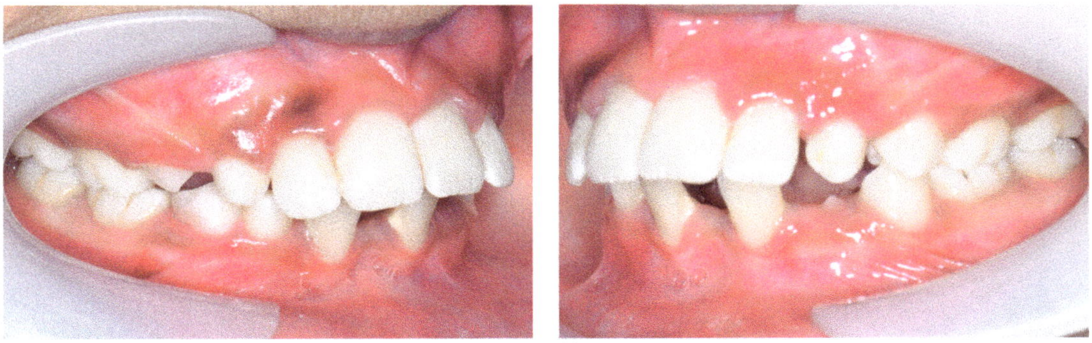

(y) (z)

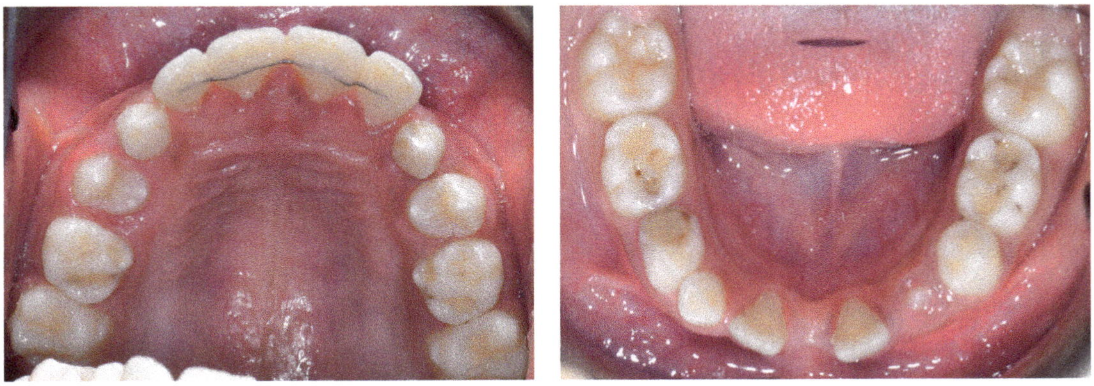

(aa) (ab)

Figure 11.2 (*Continued*)

AS

Diagnosis

A female patient (Figure 11.3) aged 12 years presented with a skeletal II profile related to mandibular retrognathia and decreased lower anterior facial height in the permanent dentition. There was a high resting position of the lower lip, resulting in isolated retroclination of the maxillary central incisors.

There was mild crowding of both dental arches, with proclination of the maxillary lateral incisors. In occlusion, molar and canine relationships were Class II bilaterally. The overjet was 3 mm to the central incisors, with a maximal overjet of 9 mm to the lateral incisors (a–h).

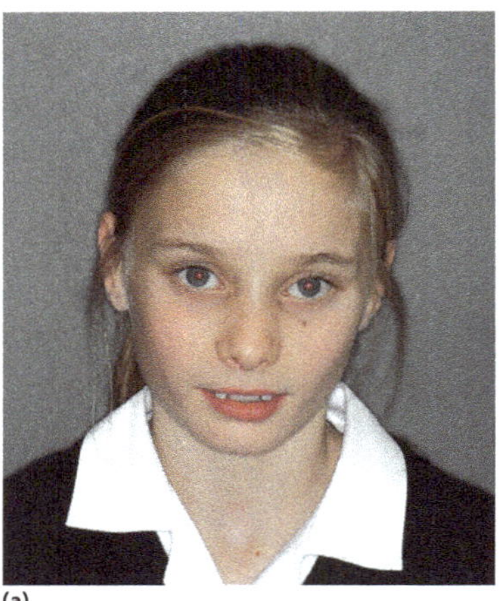
(a)

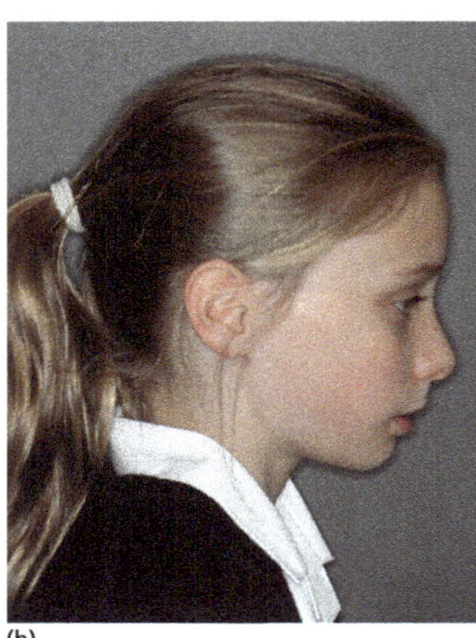
(b)

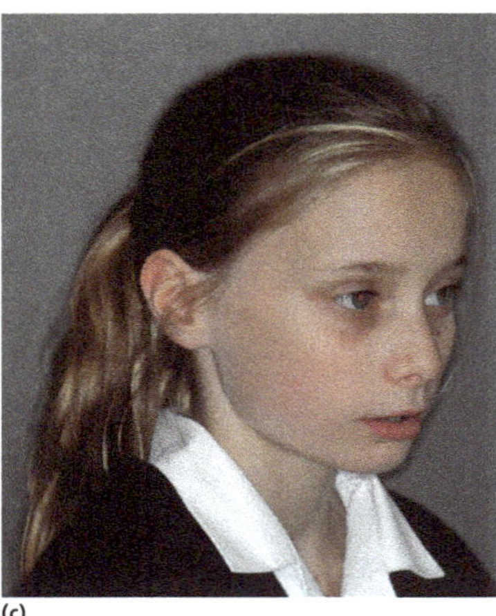
(c)

Figure 11.3

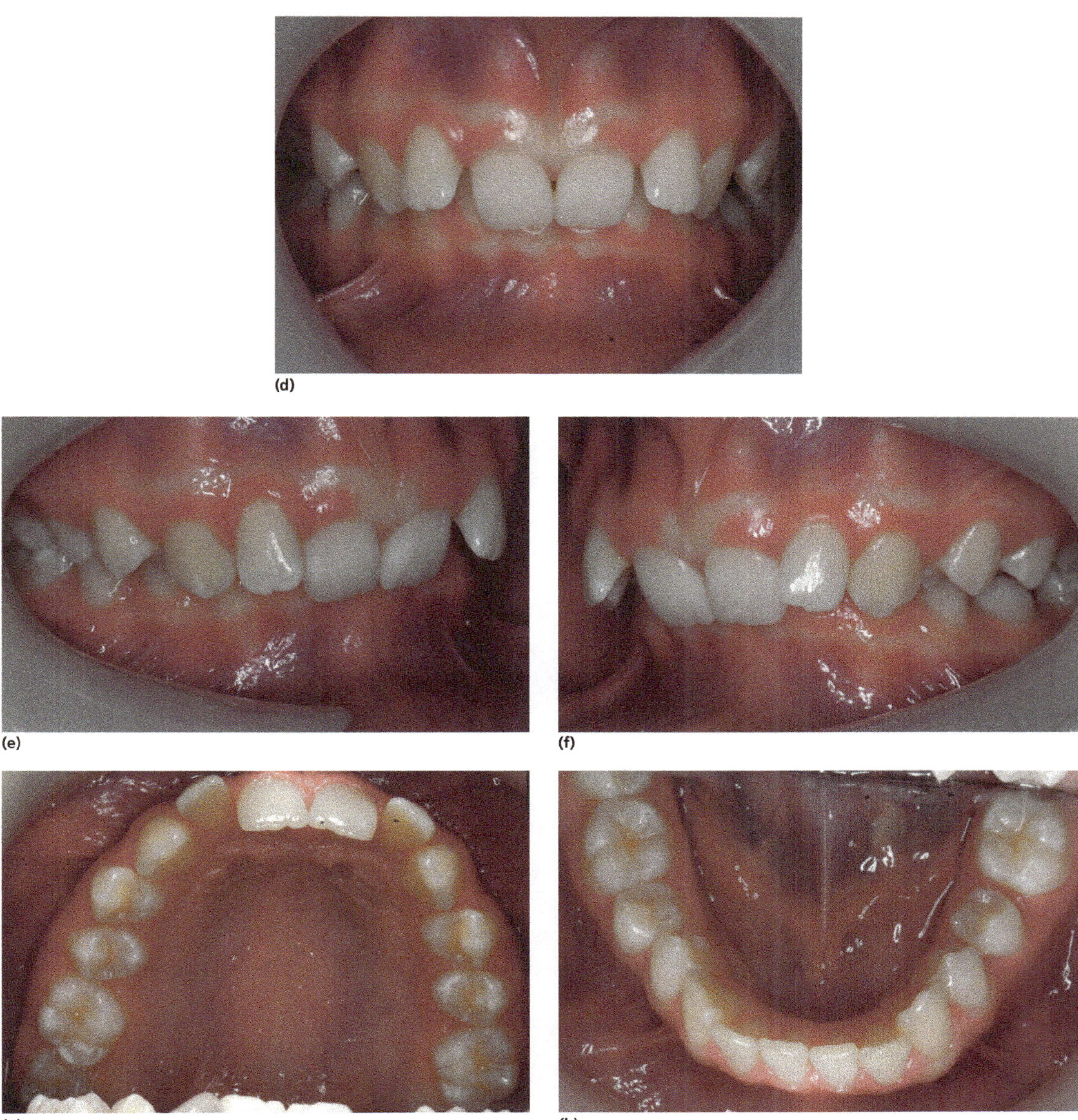

(d)

(e)

(f)

(g)

(h)

Figure 11.3 (*Continued*)

Treatment

A modified Twin Block appliance with 'T' springs to procline the maxillary central incisors was worn on a full-time basis for 12 months, resulting in full correction of the buccal segment relationships and decrease in the overbite (i–r). Following tapering of appliance wear to a nights-only basis, the lateral open bites reduced. Thereafter, fixed appliances were placed to finish and detail the occlusion, although some relapse in the overbite arose following initial alignment; this was addressed with continuous archwire mechanics, including counterforce NiTi archwires and use of Class II elastics during the fixed appliance phase (s–ak).

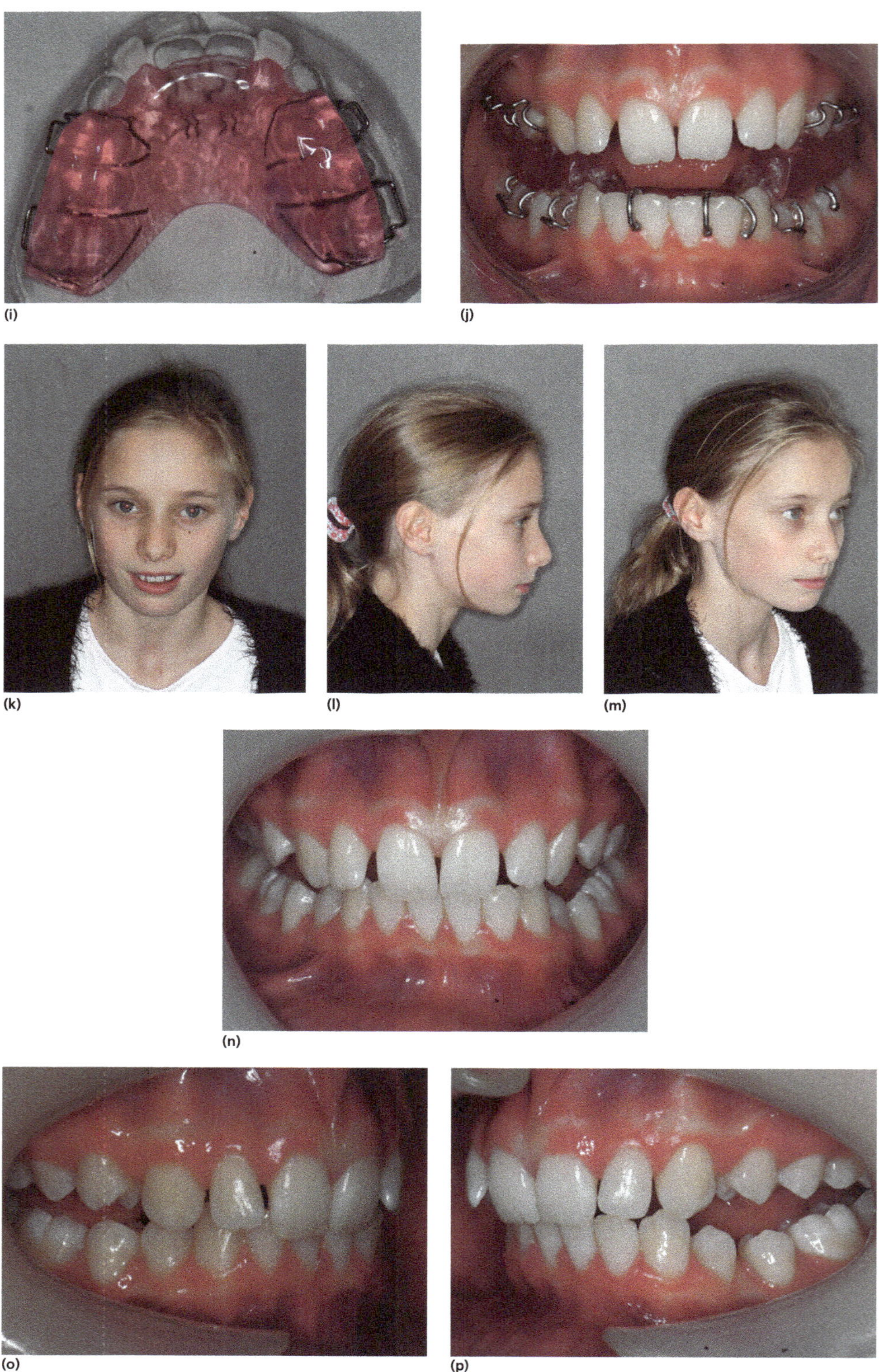

Figure 11.3 (*Continued*)

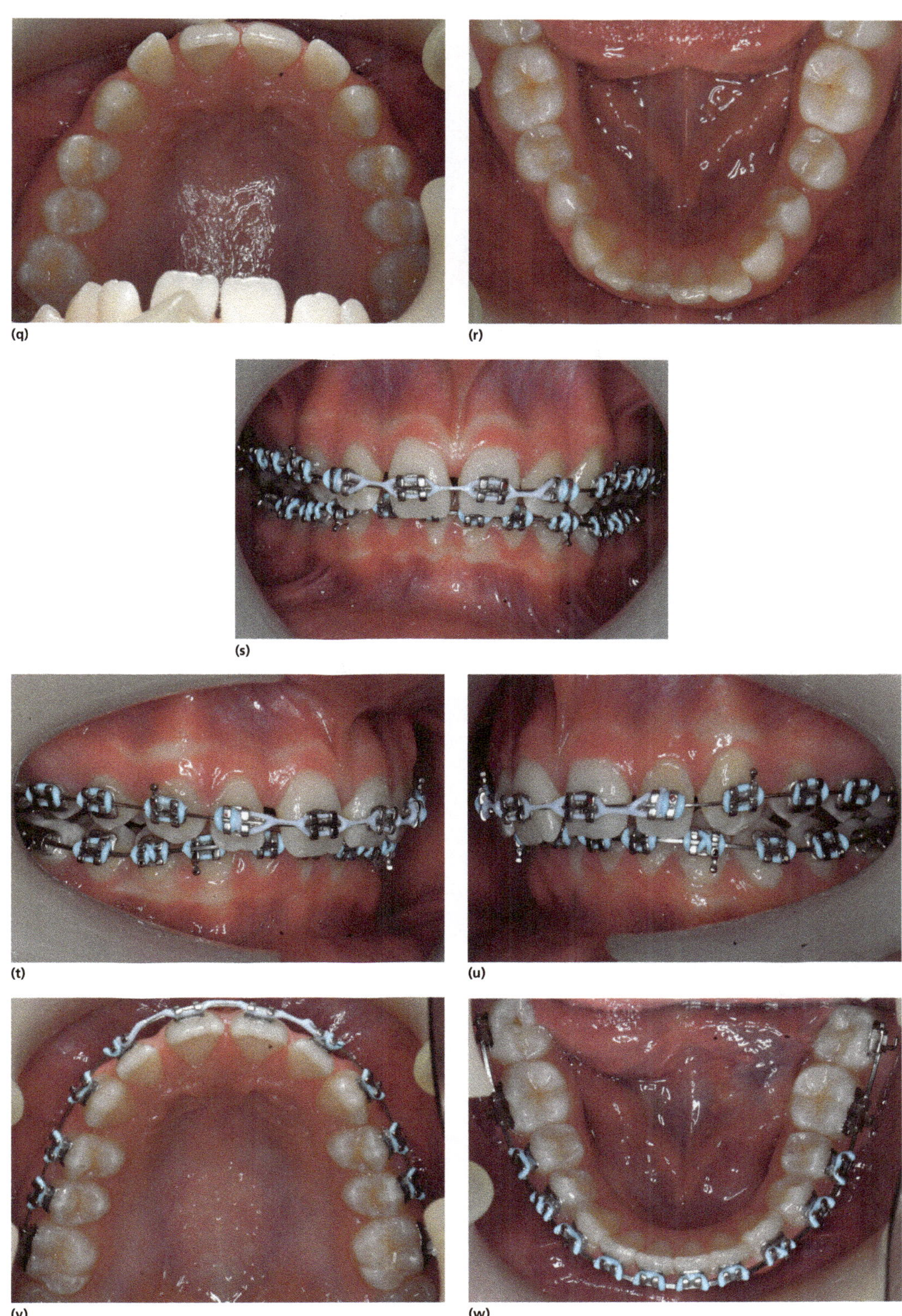

Figure 11.3 *(Continued)*

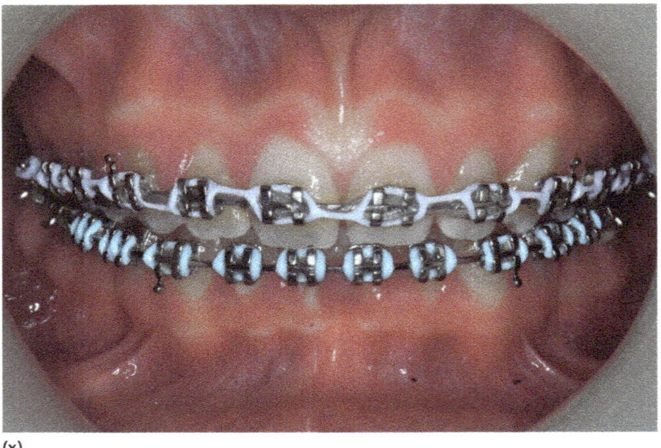
(x)

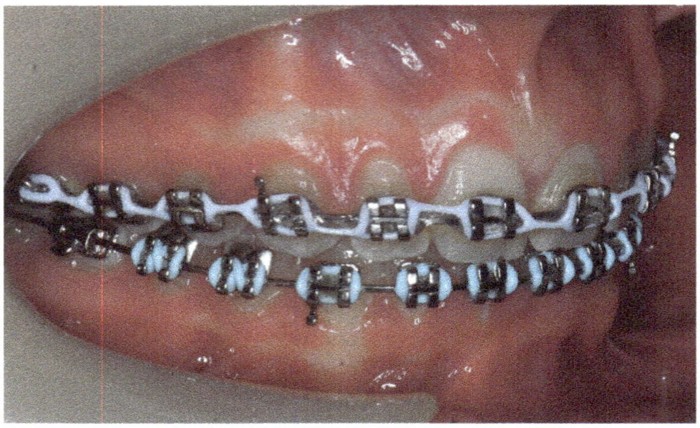

(y)

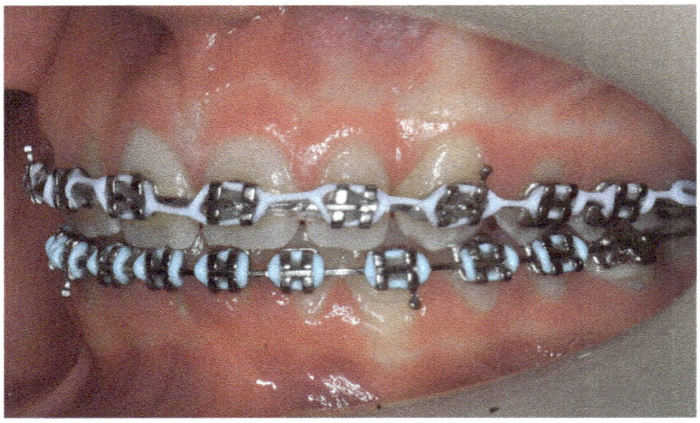

(z)

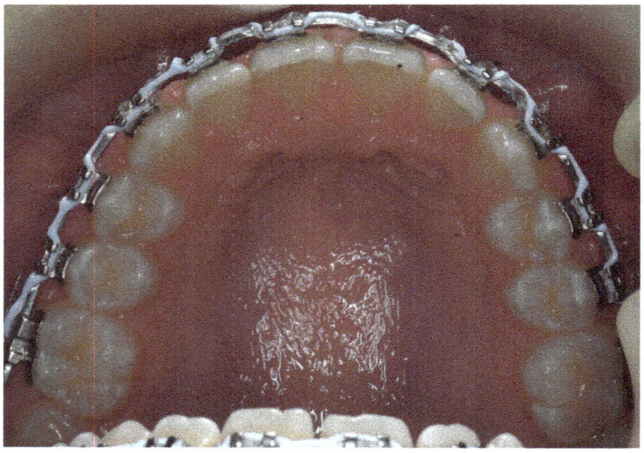

(aa)

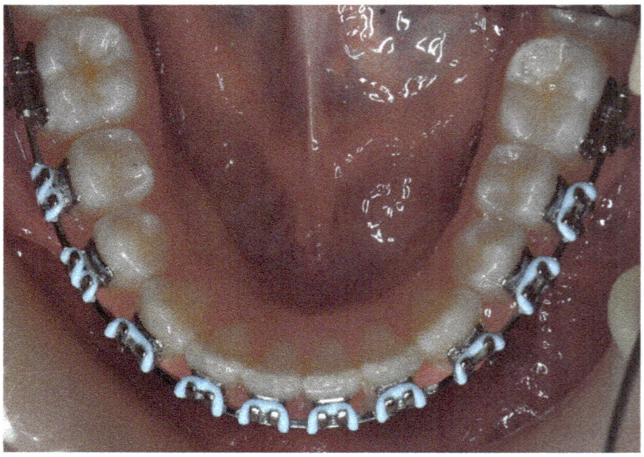

(ab)

Figure 11.3 (*Continued*)

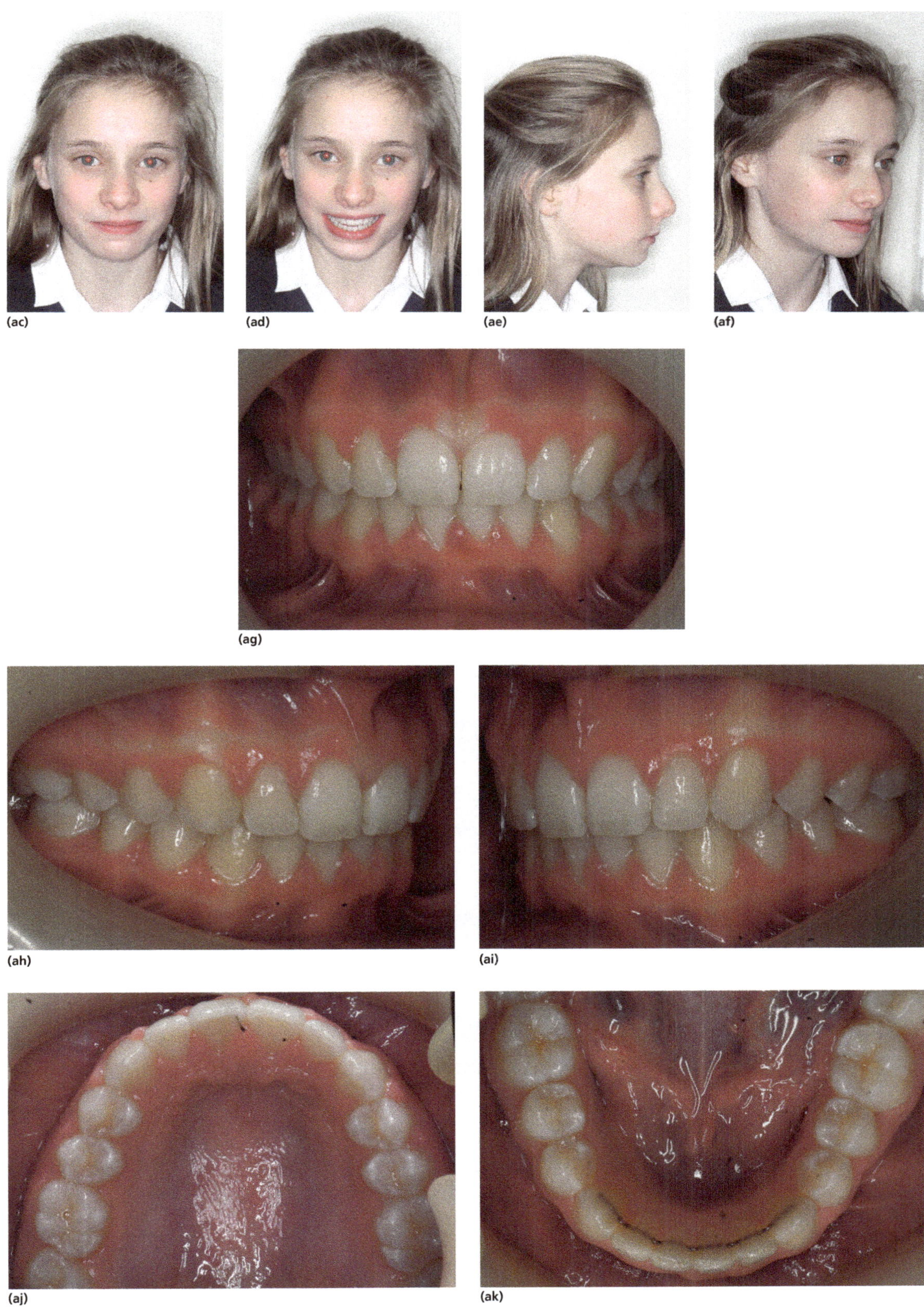

Figure 11.3 (*Continued*)

GC

Diagnosis

A male patient (Figure 11.4) aged 12 years presented with a severe skeletal II profile due to micrognathia. He had a history of a left condylar fracture in infancy, with resultant underdevelopment of the left condyle and ascending ramus. He had an associated mandibular asymmetry and a maxillary cant related to restricted vertical development of the left maxilla. The aesthetic impairment was compounded by functional issues, with a maximal inter-incisal opening of 12 mm (a–d).

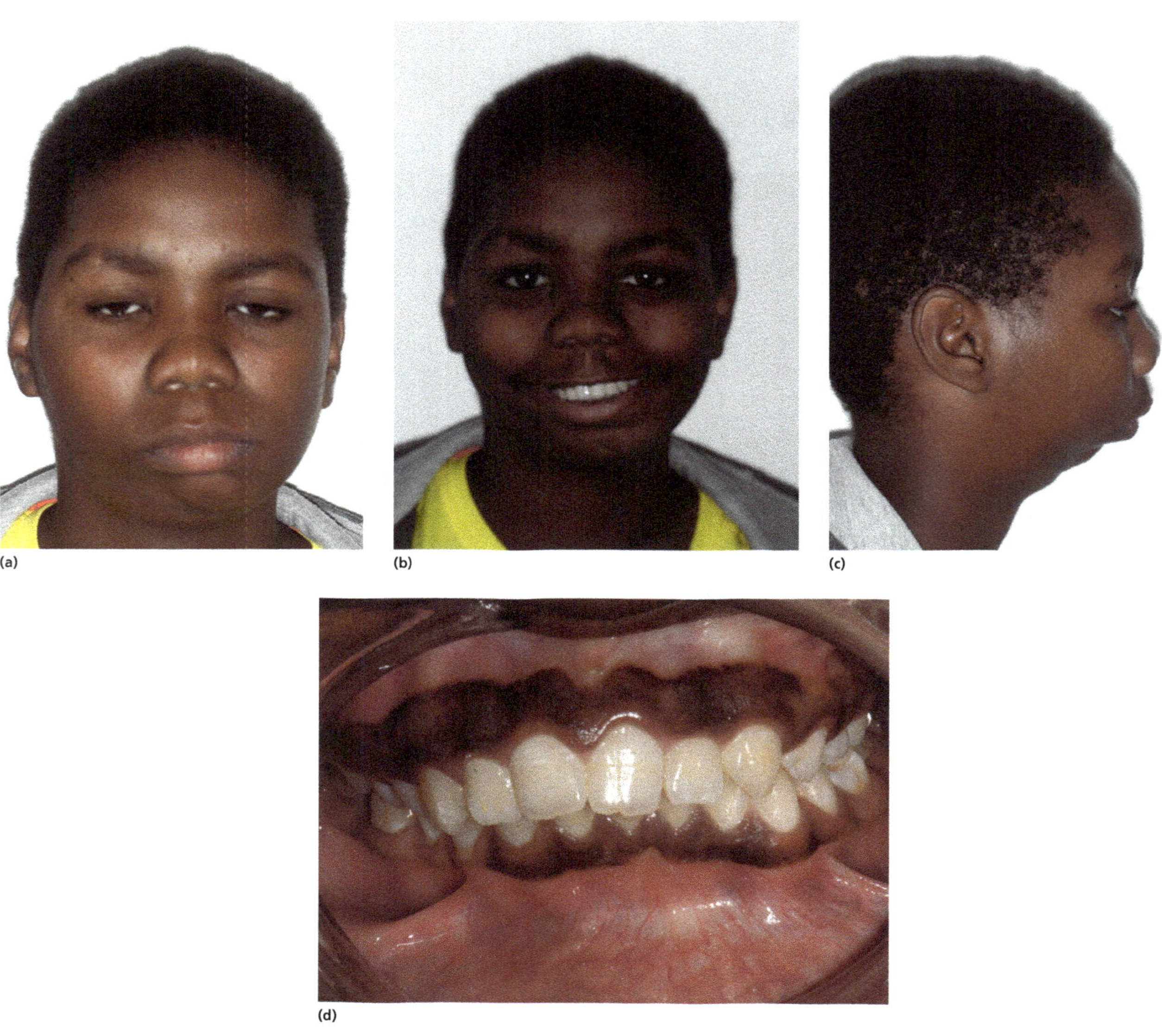

(a) (b) (c) (d)

Figure 11.4

Treatment

Distraction osteogenesis was performed on the left mandibular ramus to improve the skeletal II deformity, while restoring height to the ascending ramus (e–j). Post-surgically a hybrid activator was placed for a period of 6 months to maintain Class II correction while allowing preferential vertical development of the left maxillary segment, promoting correction of the maxillary cant (k–o). Thereafter, fixed appliances were placed to improve the occlusion. The maximal inter-incisal mouth opening increased to 26 mm. An advancement genioplasty may be considered at skeletal maturity to improve the chin prominence further (p–t).

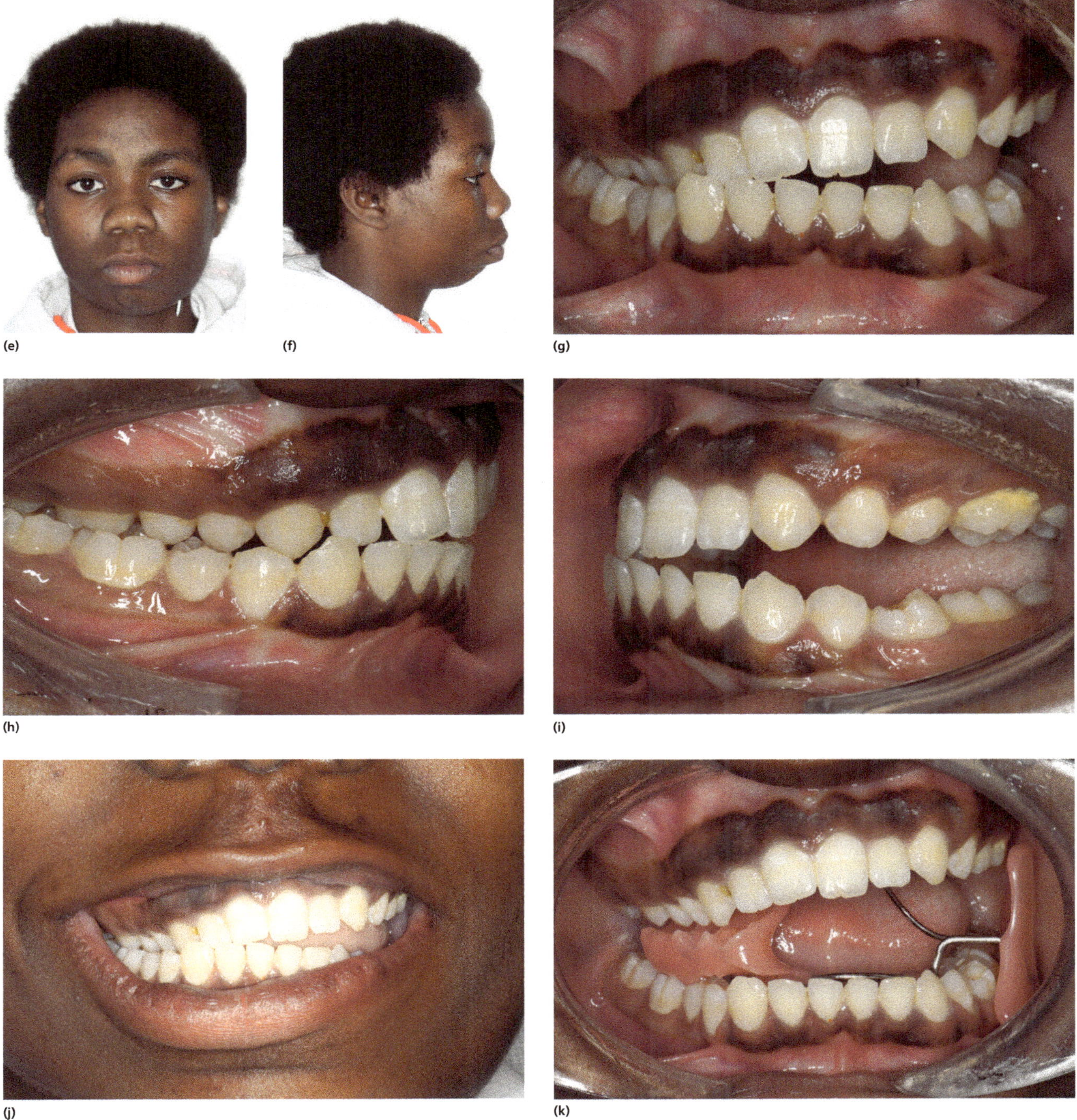

(e) (f) (g) (h) (i) (j) (k)

Figure 11.4 *(Continued)*

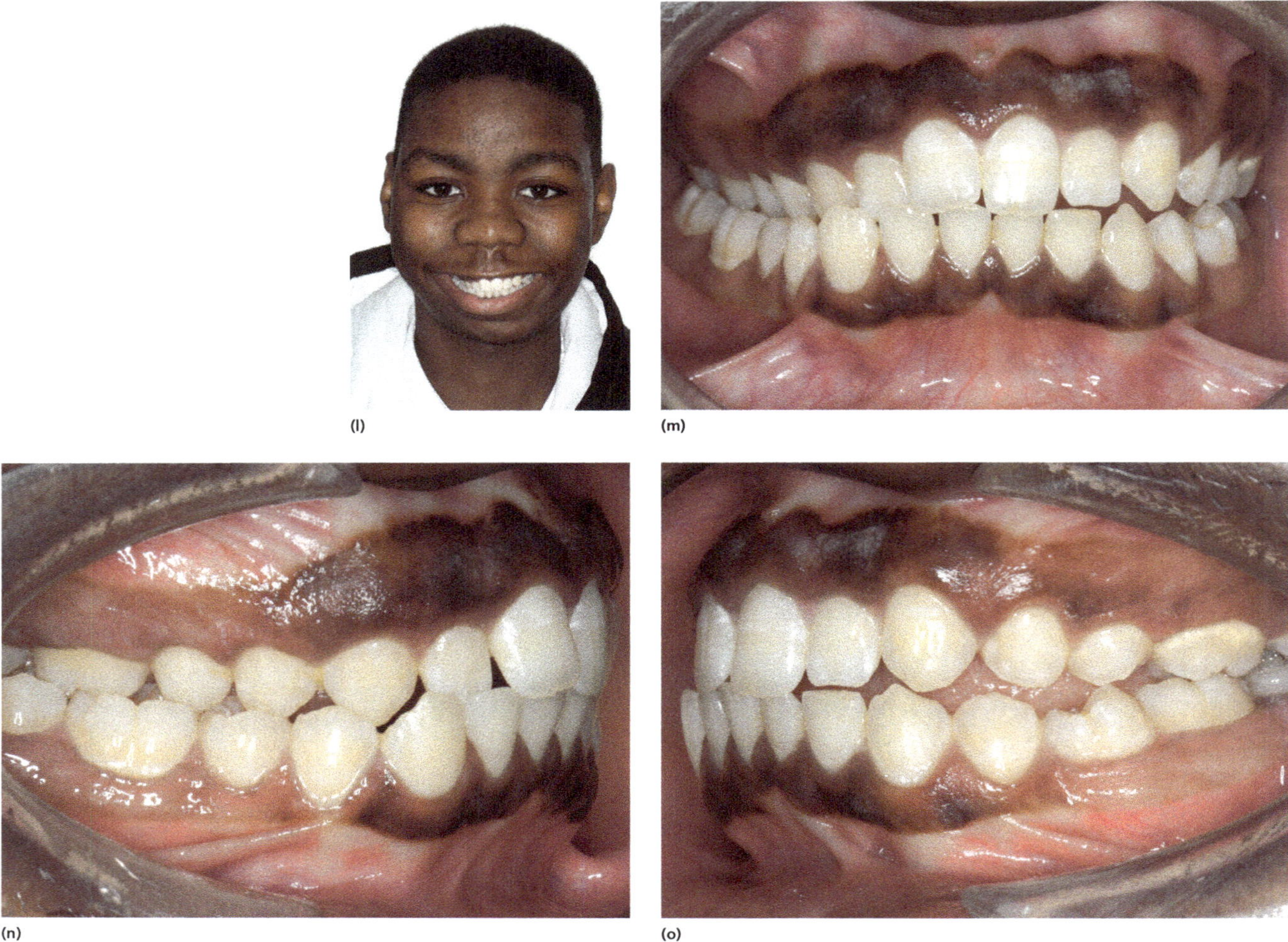

(l) (m) (n) (o)

Figure 11.4 *(Continued)*

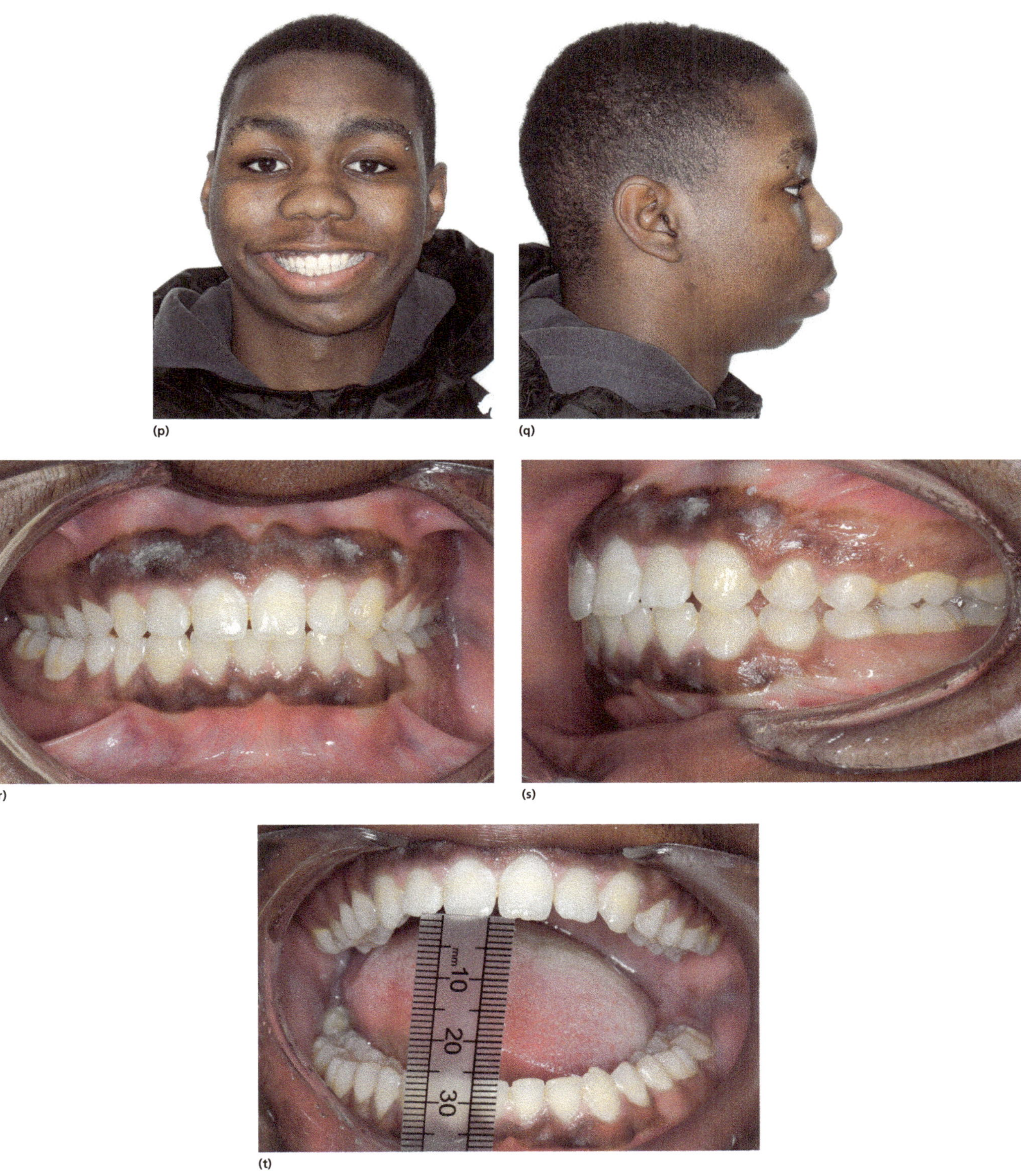

(p) (q) (r) (s) (t)

Figure 11.4 (*Continued*)

ML

Diagnosis

A female patient (Figure 11.5) aged 12 years presented with a skeletal II profile related to mandibular retrognathia and average vertical dimension in the late mixed dentition. Lips were incompetent at rest with a lower lip trap.

The arches were generally well aligned, although there was an upper midline diastema with proclined maxillary incisors. There was developmental absence of the lower right second premolar. In occlusion, molar and canine relationships were Class II bilaterally with an increased overjet of 11 mm (a–i).

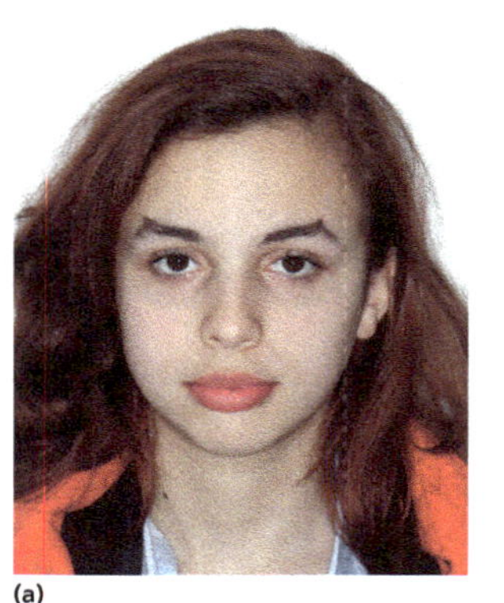
(a)

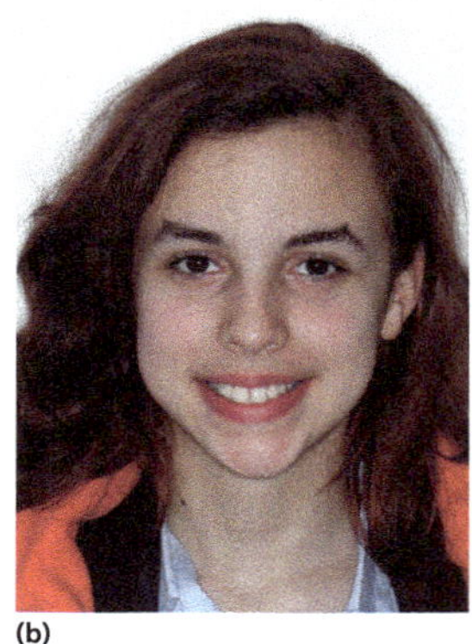
(b)

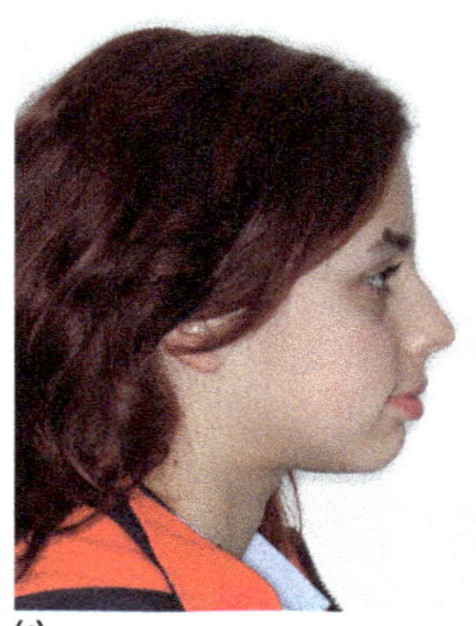
(c)

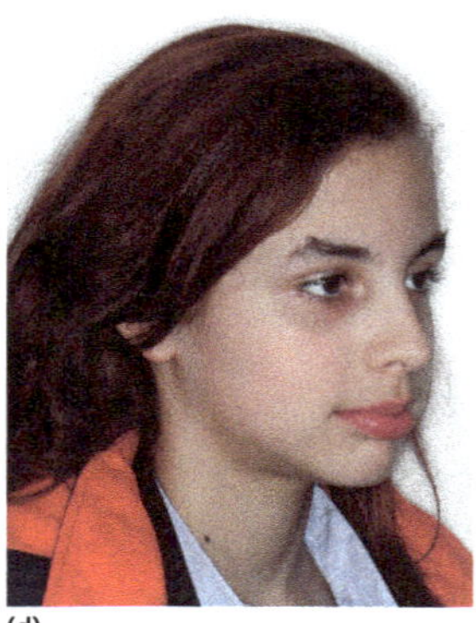
(d)

Figure 11.5

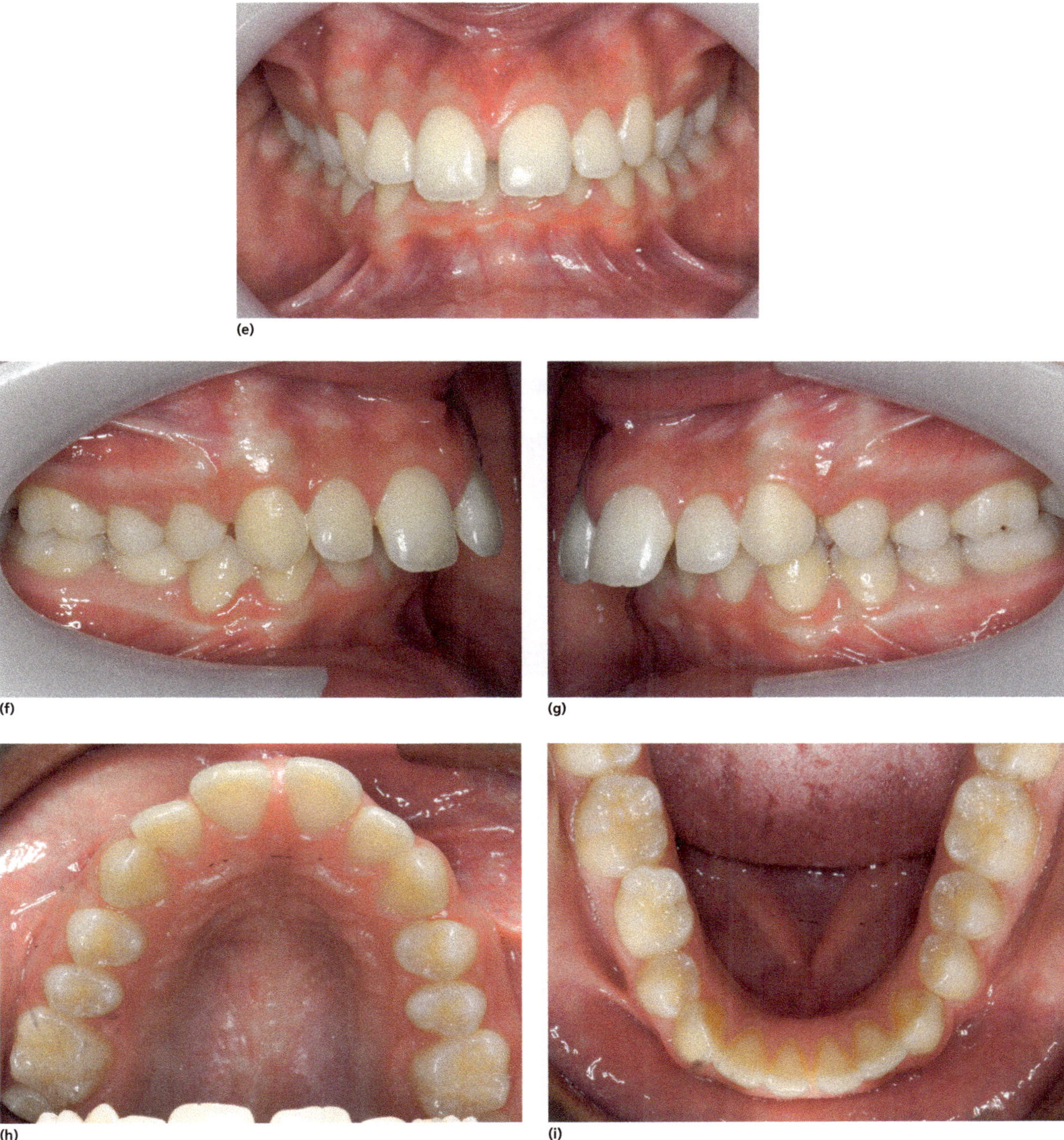

(e)

(f)

(g)

(h)

(i)

Figure 11.5 *(Continued)*

Treatment

A modified Twin Block appliance was worn on a full-time basis for 12 months, resulting in full correction of the malocclusion and improvement in the skeletal pattern. Thereafter, fixed appliances were placed to finish and detail the occlusion, with indefinite retention of the lower right second primary molar (j–y).

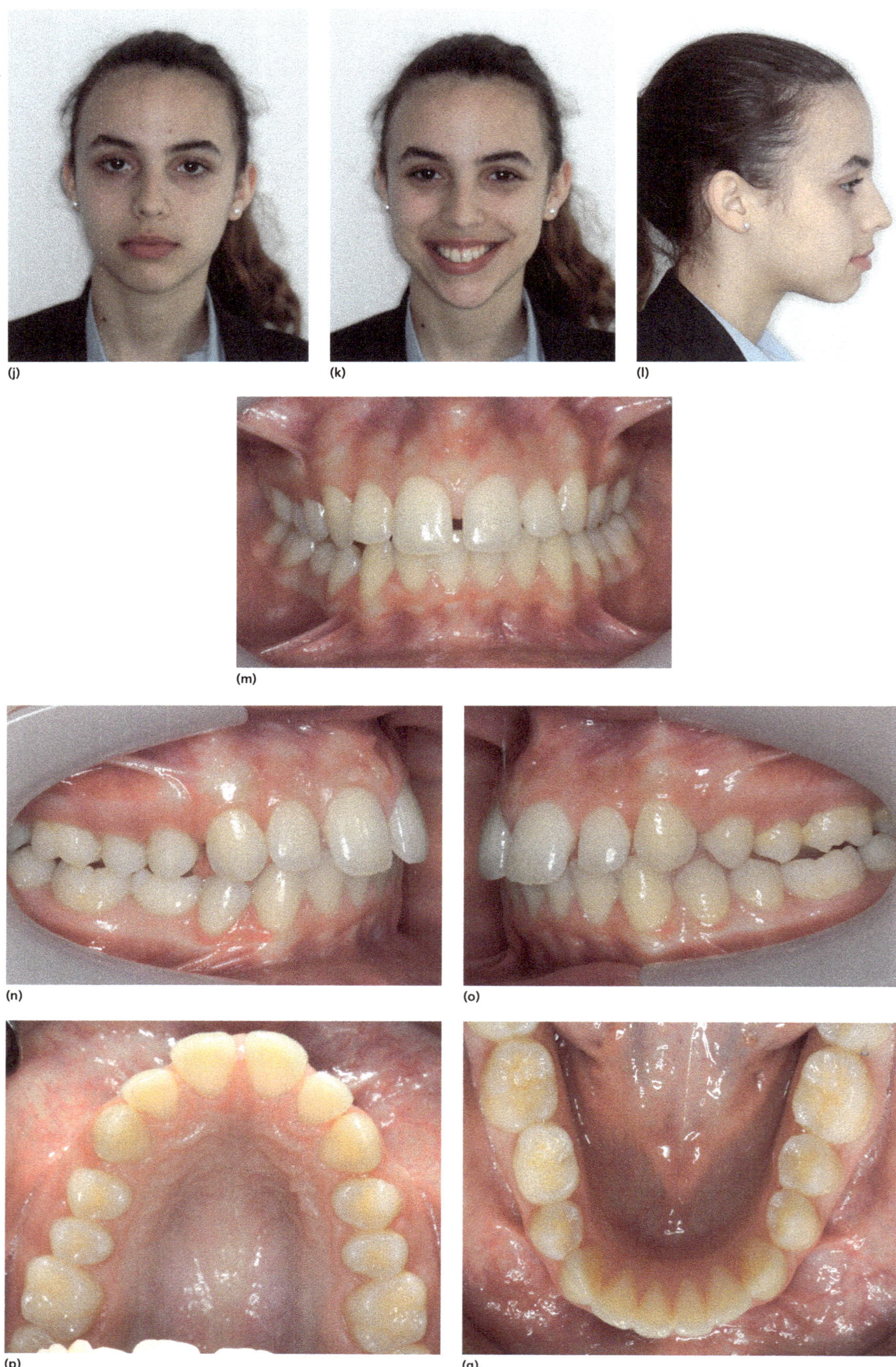

Figure 11.5 (*Continued*)

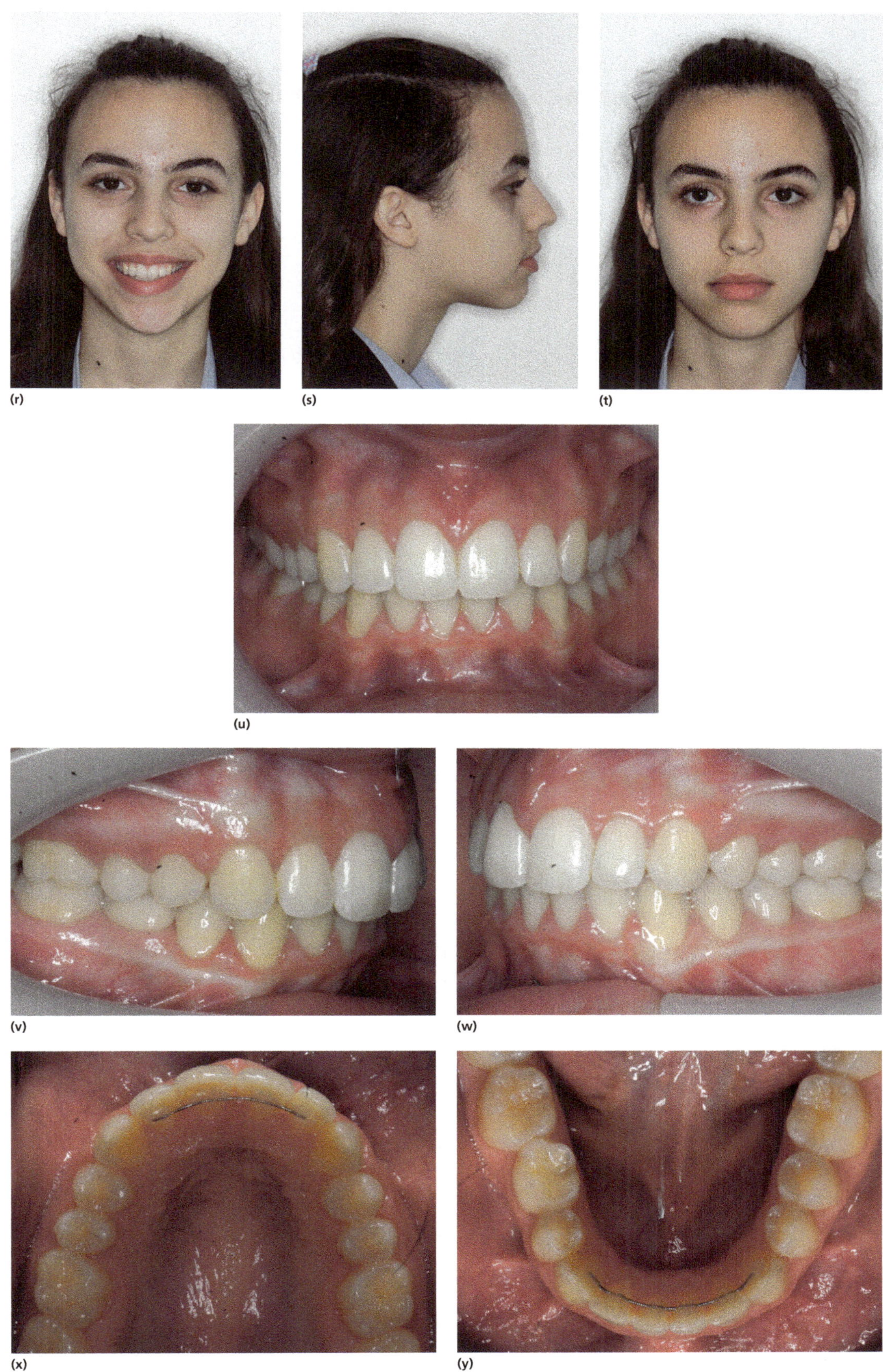

Figure 11.5 (*Continued*)

HF

Diagnosis

A female patient (Figure 11.6) aged 12 years presented with a mild skeletal III profile in the early permanent dentition. There was a mild degree of both mandibular prognathism and maxillary retrusion. She could achieve an edge-to-edge incisor relationship, displacing anteriorly on closure into a frank reverse overjet.

The mandibular arch was spaced, while the upper arch was crowding, with space loss subsequent to premature loss of the maxillary right second primary molar. There was a reversed overjet of 3 mm in the displaced position (a–g).

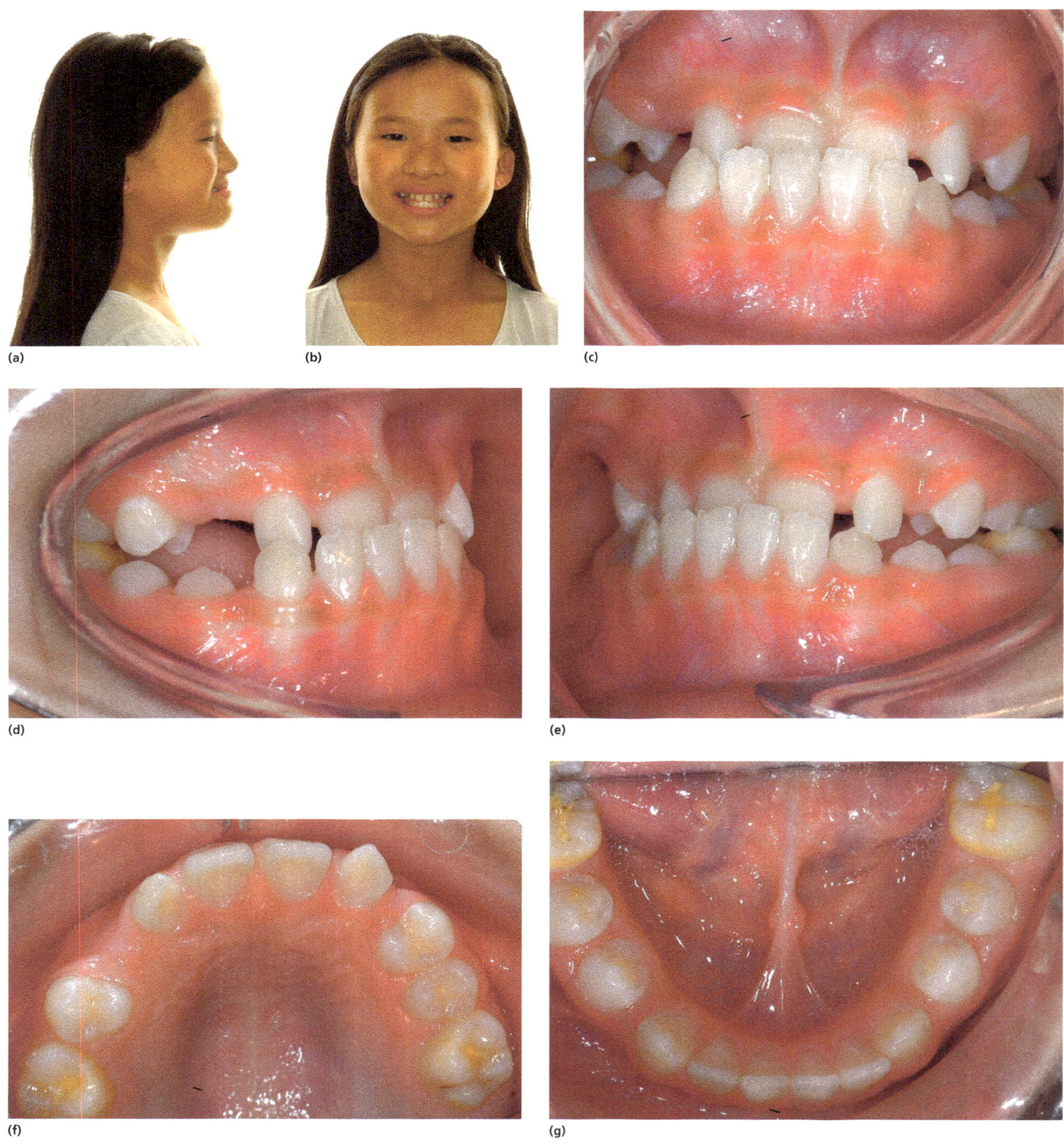

(a) (b) (c) (d) (e) (f) (g)

Figure 11.6

Treatment

A reverse Twin Block appliance was used for a period of 9 months to correct the incisor relationship, establishing a positive overjet and overbite with lateral open bites developing in the posterior regions bilaterally (h–m). Thereafter, fixed appliances were placed on a non-extraction basis, with space re-creation in the upper right side to facilitate eruption of the impacted second premolar. Following treatment, facial harmony, dental aesthetics and good interdigitation were achieved (n–v).

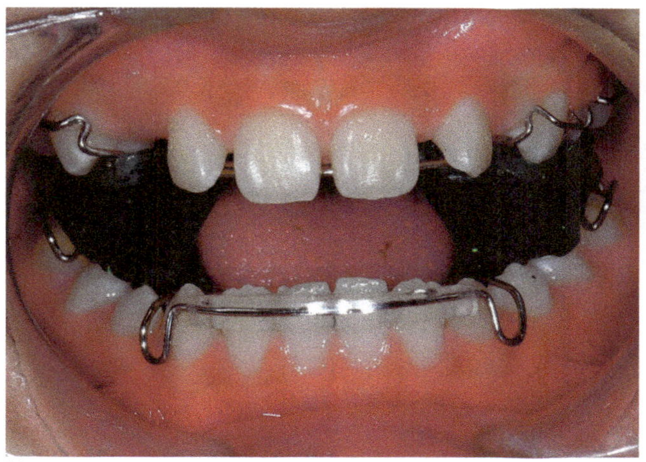

(h)

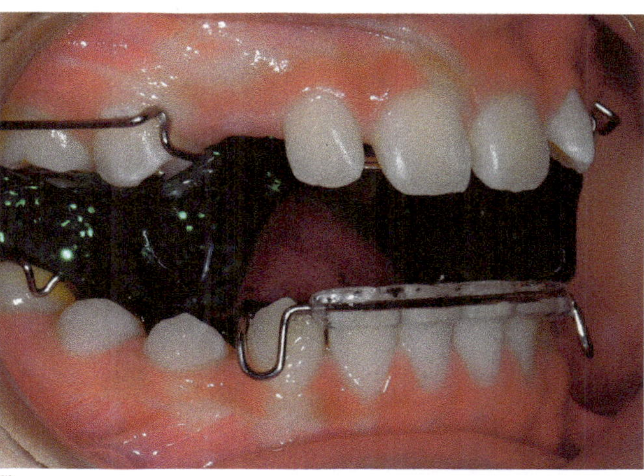

(i)

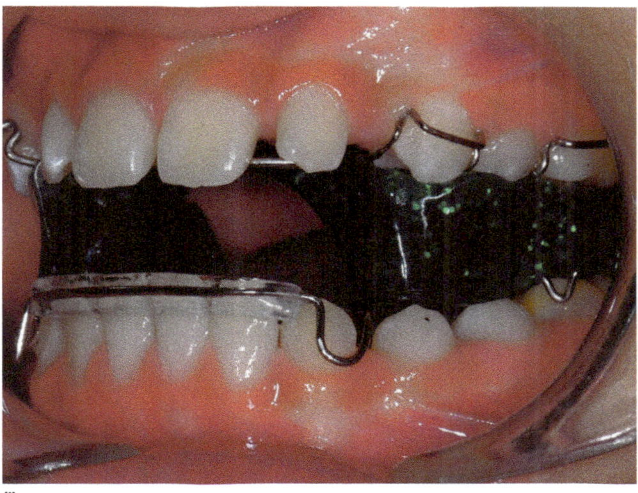

(j)

Figure 11.6 *(Continued)*

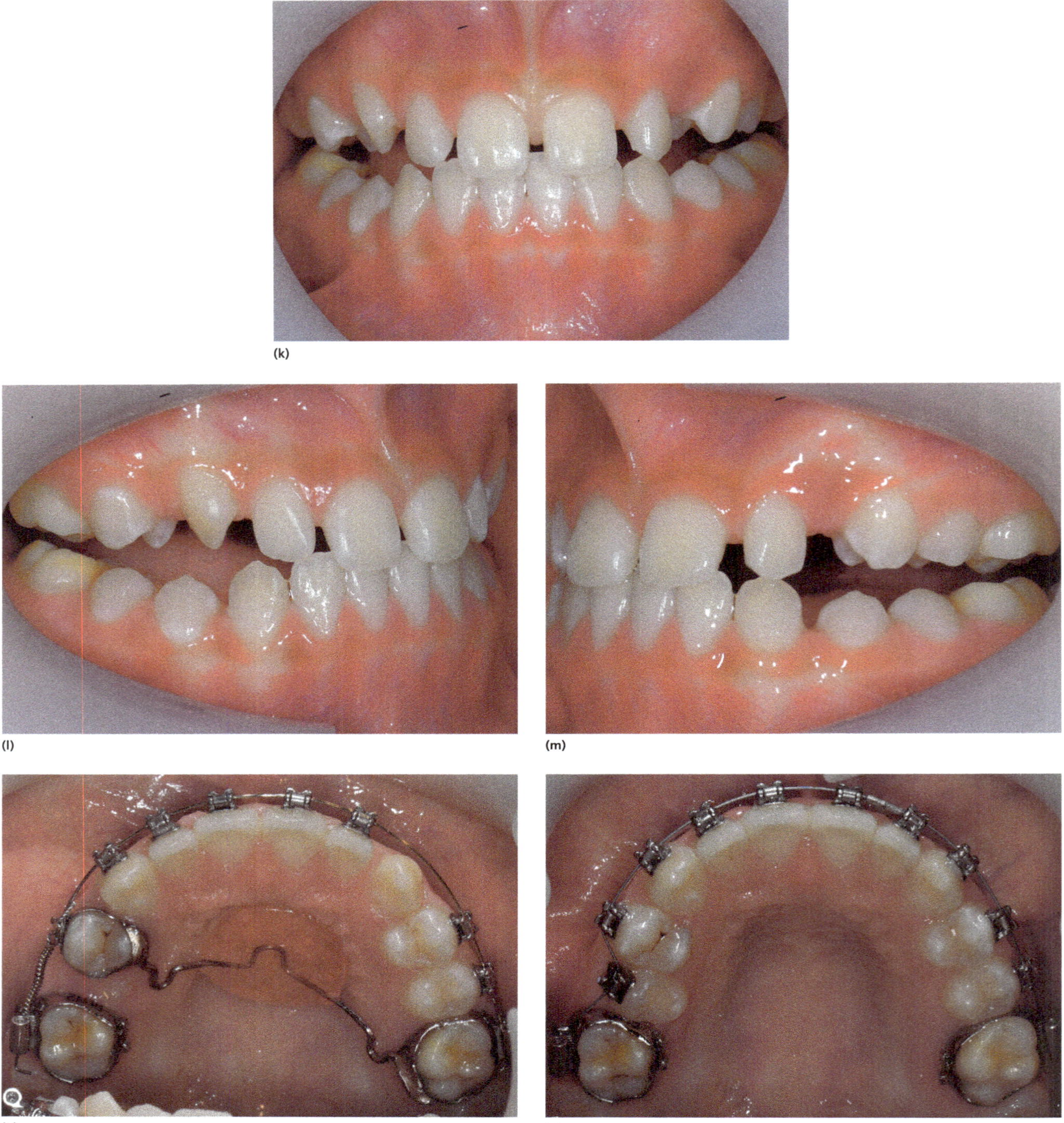

Figure 11.6 (*Continued*)

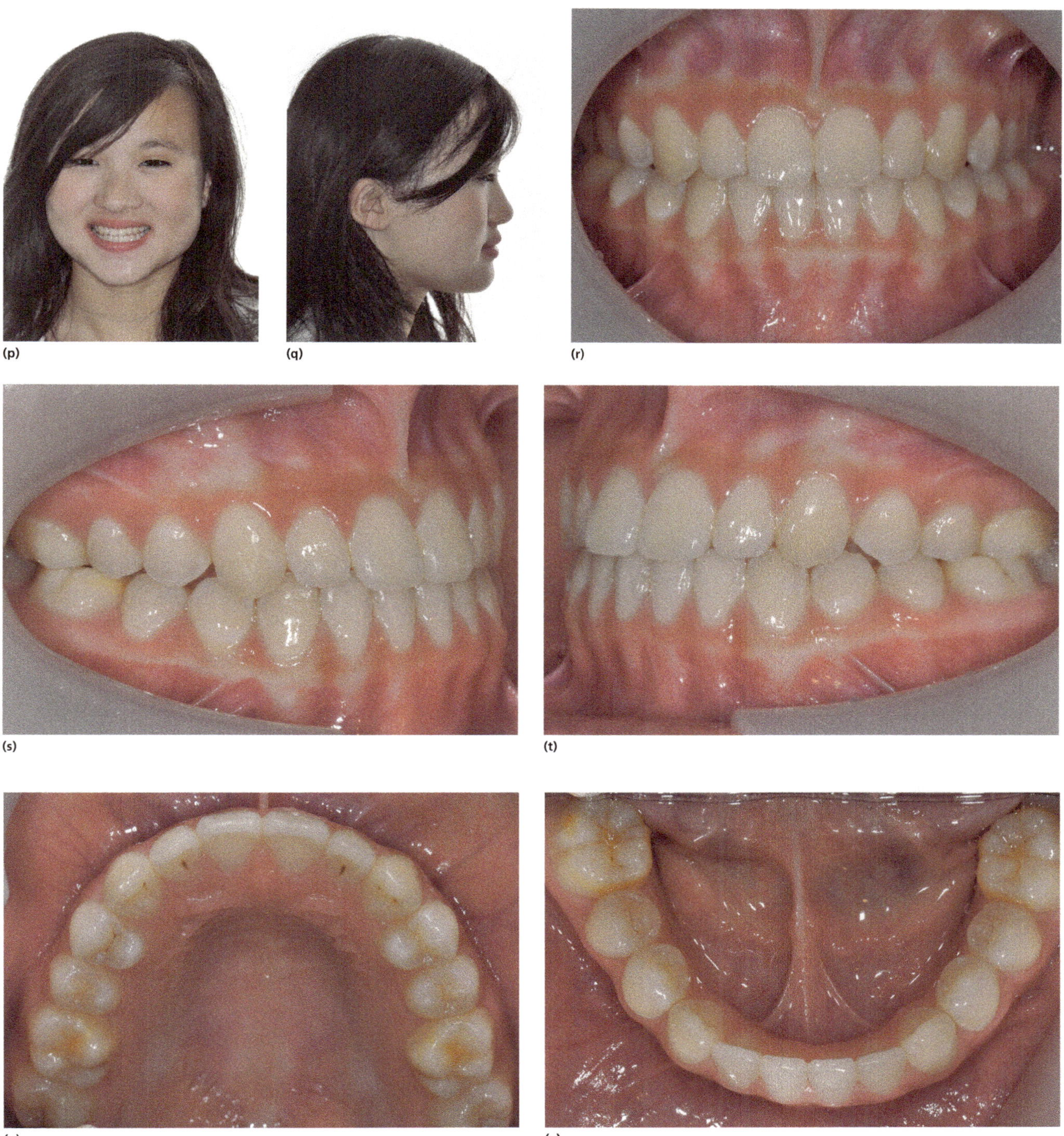

(p) (q) (r) (s) (t) (u) (v)

Figure 11.6 (*Continued*)

Index

Page References in *italics* refer to Figures; those in **bold** refer to Tables

Orthodontic Functional Appliances: Theory and Practice, First Edition. Padhraig Fleming and Robert Lee.

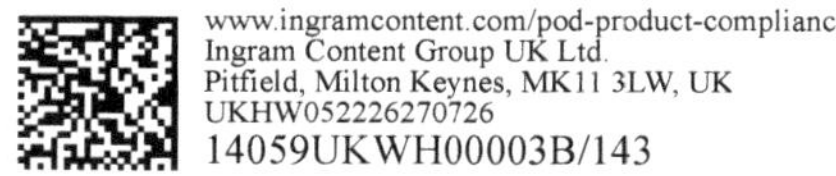
www.ingramcontent.com/pod-product-compliance
Ingram Content Group UK Ltd.
Pitfield, Milton Keynes, MK11 3LW, UK
UKHW052226270726
14059UKWH00003B/143